Lymphoma

Edited by Yusuf Tutar

Published in London, United Kingdom

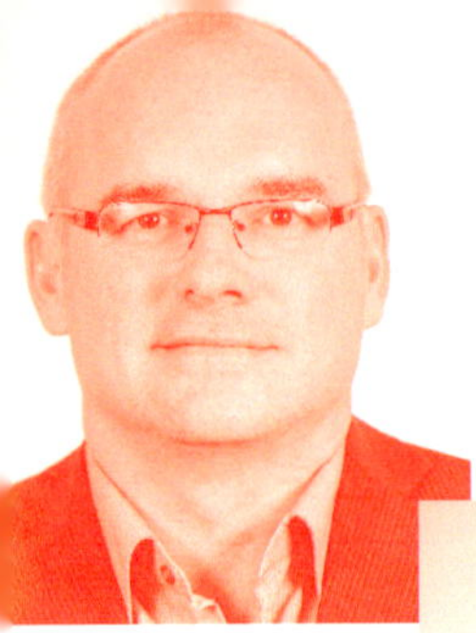
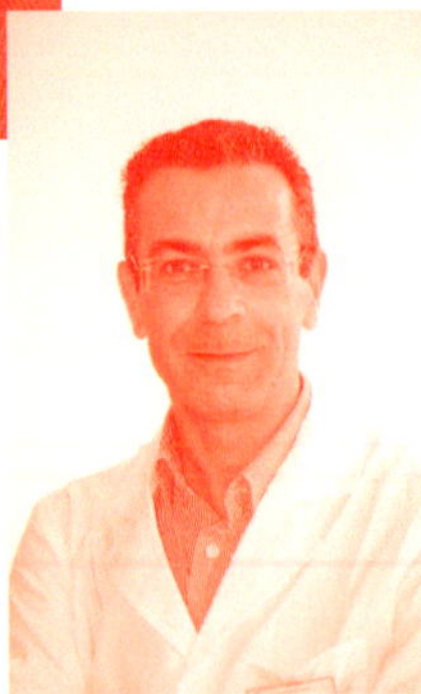
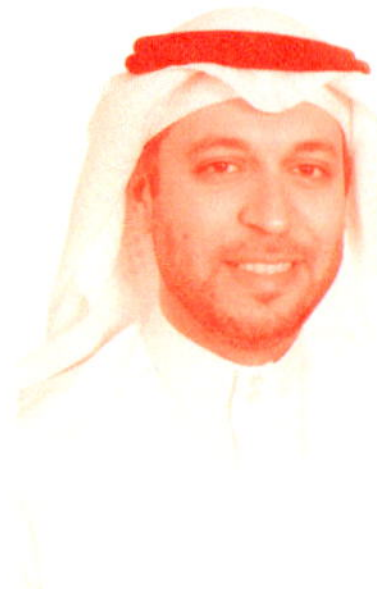
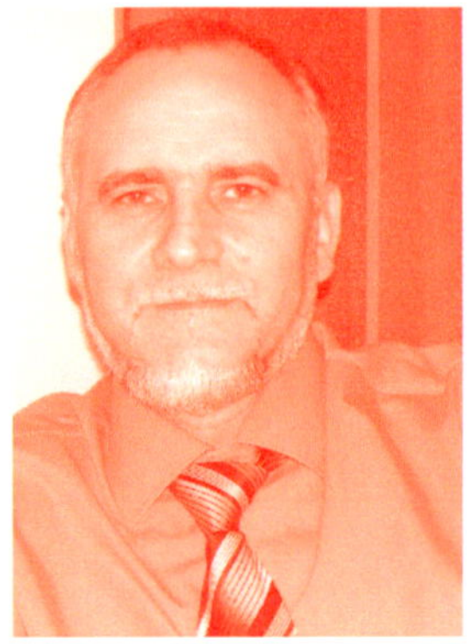
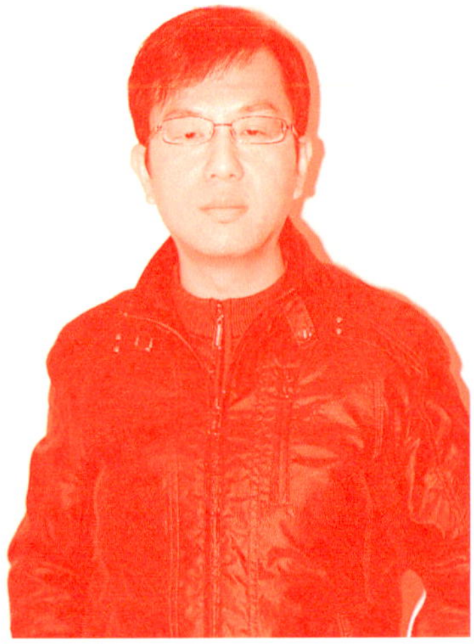
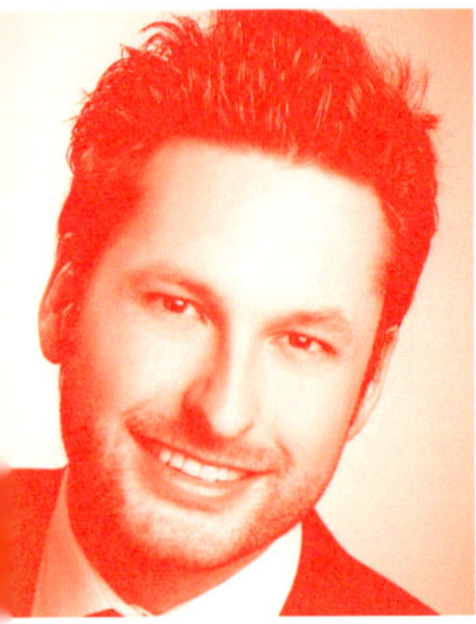
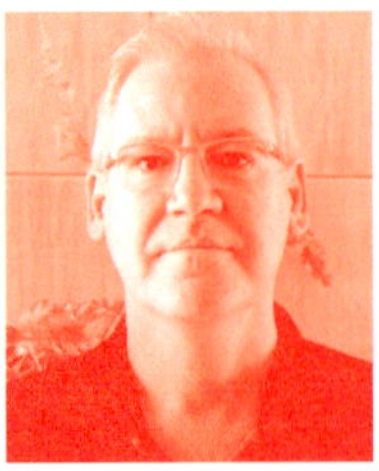

IntechOpen

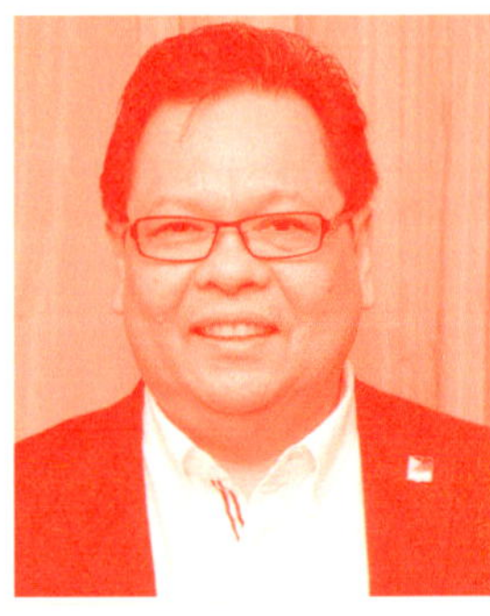
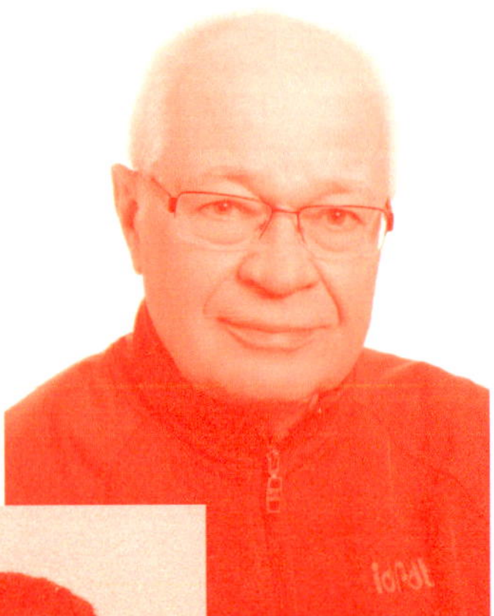
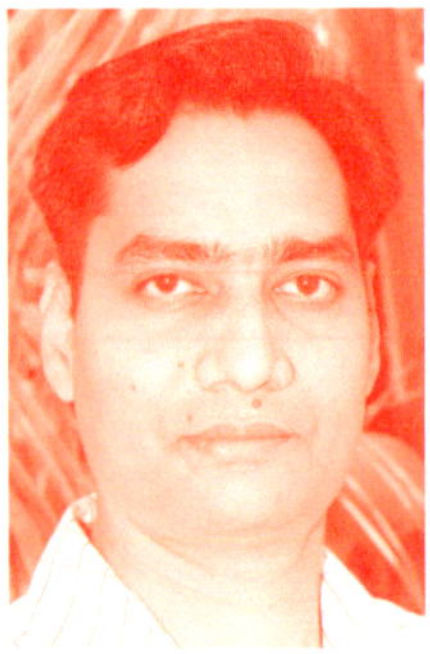
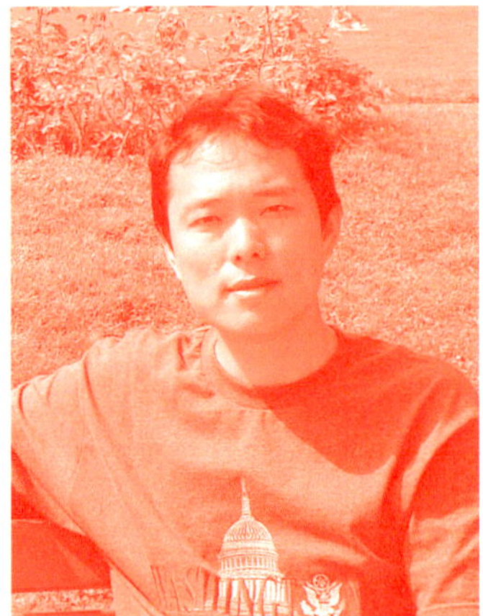
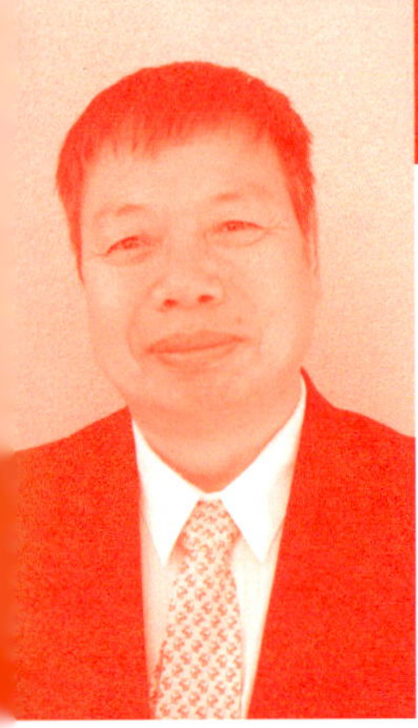
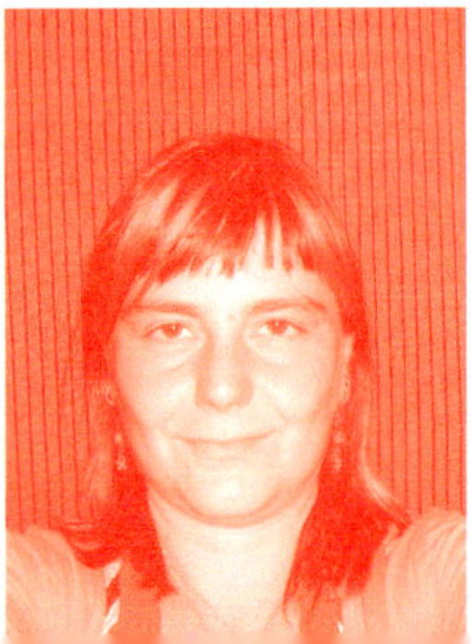

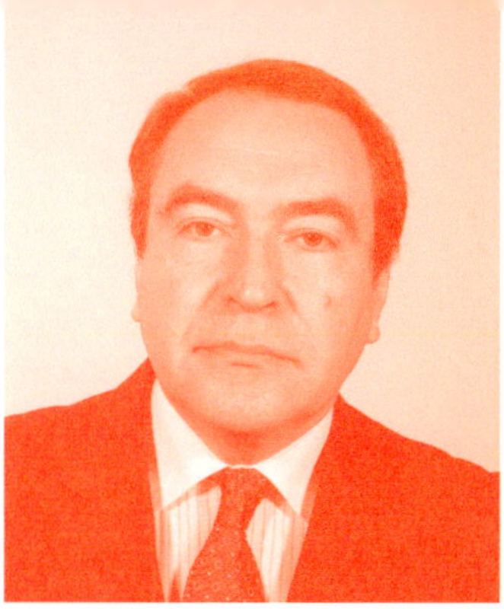
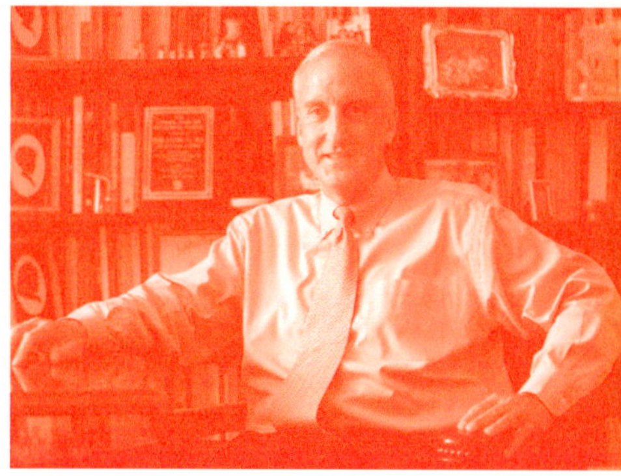
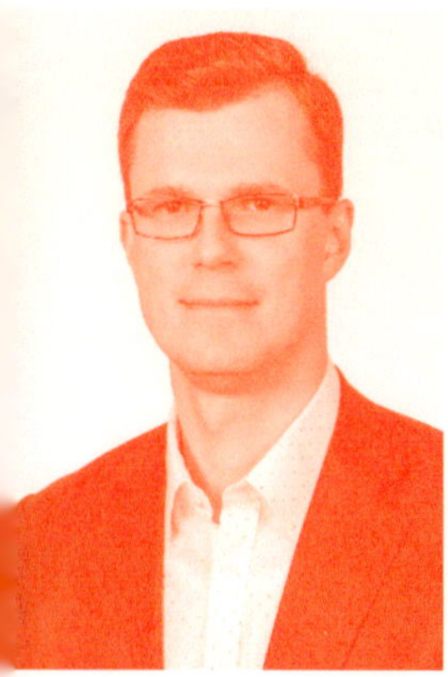
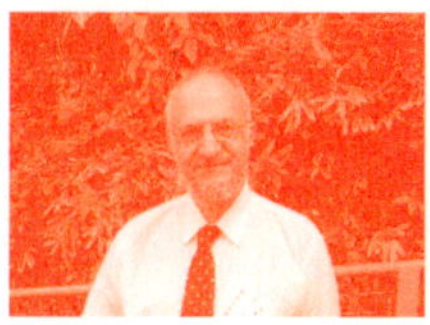
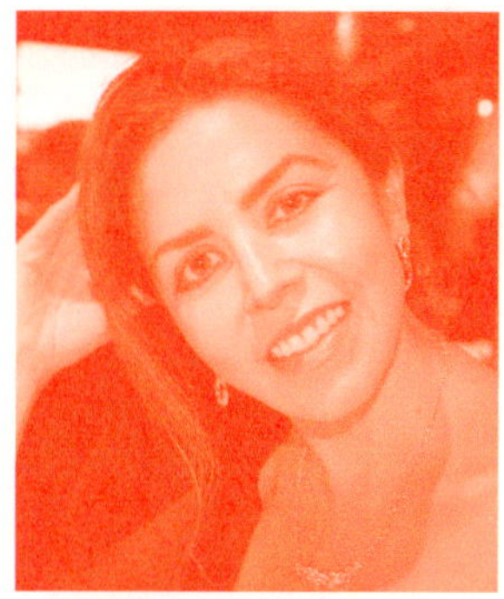

Supporting open minds since 2005

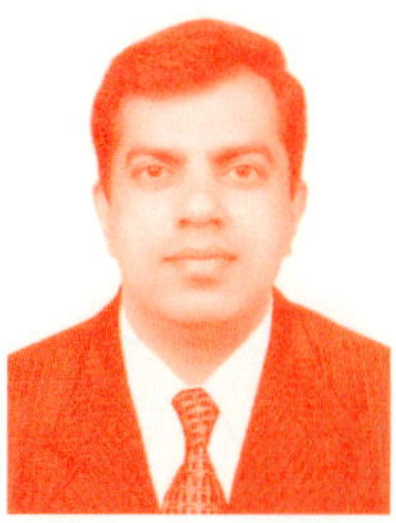
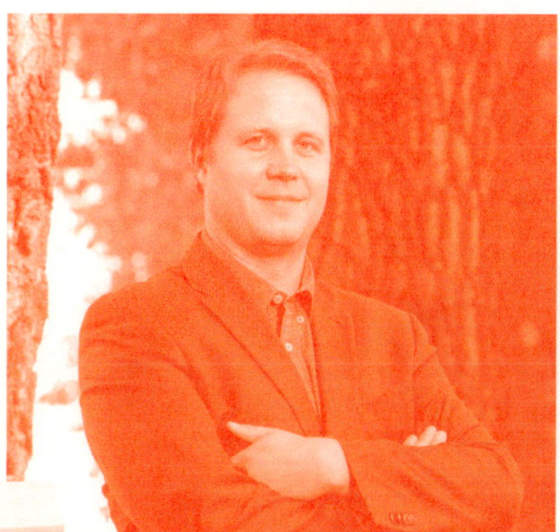
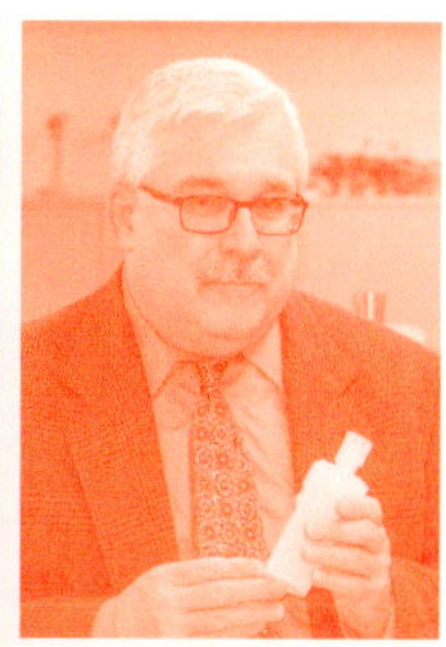
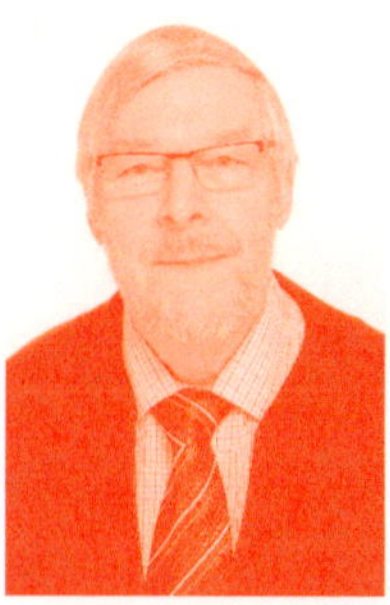
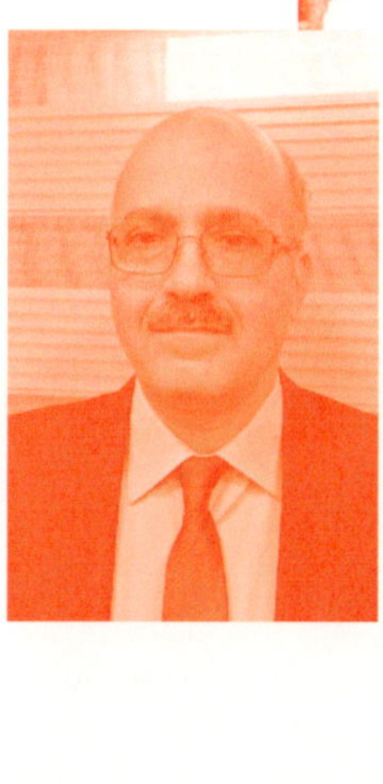
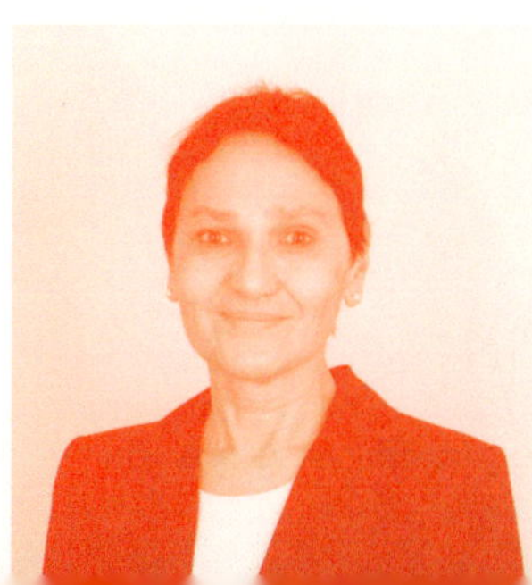
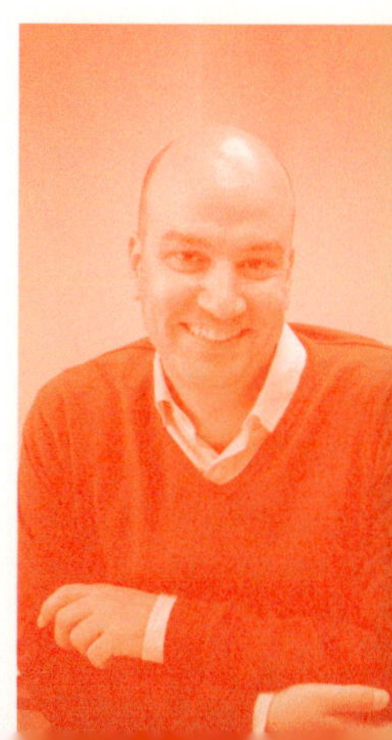

Lymphoma
http://dx.doi.org/10.5772/intechopen.94816
Edited by Yusuf Tutar

Contributors
Fernando Collado-Mesa, Alberto Artiles Medina, Javier Lorca Álvaro, Ines Laso-Garcia, César Mínguez Ojeda, Marina Mata Alcaraz, Marta Santiago González, Mariam Bajawi Carretero, Juan José Gordillo Perdomo, Victoria Gómez Dos Santos, Francisco Javier Burgos-Revilla, Ahed Khatib, Victor E. Nava, Parastou Tizro, Anita Aggarwal, Aaron Auerbach, Rami Abdulbaki, Ramiz Bayramov, Ramila Abdullayeva, Carmen Ximena Gallegos Riofrio, Juan Daniel Garzon Gallegos, Ranjit Kumar Sahoo, Praful Pandey, Saphalta Baghmar, Mukesh Patekar, Ahitagni Biswas, Aminat Magomedova, Anna Misyurina, Sergey Kravchenko, Fatima Babaeva, Andrey Vorobiev, Gopila Gupta, Vikas Garg, Barbara Iaccheri, Alessandro Lupi, Davide Tucci, Carlo Cagini, Tito Fiore, Yusuf Tutar, Kubra Acikalin Coskun, Mervenur Al, Nazlican Yurekli, Elif Cansu Abay, Merve Tutar

First published in London, United Kingdom, 2022 by IntechOpen
IntechOpen is the global imprint of INTECHOPEN LIMITED, registered in England and Wales, registration number: 11086078, 5 Princes Gate Court, London, SW7 2QJ, United Kingdom
Printed in Croatia

British Library Cataloguing-in-Publication Data
A catalogue record for this book is available from the British Library

Additional hard and PDF copies can be obtained from orders@intechopen.com

Lymphoma
Edited by Yusuf Tutar
p. cm.
Print ISBN 978-1-83968-111-0
Online ISBN 978-1-83968-112-7
eBook (PDF) ISBN 978-1-83968-117-2

For EU product safety concerns:
IN TECH d.o.o., Prolaz Marije Krucifikse Kozulić 3, 51000 Rijeka, Croatia, info@intechopen.com or visit our website at intechopen.com.

Meet the editor

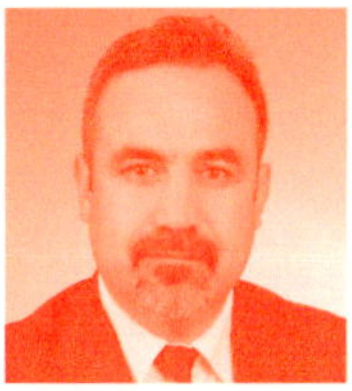

Prof. Dr. Yusuf Tutar conducts his research at Hamidiye Faculty of Pharmacy, Department of Basic Pharmaceutical Sciences, Division of Biochemistry, University of Health Sciences, Turkey. He is also a faculty member in the Molecular Oncology Program. He obtained his MSc and Ph.D. at Oregon State University and Texas Tech University, respectively. He pursued his postdoctoral studies at Rutgers University Medical School and the National Institutes of Health (NIH/NIDDK), USA. His research focuses on biochemistry, biophysics, genetics, molecular biology, and molecular medicine with specialization in the fields of drug design, protein structure function, protein folding, prions, microRNA, pseudogenes, molecular cancer, epigenetics, metabolites, proteomics, genomics, protein expression, and characterization by spectroscopic and calorimetric methods.

Contents

Preface

Lymphoma is a group of malignant diseases caused by the clonal proliferation of lymphocytes. Current treatment options include chemotherapy, radiotherapy, and bone marrow/stem cell transplantation. Development of new treatment options for cancer medications include small molecules and monoclonal antibodies for immunotherapy. In addition, the discovery of new phytochemical agents used in complementary and alternative medicine adds perspective to the treatment of lymphoma. Chapter 1, "Drugs and Drug Candidates for the Treatment of Lymphoma", highlights recent developments in the field.

Chapter 2, "Follicular Lymphoma", elaborates on general knowledge of follicular lymphoma, which is one of the most common types of indolent non-Hodgkin's lymphoma. Follicular lymphoma presents with lymphadenopathy and/or bone marrow involvement. It is a slow-growing tumor with frequent remission and relapses. Early-stage disease is usually treated with radiotherapy. Management of advanced stage depends on disease burden. Patients with advanced-stage disease may be observed in the case of low-burden disease and those with high disease load require treatment with chemo-immunotherapy. Chapter 3, "Primary Gastrointestinal Lymphoma", contributes to our understanding of a rare disease. Different regions of the gastrointestinal tract are involved in different subtypes of primary gastrointestinal lymphoma with various frequency that reflects the diversity of the causative agents and predisposing factors for each site and the subtype of primary gastrointestinal lymphoma. This chapter discusses the epidemiology of all subtypes of primary gastrointestinal lymphoma, factors and disorders contributing to their development, non-inherited and inherited conditions associated with a higher risk of the disease, diagnostic difficulties and pitfalls, and novel treatment strategies.

Chapter 4, "Splenic B-Cell Lymphoma/Leukemia, Unclassifiable", discusses the low-grade B-cell lymphoproliferative disorders that do not fit into any other splenic lymphoid neoplasm at two provisional entities: splenic diffuse red pulp small B-cell lymphoma and hairy-cell leukemia. Chapter 5, "Testicular Lymphoma: Primary and Secondary Involvement", explores testicular involvement in lymphoma and covers the epidemiology, diagnosis, treatment, and prognosis of primary testicular lymphoma. Furthermore, the chapter addresses the epidemiology and management of secondary involvement of the testis by lymphoma. Chapter 6, "Hydroa Vacciniforme-Like Cutaneous T-Cell Lymphoma", discusses a controversial skin pathology. Hydroa vacciniforme-like cutaneous T-cell lymphoma appears to be just like a vacciniform hydroa but others progress to cutaneous T-cell lymphoma, with or without angiocentricity. They are usually associated with infections by Epstein-Barr viruses and NK cell lymphomas. Clinical management can be difficult and accompanied by a high index of malignancy, thus early diagnosis is essential. Chapter 7, "Clinical and Laboratory Data Which Are Not Typical of De Novo Diffuse Large B-Cell Lymphoma", discusses this heterogeneous group of diseases of the lymphatic system, which are represented by *de novo* and secondary tumors resulting from the transformation of indolent lymphomas. In the absence of a long history of the disease at the stage of histological transformation, it is difficult to distinguish between *de novo* and secondary diffuse large B-cell lymphoma. The chapter provides a key analysis of diffuse large B-cell lymphoma. Chapter 8, “Primary Intraocular Lymphoma: The Masquerade Syndrome”, provides a comprehensive overview of primary intra-ocular lymphoma and a correct clinical approach towards this rare condition to avoid delays in diagnosis, which is considered the most important prognostic factor. In fact, a primary intra-ocular lymphoma arises with no specific symptoms and can mimic both inflammatory and non-inflammatory ocular conditions. This ocular malignant condition has a strong bond with primary central system lymphoma. Diagnosis is achieved through cytology, flow cytometry, immunohistochemistry, molecular analysis, and cytokines assay. Treatment of this condition has been completely revolutionized with the introduction of monoclonal antibodies directed against specific proteins present on the surface of lymphomatous cells.

The next three chapters are part of a section on special topics.

Chapter 9, “Primary Central Nervous System Lymphoma: Focus on Indian Perspective”, investigates treatment methods for primary CNS lymphoma. Early suspicion, withholding steroids, stereotactic biopsy, and high-dose methotrexate are essential for the treatment of this disease, making its management in lower-middle income countries challenging. Novel radiological methods, clinician awareness about the disease, and utilization of drugs like thiotepa and ibrutinib, which can be given on an outpatient basis, may allow better management of these patients in resource-poor settings. The aforementioned challenges combined with the late-presenting demographic results in poorer treatment outcomes in the Indian subcontinent as compared to its western counterparts. This chapter presents the current standard of care for primary CNS lymphoma as well as potential modifications or research areas that may potentially improve outcomes in lower-middle income countries. Chapter 10, “Breast Implant-Associated Anaplastic Large Cell Lymphoma (BIA-ALCL): Breast Imaging Perspective”, examines this rare disease. Most cases present with rapid and dramatic breast swelling resulting from the peri-implant fluid collection. Palpable mass, pain, and skin lesions also occur. The combination of clinical history, physical exam findings, and appropriate imaging workup can lead to a timely and accurate diagnosis. The disease has an excellent prognosis when it is diagnosed at an early stage and complete surgery is performed. Radiologists, particularly those involved in breast imaging, play an essential role in early diagnosis. This chapter presents an overview of the disease, including relevant imaging findings. Finally, Chapter 11, “Lymphoma and the Microenvironmental Cross-Talk between Sex Hormone Receptors and Epstein-Barr Virus in Predicting Lymphoma Clinical Status”, covers lymphoma in general with a focus on unique features linking the interaction of Epstein-Barr virus with sex steroid hormones in lymphoma cells.

Yusuf Tutar
Department of Basic Pharmaceutical Sciences,
Division of Biochemistry,
Hamidiye Faculty of Pharmacy,
University of Health Sciences-Turkey,
Istanbul, Turkey

Section 1

General Perspectives

Chapter 1

Drugs and Drug Candidates for the Treatment of Lymphoma

Kubra Acikalin Coskun, Merve Tutar, Elif Cansu Abay, Nazlican Yurekli, Mervenur Al and Yusuf Tutar

Abstract

Cancer is the biggest health problem worldwide due to its high mortality rate. Lymphoma is defined as a group of malignant diseases that is caused by clonal proliferation of lymphocytes and is classified under two major groups: Hodgkin lymphoma and non-Hodgkin lymphoma. Genetic predisposition and some environmental factors constitute risk factors. Symptoms of the disease include unexplained fever, swelling of lymph glands, swollen abdomen, tiredness, loss of appetite, frequent infections, and weight loss. Positron emission tomography (PET) and computed tomography (CT) scans, along with MRI, are widely used for the diagnosis of lymphoma. Advanced blood and lymph node biopsy tests are used to evaluate treatment effect on blood cells and to confirm the diagnosis of lymphoma, respectively. Current treatment options include chemotherapy, radiotherapy, and bone marrow/stem cell transplantation. Development of new treatment options for cancer medications includes small molecules and monoclonal antibodies for immunotherapy. In addition, the discovery of new phytochemical agents used in complementary and alternative medicine adds perspective to the treatment of lymphoma.

Keywords: lymphoma, small molecule inhibitor, alternative medicine, herbal treatment, cancer treatments

1. Introduction

Lymphoma is lymphoid system malignancy developed from lymphocytes of the immune system with diverse morphologic and distinct clinical findings. Three classes of lymphocytes are natural killer cells (NK), T cells, and B cells. They function in cytotoxic innate immunity, cytotoxic adaptive immunity, and humoral antibody-driven adaptive immunity, respectively. The lymphatic system (lymph, lymph nodes, lymphatic vessels, collecting ducts) is a network of tissues, vessels, and organs (spleen, thymus, tonsils and adenoid, bone marrow, Peyer's patches, appendix), and lymphoma can develop in these organs. However, lymphoma is classified into two classes: Hodgkin lymphoma (HL) and non-Hodgkin lymphoma (NHL). Non-Hodgkin lymphomas are more frequently seen, approximately 8 times more, than the others. Distinct lymphomas arise from immune system cells at different stages of differentiation. In addition, all groups are divided into different types within themselves. Each one of these have different clinical course, response to treatment, and drugs used in their treatment [1–3].

To treat lymphomas, different treatment approaches have been developed, including chemotherapies, radiotherapies, and bone marrow transplantation. Radiotherapies create extensive damage and leave permanent effects on cancer patients even they are effective in treatment of lymphomas. Further, bone marrow transplantation is a challenging way due to suppressed immunity and may lead rising of infectious diseases in the patients. However, in certain cases, immunotherapies (i.e. with rituximab antibody which binds cell surface protein CD20) can lead to complete responses in lymphomas with minimal side effects. Nevertheless, to benefit from the effect of metabolites from plants several studies are underway to find a better therapeutic approach [2].

1.1 Plants in the treatment of lymphoma

Several approaches in the treatment of these diseases resulted in successful outcomes and yet some have adverse effects. Plants ingredients constitute more than 90% of commercial medical drugs and different plants may be employed for treating distinct malignant diseases [3].

1.1.1 Quercetin

This agent has anti-malignant effects and it possesses a cytotoxic effect over transformed lymphoid cells by targeting key pathways such as PI3K and Wnt. Synergetic and/or additive effects of quercetin in combination with other drugs are underway to display its therapeutic effects in various lymphoma types [4].

1.1.2 Salvianolic acid from Salvia miltiorrhiza *extracts*

The phenolic salvianolic acid A display anti-tumoral activity. Diffuse B cell lymphoma treatment options are limited and the activity is used against diffuse B cell lymphoma cells. The salvianolic acid inhibited the viability of the cells by inducing apoptosis. The apoptotic pathway induces by upregulation of Bax and cleavage of PARP. *In vivo* xerograph models also displayed tumor growth suppression with salvianolic acid A and the agent showed promising anti-tumoral activity for diffuse large B cell lymphoma (DLBCL) [5].

1.1.3 Annona muricata *Linn leaf extracts*

The activity of the leaf extracts is attributed to the secondary metabolites (phenols, flavonoids, alkaloids, acetogenins). The extracts were tested against Dalton's Lymphoma Ascites (DLA) and Ehrlich Ascites Carcinoma (EAC) cells and anti-tumoral effects compared to cisplatin. Cytotoxic studies indicated poor outcomes at lower microgram concentration per milliliter but tumor burden is decreased in dose-dependent manner and tumor volume is reduced significantly with a prolonged lifespan [6].

1.1.4 Amomum subulatum

Methanolic extracts of *Amomum subulatum* dry fruits administration induces apoptosis on Dalton's Lymphoma Ascites cells both *in vitro* and *in vivo*. The extracts further increase mouse life span through regulation of pro-inflammatory cytokines and NF-κB pathway by promoting apoptosis of cancer cells. The research employed cyclophosphamide drug as positive control and the extracts displayed better activity compared to the drug. Therefore, the study proposed *A. subulatum* as a potential nutraceutical (nutrition-based therapeutic) against cancer [7].

1.1.5 Gymnopilus purpureosquamulosus *extracts*

The extract activates apoptosis indicated by annexin V-positive cells and further, production of reactive oxygen species, PARP1 cleavage, and mitochondrial membrane potential decrease upon extract treatment. The extract also displayed apoptosis in lymphoma patient cells but not in healthy patient cells [8].

1.1.6 Ingenol mebutate extract

A new therapeutic agent from *ingenol mebutate extract* displayed apoptotic activity against cutaneous T-cell lymphoma. The agent activated caspase by downregulating c-FLIP and XIAP and can be employed as a potential drug candidate [9].

1.1.7 Cucurbitacin B

Primary effusion lymphoma (PEL) is an aggressive B cell non-Hodgkin lymphoma that has been seen in immunocompromised patients. Cucurbitaceae B is a triterpene extracted from *Cucurbitaceae* plant that has several anti-cancer activities. The effect of Cucurbitaceae B was examined at distinct PEL cell lines. The agent inhibited cell proliferation of PEL cell lines Further, a xenograft model was also employed and the agent suppressed solid tumor growth. The reports proposed that Cucurbitaceae B is a promising agent as an antitumoral activity for PEL [10].

1.1.8 Achyranthes aspera *L. leaf extract*

The extract was tested against Dalton's lymphoma (DL) both *in vitro* and *in vivo*. The extract suppresses DL through attenuation of the PKCα signaling pathway and mitochondrial apoptosis [11].

Therefore, several metabolites from plant extracts potentially display anti-tumoral activity and can be used both for nutraceutical and drug design for lymphoma treatment but further research is required to optimize these agents for drug development.

1.2 Small molecule inhibitors in lymphoma

Small molecule inhibitors are usually analogs of target protein substrates like ATP or phosphotyrosine. Due to their small size, these inhibitors effectively reach and interact with their targets that are extracellular receptors, cell surface ligand-binding receptors, and intracellular proteins which include anti-apoptotic proteins known for playing an important role in transducing downstream signaling for cell growth and metastasis progression. Anti-cancer small molecule inhibitors are therapeutic agents that target key proteins in pathways involved in cell proliferation and differentiation [12].

Small molecular inhibitors (SMIs) are able to target tumor cells due to the disturbed cellular architecture [13]. Disturbed architecture is an advantage for SMIs to diffuse in the gaps between the tumor cells and reach their targets [14]. With the help of this advantage, SMIs are promising approach for the treatment of multiple tumors. Therefore, researchers develop target-specific SMIs targeting critical malignant pathways. The combination of SMIs with clinical chemotherapy agents may increase treatment efficiency [15, 16].

In the case of lymphoma, similar to other cancer cells, many of the proteins associated with the survival, angiogenesis, and metastasis of cancer cells are hyperactivated. To suppress the hyperactivation, specific proteins in lymphoma are targeted namely Bruton tyrosine kinase, PI3K, HDACs, and proteasomal system proteins [17].

1.3 FDA approved and non-approved small molecule drugs in treatment of lymphoma

The number of drugs for the treatment of lymphoma has increased with the findings of new agents. Regulatory agencies have approved many novel drugs for the treatment of various forms of lymphoid malignancies over the last two decades. Several drugs for the treatment of lymphoma include the B-cell receptor signaling inhibitor ibrutinib, the antibody-drug conjugate brentuximab vedotin, the PI3K-δ inhibitor idelalisib, the novel glycoengineered anti-CD20 antibody obinutuzumab, and the immunomodulatory drug lenalidomide [18].

The majority of novel treatments for NHL were approved for follicular B cell lymphoma. On the other hand, there are only two drugs for relapsed diffuse large B cell lymphoma in the past three decades. In some cases, a unique molecular mechanism is targeted by approved drugs while in others, multiple agents targeted the same oncogenic pathway, including the PI3 kinase pathway and Bruton tyrosine kinase (BTK). Furthermore, there are many investigational agents that target the intracellular mechanisms have studied [19].

Several antibody-drug conjugates and the BCL2 inhibitor venetoclax are some examples of unapproved targeted drugs that have shown promising efficacy. Additionally, various immunotherapies, such as mono- and bispecific antibodies, immune-checkpoint inhibitors, and engineered chimeric antigen receptor (CAR) T cells, have also shown efficacy in lymphoma patients [18]. Therefore, in view of the multitude of new agents, the finding of drugs for the treatment of lymphoma has grown, demanding the efficient prioritization of drugs for faster development. Here, additional focus will be given to overview of the U.S. Food and Drug Administration (FDA) approved drugs for the treatment of lymphoma and drug development at new targets.

1.3.1 Bruton tyrosine kinase (BTK) inhibitors

BTK is an important therapeutic target for B-cell NHL because it plays a crucial role in the BCR signaling pathway [20]. Ibrutinib is a BTK inhibitor, that binds to BTK's Cysteine 481 (C481) site in an irreversible manner, disrupting the antigen-dependent active BCR signaling pathway [21]. This inhibitor is approved by the FDA for the treatment of chronic lymphocytic leukemia (CLL), mantle-cell lymphoma (MCL), and Waldenstrom macroglobulinemia (WM) [22].

Ibrutinib resistance has been shown to be conferred by acquired mutations in the C481 binding site, as well as gain-of-function mutations in the downstream PLCγ2 kinase increasing BCR signaling [23]. In order to overcome ibrutinib resistance by inhibiting both wild-type and C481-mutated BTK non-covalently, novel highly selective BTK inhibitors are currently being investigated [24]. Ibrutinib was approved by the US FDA-approved for the treatment of WM demonstrating a 90.5% overall response rate (ORR) [25]. Ibrutinib is also FDA approved inhibitor for MCL after ≥1 prior line of therapy and for MZL after ≥1 prior anti-CD20-directed therapy [26, 27]. Because of its capacity to permeate the blood-brain barrier, ibrutinib has shown a promising effect on primary central nervous system (CNS) lymphoma [28]. Combining therapies, ibrutinib with venetoclax, lenalidomide, second-generation anti-CD20 mAbs, immune checkpoint inhibitors, and chimeric antigen receptor (CAR) T-cell therapy are still investigating in different NHLs [22].

Acalabrutinib is another BTK inhibitor and when it is compared to ibrutinib, it has less off-target kinase inhibition and a better safety profile. Patients with severe liver disease, as well as those using powerful CYP3A inhibitors and inducers or proton pump inhibitors, should avoid acalabrutinib. According to a phase II trial that demonstrates 81% ORR, acalabrutinib was approved by FDA for MCL [29]. In addition, zanubrutinib is FDA BTK inhibitor for MCL ≥1 prior line of therapy. Patients with severe liver disease or who are taking CYP3A inhibitors and inducers at the same time should alter their doses [30].

1.3.2 Immunomodulatory drugs (IMiDs)

Immunomodulators (IMiDs) bind cereblon E3 ubiquitin ligase complex that degrades the transcription factors of Aiolos and Ikraos. In this way, it results in the direct death of malignant B cells as well as overexpression of IL-2, which leads to T and NK cell activation [31]. Teratogenicity, cytopenias, infection, thrombosis, secondary malignancy, and rash are all side effects of the IMiD class [32].

Lenalidomide is a second-generation IMiD that is given at a daily dose of 20–25 mg for the first 21 days of a 28-day therapy cycle. Despite, lenalidomide's single-agent ORR for relapsed indolent lymphoma is low (23%), this drug is still used in combination with rituximab (R) (anti-CD20 monoclonal antibody (mAb)) for relapsed/refractory follicular lymphoma (FL) and marginal zone lymphoma (MZL) treatment. In addition, lenalidomide has shown activity in patients with relapsed/refractory MCL with an ORR of 28%. In a randomized phase II trial, relapsed MCL patients who got single-agent lenalidomide had a better ORR than those who received other single agents (40% vs. 11%). Lenalidomide was approved by the FDA in the United States for relapsed/refractory MCL after ≥2 prior therapies, including bortezomib [22].

1.3.3 Phosphoinositide 3-kinase (PI3K) inhibitors

PI3K activates AKT and mTOR via the B-cell receptor signaling pathway, resulting in enhanced cell survival. Class 1 PI3K has four distinct isoforms: α, β, γ, and δ with significantly expressed in lymphocytes. In NHL, inhibiting this pathway with PI3K inhibitors is a key focus [22].

Idelalisib is a PI3K inhibitor that targets PI3K specifically, and it has been approved by FDA as a single-agent treatment for patients with relapsed/refractory FL [33]. Copanlisib is the other US FDA inhibitor that targets α and δ isoforms for relapsed FL. In addition, it has specificity for the α isoform that has a role in insulin and glucose metabolism. For this reason, unique toxicity of hyperglycemia, liver toxicity, diarrhea, neutropenia, and infection are observed [34]. Lastly, duvelisib is a dual PI3K FDA approval inhibitor for relapsed/refractory FL after ≥2 prior systemic therapies. Inhibition of both the γ and the δ isoforms is expected to be synergistic since it targets both B cell proliferation and survival as well as the tumor microenvironment. In a phase II clinical trial, duvelisib was tested as a single treatment in indolent NHL and exhibited an ORR of 47.3% [35].

1.3.4 Proteasome inhibitors

Proteasome inhibitors prevent ubiquitin-tagged proteins from being degraded, affecting cellular homeostasis and triggering apoptosis. Bortezomib is a proteasome inhibitor and it was approved by the FDA in the United States for the treatment of MCL based on a phase II study with an ORR of 33% [36]. Additionally, bortezomib also received U.S. FDA approval in combination with R-cyclophosphamide, doxorubicin, prednisone (R-CAP) for untreated MCL [37]. Plasmablastic lymphoma, Waldenstrom's macroglobulinemia (WM), and peripheral T cell lymphomas (PTCL) had promising activity by bortezomib [38, 39] while randomized trials showed no benefit from adding it to frontline chemoimmunotherapy for DLBCL and FL [40].

1.3.5 Histone deacetylase inhibitors

Histone deacetylase (HDAC) inhibitors work against cancer by altering the acetylation of histone and transcription factor proteins, causing cell cycle arrest and apoptosis. The inhibitor romidepsin was approved by FDA for the treatment of relapsed/refractory PTCL demonstrating ORR 25–38% in phase II studies [41]. Moreover, romidepsin is being tested for relapsed/refractory NHLs in combination with lenalidomide, the folate antagonist pralatrexate, and the immune checkpoint inhibitor pembrolizumab [22].

The other FDA-approved HDAC inhibitor is belinostat for the treatment of relapsed/refractory PTCL demonstrating a 26% ORR [42]. Vorinostat is also FDA approved HDAC inhibitor after two prior lines of systemic therapies for cutaneous T cell lymphomas (CTCL) that have progressed with a 30% ORR [43].

1.3.6 Selective nuclear export inhibitors (SINE)

Selinexor, a selective inhibitor of nuclear export (SINE) prevents tumor suppressor genes from being exported from the nucleus by inhibiting the shuttling protein exportin 1 (XPO1) [22]. Cytopenias, anorexia, nausea, vomiting, diarrhea, tiredness, hyponatremia, infections, and neurological toxicity are the most prevalent significant side effects of selinexor [33]. Selinexor is approved by U.S. FDA for the treatment of relapsed/refractory DLBCL. Moreover, it is being studied in combination with standard R-CHOP chemoimmunotherapy for the initial treatment of DLBCL, as well as in combination with venetoclax or salvage chemoimmunotherapy [22].

1.3.7 EZH2 (enhancer of zeste homolog 2) inhibitors

EZH2 is a histone-lysine N-methyltransferase enzyme; a histone methyltransferase responsible for methylation of lysine 27 of histone H3 (H3Lys27). In addition, a DNA alteration is linked to repressed transcription when it is trimethylated (H3Lys27me3). That is why, abnormal EZH2 activity that activates mutations, has been identified as an oncogenic driver [18].

In 22–29% of patients with FL, mutations in the EZH2 gene have been observed. A phase II study revealed that tazemetostat had an ORR of 69% in EZH2-mutated FL and 35% in EZH2 wild-type FL in 99 patients with relapsed/refractory FL. According to these results, tazemetostat was approved by U.S. FDA for patients with EZH2-mutated FL. Furthermore, the effect of tazemetostat in relapsed/refractory B-cell lymphomas is being investigated in a variety of early-phase studies [23].

1.4 Lymphoma drug candidates

Different approaches have been developed and applied to cure lymphoma [19]. There are few drugs approved by FDA. However, efficient therapeutics to treat lymphomas are still under investigation. Researchers have been working on novel agents. Recent studies have discovered promising drug candidates for lymphoma cancer cells [44]. Researchers have still been working on few drug candidates [45]. These candidates can be classified according to their target signaling pathways as follows:

1.4.1 SYK inhibitors

Cerdulatinib is an inhibitor of SYK, JAK1, JAK3, and TYK2 and was investigated in phase 1 experiments. Preclinical and clinical research showed that cerdulatinib inhibits SYK/JAK signaling cascade activity and showed promising effects on diffuse large B cell lymphoma. In a research report, a phase 1 dose study of cerdulatinib drug in 43 patients with r/r CLL and NHL was completed in 2016 and according to results, SYK and JAK inhibition was well tolerated and antitumor activity of the drug was proved in CLL and FL patients [45].

Entospletinib is a small-molecule inhibitor that specifically binds and inhibits the SYK activity. Phase 2 studies showed that usage of the inhibitor with other drugs as a combined therapy resulted in inhibition of BCL signaling activity [46].

Fostamatinib: Phase 1/2 clinical trial of fostamatinib disodium drug which is classified as the first clinically available oral SYK inhibitor was applied in patients with recurrent B-cell non-Hodgkin lymphoma (B-NHL). Results showed that the drug has ability to induce apoptosis by inhibition of SYK [47].

Mivavotinib TAK659: Last drug that inhibits SYK activity to block BCL signaling pathway and results in inhibition of activation, adhesion, and proliferation of B-cell. Phase 1 study is completed, however, phase 2 study was not completed due to the lack of step 1 in the designed experiments [48].

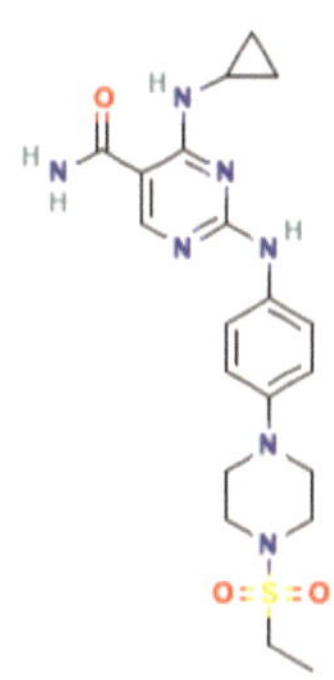

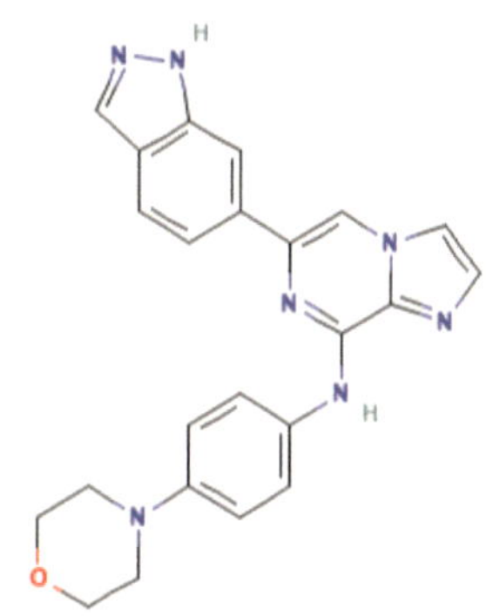

Cerdulatinib (PubChem CID: 44595079) Entospletinib (PubChem CID: 59473233)

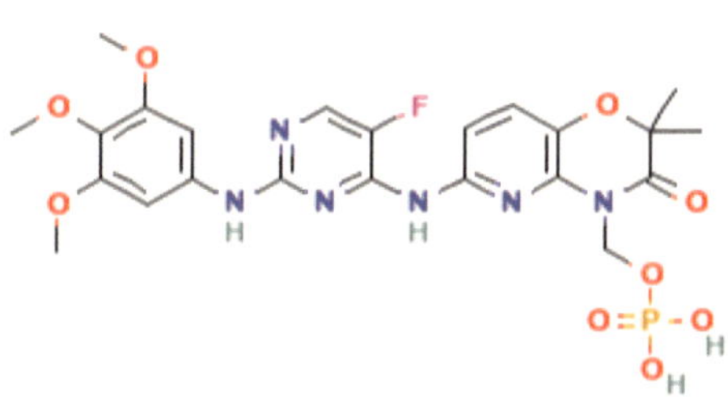

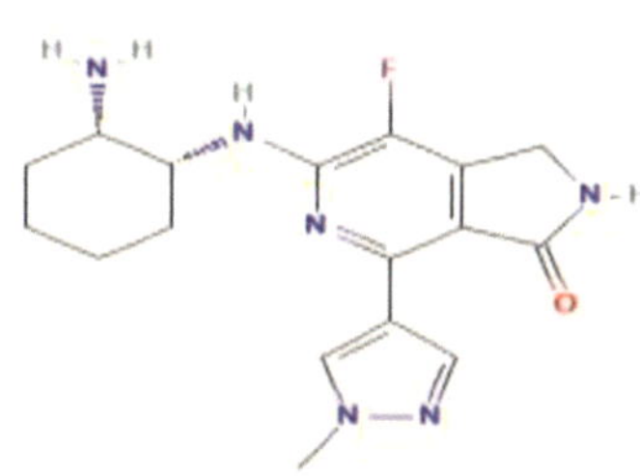

Fostamatinib (PubChem CID: 11671467) Mivavotinib TAK659(PubChem CID:53252276)

1.4.2 IMID inhibitors

Avadomide CC-122 is cereblon-modulating agent that has a potential antineoplastic, antiangiogenic and immunomodulatory activity in the cell. Avadomide has a role in the ubiquitination and rapid proteasomal degradation of Aiolos and Ikaros proteins which are the hematopoietic transcriptional factors and induce apoptosis of DLBCL. Treatment including avadomide with another anti-lymphoma drugs combination is suggested for the best results [49].

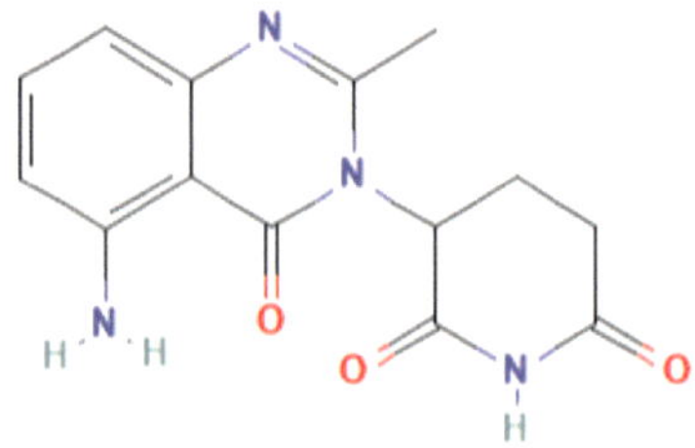

Avadomide CC-122(PubChem CID:24967599)

1.4.3 PI3K/PI3Kδ-pan PI3K inhibitors

Acalisib (GS-9820, 6-fluoro-3-phenyl-2-[(1S)-1-(9Hpurin-6-ylamino) ethyl]-4(3H)-quinazolinone): acalisib is a drug candidate for all lymphoma types including CLL, NHL. Phase 1 research showed in a human basophil activation experiment that Acalisib molecule suppresses IgE receptor by PI3Kδ-mediated CD63 expression [50].

Fimepinostat CUDC-907: a small molecule inhibits HDAC/PI3K. According to the researchers, at phase 1 experiments, dual HDAC/PI3K inhibition with fimepinostat CUDC-907 showed a well-tolerated activity in suppression of target protein activities and further, low toxicity profile was observed [48].

Umbralisib is an oral inhibitor of PI3K-delta and CK1-epsilon. Cellular functions of the PI3K-delta include cell proliferation and survival, cell differentiation, intracellular trafficking, and immunity. CK1-epsilon regulates oncoprotein regulation and the process drives the growth and survival of lymphoma. The inhibitor is in phase 2b and phase 3 trials in NHL and CLL patients. In the phase 1 study, side effects are observed in the lymphoma patients including diarrhea, nausea, and fatigue [51].

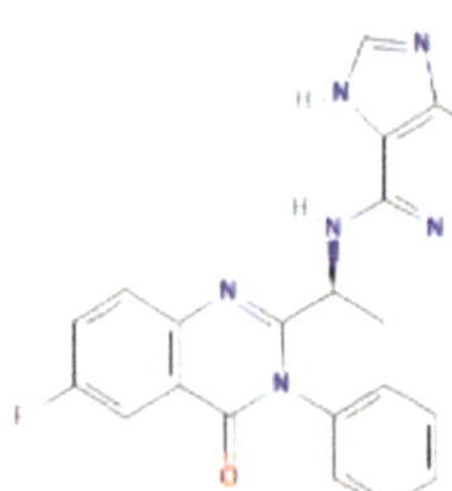

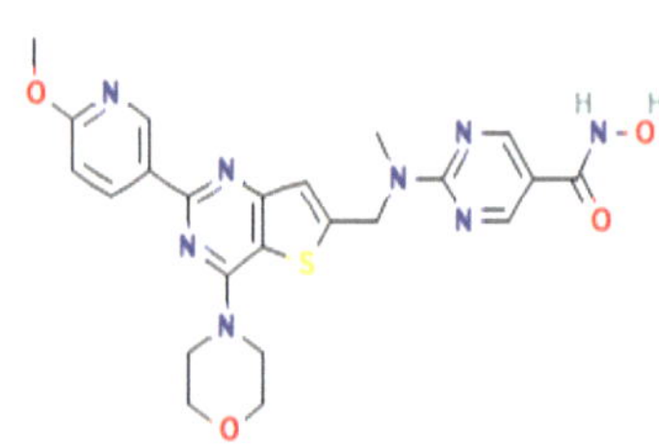

Acalisib (GS-9820) (PubChem CID:11618268) Fimepinostat CUDC-907 (PubChem CID:54575456)

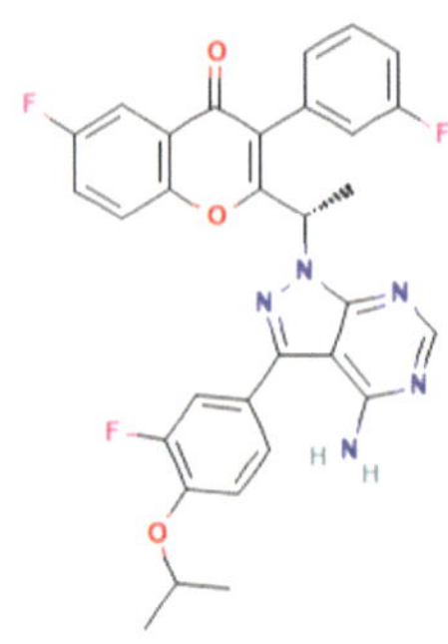

Umbralisib (PubChem CID:72950888)

1.4.4 mTOR inhibitors

Everolimus is an oral mTOR inhibitor and is used against relapsed lymphomas. A recent phase 2 study have shown that everolimus dramatically increases the efficiency of treatment in lymphoma patients when it is combined with other anti-lymphoma drugs [52].

Temsirolimus is an mTOR inhibitor that inhibits the synthesis of the proteins such as VEGF (vascular endothelial growth factor) that have role in cell proliferation and survival in mantle-cell lymphoma [53].

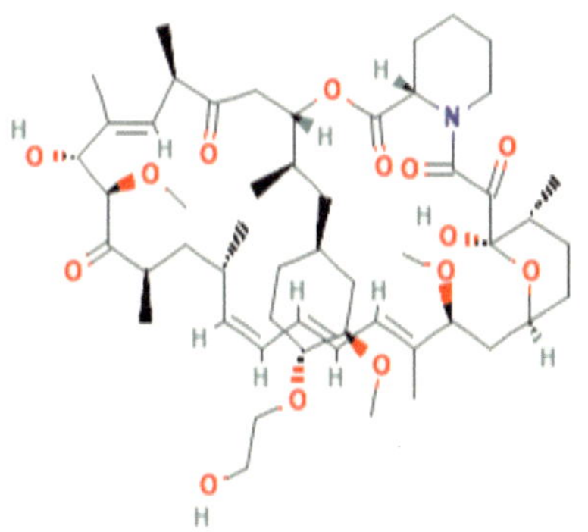

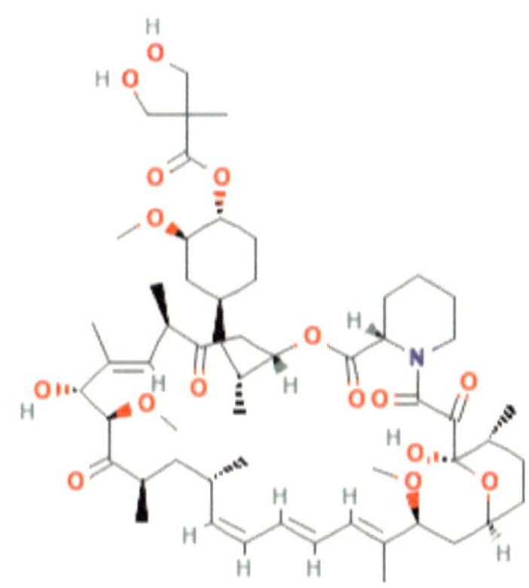

Everolimus (PubChem CID: 6442177) Temsirolimus (PubChem CID: 6918289)

1.4.5 HDAC (histone deacetylase) inhibitors

Mocetinostat MGCD0103 is classified as a HDAC inhibitor. Phase 2 study showed that a combination of mocetinostat with other anti-lymphoma agents resulted in higher efficiency in the treatment of lymphomas compared to the application of mocetinostat alone [54].

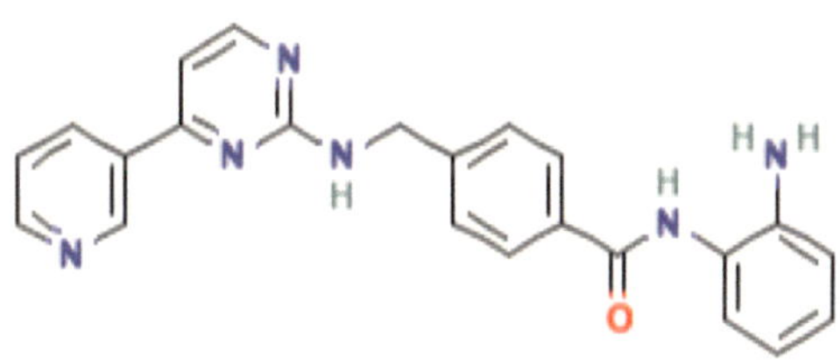

Mocetinostat MGCD0103 (PubChem CID: 9865515)

1.4.6 Aurora A kinase inhibitors

Alisertib is an Aurora A kinase inhibitor. This inhibitor leads to abnormal mitotic spindle formation that causes mitotic cell accumulation and lowers tumor cell proliferation upon treatment of malignant cells. Since Aurora A kinase has a mitotic role in the cancer cells, anti-mitotic agents may have benefits to treat lymphoma [55, 56].

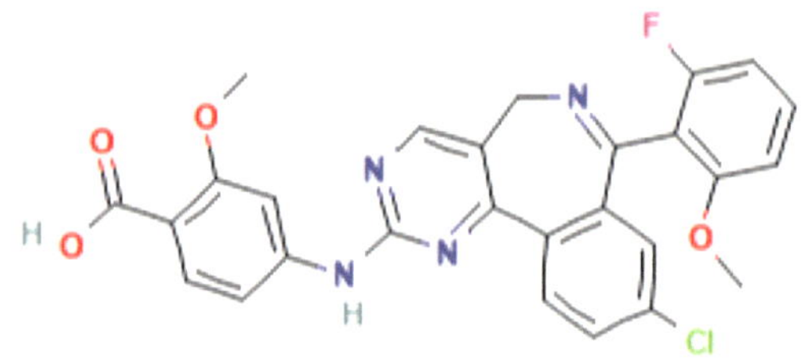

Alisertib (PubChem CID: 24771867)

1.4.7 BCL2 inhibitors

Venetoclax is a BLC2 inhibitor and BCL2 is highly expressed at CLL. The protein helps CLL cancer cells to survive and provide resistance to drugs. Venotoclax binds CLL to slow down the progression. Treatment of venetoclax with the other anti-lymphoma agents like ibrutinib displayed higher drug efficiency in patients at phase 2 trials. In the light of phase 2 results, researchers combine venetoclax with anti-lymphoma agents in phase 3 trials [57]. Combination drug treatment of venetoclax with obinutuzumab is FDA approved treatment and currently used against lymphomas [58].

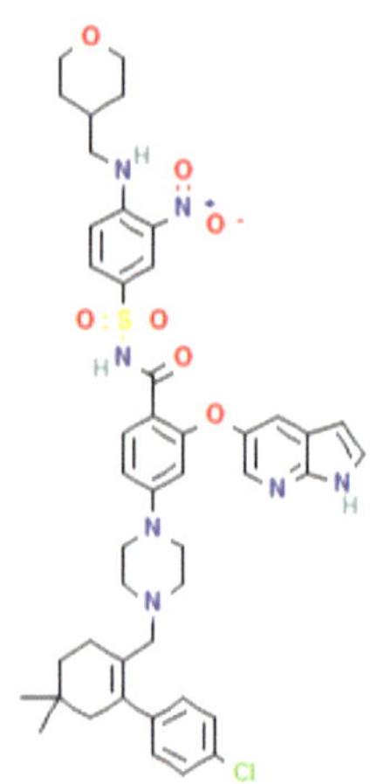

Venetoclax (PubChem CID: 49846579)

2. Conclusion

Cancer with all of its different types is a big health issue for everyone around the world. Lymphoma is one of the most common types of cancer [1]. Like all other cancer types, it has its own risk factors, causes, and treatments that are still open to discovery. Besides other cancer types, lymphoma is defined as cancer transformation of lymphoid cells. Hodgkin lymphoma and non-Hodgkin lymphoma are the main subtypes of lymphoma [1].

The treatment options for lymphoma include chemotherapy, radiotherapy, and bone marrow transplantation but research to develop the treatment options are still underway. As mentioned above, small molecule inhibitor agents are new perspectives found for the traditional treatment options for lymphoma.

The drugs and potential anticancer agents for lymphoma are mentioned in detail in this review.

Acknowledgements

Mervenur Al acknowledges YOK 100/2000 Scholarship.

Author details

Kubra Acikalin Coskun[1], Merve Tutar[2], Elif Cansu Abay[3], Nazlican Yurekli[3], Mervenur Al[4] and Yusuf Tutar[5,6,7]*

1 Division of Medicinal Biology, Department of Basic Sciences, Faculty of Medicine, Istanbul Aydin University, Turkey

2 Department of Molecular Biology and Genetics, Bilkent University, Ankara, Turkey

3 Division of Medicinal Biology, Department of Basic Sciences, Hamidiye Faculty of Medicine, University of Health Sciences-Turkey, Istanbul, Turkey

4 Division of Medicinal Biochemistry, Department of Basic Sciences, Hamidiye Faculty of Medicine, University of Health Sciences-Turkey, Istanbul, Turkey

5 Division of Biochemistry, Department of Basic Pharmaceutical Sciences, Hamidiye Faculty of Pharmacy, University of Health Sciences-Turkey, Istanbul, Turkey

6 Division of Molecular Oncology, Hamidiye Health Sciences Institutes, University of Health Sciences-Turkey, Istanbul, Turkey

7 Validebağ Research Center, University of Health Sciences-Turkey, Istanbul, Turkey

*Address all correspondence to: yusuf.tutar@sbu.edu.tr

References

[1] Vanneman M, Dranoff G. Combining immunotherapy and targeted therapies in cancer treatment. Nature Reviews. Cancer. 2012;**12**(4):237-251. DOI: 10.1038/nrc3237

[2] Seca AML, Pinto DCGA. Plant secondary metabolites as anticancer agents: Successes in clinical trials and therapeutic application. International Journal of Molecular Sciences. 2018;**19**(1):263. DOI: 10.3390/ijms19010263

[3] Williams KM, Gress RE. Immune reconstitution and implications for immunotherapy following haematopoietic stem cell transplantation. Best Practice & Research. Clinical Haematology. 2008;**21**(3):579-596. DOI: 10.1016/j.beha.2008.06.003

[4] Soofiyani SR, Hosseini K, Forouhandeh H, Ghasemnejad T, Tarhriz V, Asgharian P, et al. Quercetin as a novel therapeutic approach for lymphoma. Oxidative Medicine and Cellular Longevity. 2021;**2021**:3157867. DOI: 10.1155/2021/3157867

[5] Li S, Fang J, Si T, Lu Y, Jiang L. Salvianolic acid A inhibits the growth of diffuse large B-cell lymphoma through MAPK pathways. Experimental Hematology. 2021;**94**:60-68.e2. DOI: 10.1016/j.exphem.2020.11.007. Epub 2020 Dec 2

[6] Naik AV, Dessai SN, Sellappan K. Antitumour activity of *Annona muricata* L. leaf methanol extracts against Ehrlich ascites carcinoma and Dalton's lymphoma ascites mediated tumours in Swiss albino mice. Libyan Journal of Medicine. 2021;**16**(1):1846862. DOI: 10.1080/19932820.2020.1846862

[7] Sudarsanan D, Suresh Sulekha D, Chandrasekharan G. *Amomum subulatum* induces apoptosis in tumor cells and reduces tumor burden in experimental animals via modulating pro-inflammatory cytokines. Cancer Investigation. 2021;**39**(4):333-348. DOI: 10.1080/07357907.2021.1878529. Epub 2021 Feb 1

[8] Dulay RM, Valdez BC, Li Y, Chakrabarti S, Dhillon B, Kalaw SP, et al. Cytotoxicity of *Gymnopilus purpureosquamulosus* extracts on hematologic malignant cells through activation of the SAPK/JNK signaling pathway. PLoS One. 2021;**16**(5):e0252541. DOI: 10.1371/journal.pone.0252541

[9] Sumarni U, Reidel U, Eberle J. Targeting cutaneous T-cell lymphoma cells by ingenol mebutate (PEP005) correlates with PKCδ activation, ROS induction as well as downregulation of XIAP and c-FLIP. Cell. 2021;**10**(5):987. DOI: 10.3390/cells10050987

[10] Ueno M, Kariya R, Sittithumcharee G, Okada S. Cucurbitacin B induces apoptosis of primary effusion lymphoma via disruption of cytoskeletal organization. Phytomedicine. 2021;**85**:153545. DOI: 10.1016/j.phymed.2021.153545. Epub 2021 Mar 10

[11] Singh RK, Verma PK, Kumar A, Kumar S, Acharya A. *Achyranthes aspera* L. leaf extract induced anticancer effects on Dalton's lymphoma via regulation of PKCα signaling pathway and mitochondrial apoptosis. Journal of Ethnopharmacology. 2021;**274**:114060. DOI: 10.1016/j.jep.2021.114060. Epub 2021 Mar 23

[12] Wang L, Li LR, Zhang L, Wang JW. The landscape of new drugs in extranodal NK/T-cell lymphoma. Cancer Treatment Reviews. 2020;**89**:102065. DOI: 10.1016/j.ctrv.2020.102065. Epub 2020 Jul 2

[13] Abdel-Wahab O, Levine RL. Recent advances in the treatment of acute

myeloid leukemia. F1000 Medicine Reports. 2010;**2**:55. DOI: 10.3410/M2-55

[14] Shi Y, van der Meel R, Chen X, Lammers T. The EPR effect and beyond: Strategies to improve tumor targeting and cancer nanomedicine treatment efficacy. Theranostics. 2020;**10**(17): 7921-7924. DOI: 10.7150/thno.49577

[15] Al-Hussaini M, DiPersio JF. Small molecule inhibitors in acute myeloid leukemia: From the bench to the clinic. Expert Review of Hematology. 2014;**7**(4):439-464. DOI: 10.1586/17474086.2014.932687

[16] Sweta J, Khandelwal R, Srinitha S, Pancholi R, Adhikary R, Ali MA, et al. Identification of high-affinity small molecule targeting IDH2 for the clinical treatment of acute myeloid leukemia. Asian Pacific Journal of Cancer Prevention. 2019;**20**(8):2287-2297. DOI: 10.31557/APJCP.2019.20.8.2287

[17] Makita S, Hosoba R, Tobinai K. Safety considerations with targeted therapy drugs for B-cell non-Hodgkin lymphoma. Expert Opinion on Drug Safety. 2020;**19**(9):1105-1120. DOI: 10.1080/14740338.2020.1802424. Epub 2020 Aug 25

[18] Younes A, Ansell S, Fowler N, Wilson W, de Vos S, Seymour J, et al. The landscape of new drugs in lymphoma. Nature Reviews. Clinical Oncology. 2017;**14**(6):335-346. DOI: 10.1038/nrclinonc.2016.205. Epub 2016 Dec 29

[19] Younes A. New drugs for new targets in lymphoma. Hematological Oncology. 2019;**37**(Suppl. 1):105-109. DOI: 10.1002/hon.2592

[20] Pal Singh S, Dammeijer F, Hendriks RW. Role of Bruton's tyrosine kinase in B cells and malignancies. Molecular Cancer. 2018;**17**(1):57. DOI: 10.1186/s12943-018-0779-z. Erratum in: Molecular Cancer. 2019;**18**(1):79

[21] Fowler N, Davis E. Targeting B-cell receptor signaling: Changing the paradigm. Hematology. American Society of Hematology. Education Program. 2013;**2013**:553-560. DOI: 10.1182/asheducation-2013.1.553

[22] Manji F, Puckrin R, Stewart DA. Novel synthetic drugs for the treatment of non-Hodgkin lymphoma. Expert Opinion on Pharmacotherapy. 2021;**22**(11):1417-1427. DOI: 10.1080/14656566.2021.1902988. Epub 2021 Mar 25

[23] Woyach JA, Ruppert AS, Guinn D, Lehman A, Blachly JS, Lozanski A, et al. BTK^{C481S}-mediated resistance to ibrutinib in chronic lymphocytic leukemia. Journal of Clinical Oncology. 2017;**35**(13):1437-1443. DOI: 10.1200/JCO.2016.70.2282. Epub 2017 Feb 13

[24] Mato MD, Anthony R. LOXO-305, a next generation, highly selective, non-covalent BTK inhibitor in previously treated CLL/SLL: Results from the phase 1/2 BRUIN study. Blood. 2020;**136**:35-37

[25] Treon SP, Tripsas CK, Meid K, Warren D, Varma G, Green R, et al. Ibrutinib in previously treated Waldenström's macroglobulinemia. The New England Journal of Medicine. 2015;**372**(15):1430-1440. DOI: 10.1056/NEJMoa1501548

[26] Dreyling M, Jurczak W, Jerkeman M, Silva RS, Rusconi C, Trneny M, et al. Ibrutinib versus temsirolimus in patients with relapsed or refractory mantle-cell lymphoma: An international, randomised, open-label, phase 3 study. Lancet. 2016;**387**(10020):770-778. DOI: 10.1016/S0140-6736(15)00667-4. Epub 2015 Dec 7. Erratum in: Lancet. 2016;**387**(10020):750

[27] Rule S, Jurczak W, Jerkeman M, Rusconi C, Trneny M, Offner F, et al. Ibrutinib versus temsirolimus: 3-year follow-up of patients with previously

treated mantle cell lymphoma from the phase 3, international, randomized, open-label RAY study. Leukemia. 2018;**32**(8):1799-1803. DOI: 10.1038/s41375-018-0023-2. Epub 2018 Feb 2

[28] Soussain C, Choquet S, Blonski M, Leclercq D, Houillier C, Rezai K, et al. Ibrutinib monotherapy for relapse or refractory primary CNS lymphoma and primary vitreoretinal lymphoma: Final analysis of the phase II 'proof-of-concept' iLOC study by the Lymphoma study association (LYSA) and the French oculo-cerebral lymphoma (LOC) network. European Journal of Cancer. 2019;**117**:121-130. DOI: 10.1016/j.ejca.2019.05.024. Epub 2019 Jul 3

[29] Wang M, Rule S, Zinzani PL, Goy A, Casasnovas O, Smith SD, et al. Acalabrutinib in relapsed or refractory mantle cell lymphoma (ACE-LY-004): A single-arm, multicentre, phase 2 trial. Lancet. 2018;**391**(10121):659-667. DOI: 10.1016/S0140-6736(17)33108-2. Epub 2017 Dec 11

[30] Wang W, Sun Q. Novel targeted drugs approved by the NMPA and FDA in 2019. Signal Transduction and Targeted Therapy. 2020;**5**(1):65. DOI: 10.1038/s41392-020-0164-4

[31] Gribben JG, Fowler N, Morschhauser F. Mechanisms of action of lenalidomide in B-cell non-Hodgkin lymphoma. Journal of Clinical Oncology. 2015;**33**(25):2803-2811. DOI: 10.1200/JCO.2014.59.5363. Epub 2015 Jul 20

[32] Ludwig H, Delforge M, Facon T, Einsele H, Gay F, Moreau P, et al. Prevention and management of adverse events of novel agents in multiple myeloma: A consensus of the European myeloma network. Leukemia. 2018;**32**(7):1542-1560. DOI: 10.1038/s41375-018-0040-1. Epub 2018 May 2

[33] Gavriatopoulou M, Chari A, Chen C, Bahlis N, Vogl DT, Jakubowiak A, et al. Integrated safety profile of selinexor in multiple myeloma: Experience from 437 patients enrolled in clinical trials. Leukemia. 2020;**34**(9):2430-2440. DOI: 10.1038/s41375-020-0756-6. Epub 2020 Feb 24

[34] Dreyling M, Santoro A, Mollica L, Leppä S, Follows GA, Lenz G, et al. Phosphatidylinositol 3-kinase inhibition by copanlisib in relapsed or refractory indolent lymphoma. Journal of Clinical Oncology. 2017;**35**(35):3898-3905. DOI: 10.1200/JCO.2017.75.4648. Epub 2017 Oct 4. Erratum in: Journal of Clinical Oncology. 2018;**36**(5):521

[35] Flinn IW, Miller CB, Ardeshna KM, Tetreault S, Assouline SE, Mayer J, et al. DYNAMO: A phase II study of duvelisib (IPI-145) in patients with refractory indolent non-Hodgkin lymphoma. Journal of Clinical Oncology. 2019;**37**(11):912-922. DOI: 10.1200/JCO.18.00915. Epub 2019 Feb 11. Erratum in: Journal of Clinical Oncology. 2019;**37**(16):1448

[36] Tan CRC, Abdul-Majeed S, Cael B, Barta SK. Clinical pharmacokinetics and pharmacodynamics of bortezomib. Clinical Pharmacokinetics. 2019;**58**(2): 157-168. DOI: 10.1007/s40262-018-0679-9

[37] Fisher RI, Bernstein SH, Kahl BS, Djulbegovic B, Robertson MJ, de Vos S, et al. Multicenter phase II study of bortezomib in patients with relapsed or refractory mantle cell lymphoma. Journal of Clinical Oncology. 2006;**24**(30):4867-4874. DOI: 10.1200/JCO.2006.07.9665. Epub 2006 Sep 25

[38] Dimopoulos MA, García-Sanz R, Gavriatopoulou M. Primary therapy of Waldenstrom macroglobulinemia (WM) with weekly bortezomib, low-dose dexamethasone, and rituximab (BDR): Long-term results of a phase 2 study of the European myeloma network (EMN). Blood. 2013;**122**(19): 3276-3282. DOI: 10.1182/blood-2013-05-503862

[39] Castillo JJ, Guerrero-Garcia T, Baldini F, Tchernonog E, Cartron G, Ninkovic S, et al. Bortezomib plus EPOCH is effective as frontline treatment in patients with plasmablastic lymphoma. British Journal of Haematology. 2019;**184**(4):679-682. DOI: 10.1111/bjh.15156. Epub 2018 Mar 12

[40] Davies A, Cummin TE, Barrans S, Maishman T, Mamot C, Novak U, et al. Gene-expression profiling of bortezomib added to standard chemoimmunotherapy for diffuse large B-cell lymphoma (REMoDL-B): An open-label, randomised, phase 3 trial. The Lancet Oncology. 2019;**20**(5):649-662. DOI: 10.1016/S1470-2045(18)30935-5. Epub 2019 Apr 1

[41] Smolewski P, Robak T. The discovery and development of romidepsin for the treatment of T-cell lymphoma. Expert Opinion on Drug Discovery. 2017;**12**(8):859-873. DOI: 10.1080/17460441.2017.1341487. Epub 2017 Jun 22

[42] O'Connor OA, Horwitz S, Masszi T, Van Hoof A, Brown P, Doorduijn J, et al. Belinostat in patients with relapsed or refractory peripheral T-cell lymphoma: Results of the pivotal phase II BELIEF (CLN-19) study. Journal of Clinical Oncology. 2015;**33**(23):2492-2499. DOI: 10.1200/JCO.2014.59.2782. Epub 2015 Jun 22

[43] Olsen EA, Kim YH, Kuzel TM, Pacheco TR, Foss FM, Parker S, et al. Phase IIb multicenter trial of vorinostat in patients with persistent, progressive, or treatment refractory cutaneous T-cell lymphoma. Journal of Clinical Oncology. 2007;**25**(21):3109-3115. DOI: 10.1200/JCO.2006.10.2434. Epub 2007 Jun 18

[44] Giacinti C, Giordano A. RB and cell cycle progression. Oncogene. 2006;**25**(38):5220-5227. DOI: 10.1038/sj.onc.1209615

[45] Patriarca A, Gaidano G. Investigational drugs for the treatment of diffuse large B-cell lymphoma. Expert Opinion on Investigational Drugs. 2021;**30**(1):25-38. DOI: 10.1080/13543784.2021.1855140. Epub 2020 Dec 21

[46] Barr PM, Saylors GB, Spurgeon SE, Cheson BD, Greenwald DR, O'Brien SM, et al. Phase 2 study of idelalisib and entospletinib: Pneumonitis limits combination therapy in relapsed refractory CLL and NHL. Blood. 2016;**127**(20):2411-2415. DOI: 10.1182/blood-2015-12-683516. Epub 2016 Mar 11

[47] Friedberg JW, Sharman J, Sweetenham J, Johnston PB, Vose JM, Lacasce A, et al. Inhibition of Syk with fostamatinib disodium has significant clinical activity in non-Hodgkin lymphoma and chronic lymphocytic leukemia. Blood. 2010;**115**(13):2578-2585. DOI: 10.1182/blood-2009-08-236471. Epub 2009 Nov 17

[48] Phillips TJ. A phase 2 study of TAK-659, an investigational reversible dual SYK/FLT3 inhibitor, in patients with relapsed or refractory diffuse large B-cell lymphoma. Blood. 2019;**134** (Suppl. 1):5310-5310. DOI: 10.1182/blood-2019-125650

[49] Carpio C, Bouabdallah R, Ysebaert L, Sancho JM, Salles G, Cordoba R, et al. Avadomide monotherapy in relapsed/refractory DLBCL: Safety, efficacy, and a predictive gene classifier. Blood. 2020;**135**(13):996-1007. DOI: 10.1182/blood.2019002395. Erratum in: Blood. 2021;**137**(15):2126

[50] Kater AP, Tonino SH, Spiering M, Chamuleau MED, Liu R, Adewoye AH, et al. Final results of a phase 1b study of the safety and efficacy of the PI3Kδ inhibitor acalisib (GS-9820) in relapsed/refractory lymphoid malignancies. Blood Cancer Journal. 2018;**8**(2):16. DOI: 10.1038/s41408-018-0055-x

[51] Aydin E, Faehling S, Saleh M, Llaó Cid L, Seiffert M, Roessner PM. Phosphoinositide 3-kinase signaling in the tumor microenvironment: What do we need to consider when treating chronic lymphocytic leukemia with PI3K inhibitors? Frontiers in Immunology. 2021;**11**:595818. DOI: 10.3389/fimmu.2020.595818

[52] Kim SJ, Shin DY, Kim JS, Yoon DH, Lee WS, Lee H, et al. A phase II study of everolimus (RAD001), an mTOR inhibitor plus CHOP for newly diagnosed peripheral T-cell lymphomas. Annals of Oncology. 2016;**27**(4):712-718. DOI: 10.1093/annonc/mdv624. Epub 2016 Feb 8

[53] Schulze M, Stock C, Zaccagnini M, Teber D, Rassweiler JJ. Temsirolimus. Recent Results in Cancer Research. 2014;**201**:393-403. DOI: 10.1007/978-3-642-54490-3_24

[54] Batlevi CL, Crump M, Andreadis C, Rizzieri D, Assouline SE, Fox S, et al. A phase 2 study of mocetinostat, a histone deacetylase inhibitor, in relapsed or refractory lymphoma. British Journal of Haematology. 2017;**178**(3):434-441. DOI: 10.1111/bjh.14698. Epub 2017 Apr 25

[55] Yuan CX, Zhou ZW, Yang YX, He ZX, Zhang X, Wang D, et al. Inhibition of mitotic Aurora kinase A by alisertib induces apoptosis and autophagy of human gastric cancer AGS and NCI-N78 cells. Drug Design, Development and Therapy. 2015;**9**: 487-508. DOI: 10.2147/DDDT.S74127

[56] Friedberg JW, Mahadevan D, Cebula E, Persky D, Lossos I, Agarwal AB, et al. Phase II study of alisertib, a selective Aurora A kinase inhibitor, in relapsed and refractory aggressive B- and T-cell non-Hodgkin lymphomas. Journal of Clinical Oncology. 2014;**32**(1):44-50. DOI: 10.1200/JCO.2012.46.8793

[57] Tam CS, Anderson MA, Pott C, Agarwal R, Handunnetti S, Hicks RJ, et al. Ibrutinib plus venetoclax for the treatment of mantle-cell lymphoma. The New England Journal of Medicine. 2018;**378**(13):1211-1223. DOI: 10.1056/NEJMoa1715519

[58] Combination Therapy with Venetoclax Approved for CLL. National Cancer Institute; 2019. Available from: https://www.cancer.gov/news-events/cancer-currents-blog/2019/venetoclax-obinutuzumab-fda-approval-cll-sll#CLL-treatment

Chapter 2

Follicular Lymphoma

Gopila Gupta and Vikas Garg

Abstract

Follicular lymphoma (FL) is one of the most common type of indolent non- Hodgkin's lymphoma. It originates from germinal center B cells and has characteristic translocation t(11,14) involving immunoglobulin heavy chain gene (chromosome 14q32) and Bcl2 gene (chromosome 18q21) in 90% of patients. FL presents with lymphadenopathy and/or bone marrow involvement. Diagnosis is confirmed by histological examination of lymph nodes. FL is a slow growing tumor with frequent remission and relapses. Follicular lymphoma international prognostic index (FLIPI) and progression of disease within 24 months (POD24) are most important prognostic markers. Early-stage disease is usually treated with radiotherapy. Management of advanced stage depends on disease burden. Patients with advanced stage disease may be observed in case of low burden disease and those with high disease load require treatment with chemo-immunotherapy.

Keywords: Follicular lymphoma, non-Hodgkin's lymphoma, NHL, Low grade lymphoma

1. Introduction - Epidemiology

Follicular lymphoma (FL) is one of the most common forms of indolent lymphoma constituting 20–25% of all non-Hodgkin's lymphoma (NHL) in the United States and Europe. However, it is less common in the African and Asian population accounting for 10% of all NHL [1–4]. There is no known risk factor for follicular lymphoma [5]. It is a disease of the elderly with a median age of 65 years, and the young are only rarely affected [6]. It is an indolent disease that typically manifests as asymptomatic adenopathy. Involvement of the bone marrow is frequent, occurring in up to 80% of cases. B symptoms and high serum lactate dehydrogenase (LDH) levels are observed in approximately 20% of patients. Extranodal involvement is less prevalent, occurring in about 10% of cases [7, 8].

2. Histology

On histopathologic examination, Follicular lymphoma shows densely packed follicles with attenuated mantle zones that obscure nodal architecture. The follicles consist of two major cell types, centrocytes, and centroblasts. Centrocytes are small to medium-sized with scarce cytoplasm, elongated or cleft nuclei, and small nucleoli. Centroblasts are large cells (about three times the size of a lymphocyte) with a basophilic cytoplasm ring, round to oval non-cleaved nuclei, and prominent nucleoli. Histological grading (**Table 1**) is based on the proportion of centrocytes and centroblasts present in the germinal centers. FL grades 1 to 3a is considered a low-grade

Histologic grade	Microscopic features
Grade 1 (follicular small cleaved)	Up to 5 centroblasts per HPF
Grade 2 (follicular mixed)	6–15 centroblasts per HPF
Grade 3a (follicular large cell)	More than 15 centroblasts per HPF
Grade 3b	Solid sheets of centroblasts

HPF high power field.

Table 1.
Histologic grading of follicular lymphoma.

indolent disease, whereas FL grade 3b is considered an aggressive form of lymphoma [9]. Follicular lymphoma has a paratrabecular pattern of involvement in the bone marrow, and the appearance of tumor cells is similar to that found in lymph nodes.

On immunohistochemistry (IHC) Follicular lymphoma cells express B-cell antigens (CD19, CD20, CD22, and CD79a), BCL2, BCL6, and CD10. Surface expression of immunoglobulin is observed in about one-half of cases. BCL2 overexpression is present in the majority of grade 1 FL–2 FL, however, it is less common in grade 3 FL [10]. CD 10 negative FL are commonly high grade, express IRF4/MUMI and BCL 6 but lacks BCL2 expression.

3. Pathobiology

The germinal center B cell expressing CD20 and B-cell leukemia/lymphoma 2 (BCL2) is the cell of origin for follicular lymphoma [11]. The characteristic translocation [t(14,18)] involving the BCL2 gene on chromosome 18q21.3 and immunoglobulin heavy chain gene on chromosome 14q32; q21 is observed in up to 90% of patients. It provides a survival advantage to malignant B cells by upregulation of anti-apoptotic signals [11]. However, BCL2 overexpression alone is insufficient for malignant transformation to FL, and additional hits are required [12]. KMT2D, CREBBP, EZH2, EP300, KMT2C, and ARID1A mutations are commonly identified, although their significance in FL remains unknown [13, 14].

4. Pre-treatment evaluation

The initial evaluation should entail recording a detailed history and completing a comprehensive physical examination. A biopsy of the afflicted lymph node, either excisional or incisional, is required [9, 15]. Biopsy samples should be evaluated by an expert haemato-pathologist. For baseline staging, either contrast-enhanced computed tomography (CECT) of the neck, chest, and abdomen or whole-body positron emission tomography (PET) with computed tomography, should be performed [16, 17]. PET is preferable in early-stage patients and for assessing response at the end of treatment (EOT) [10, 18]. All individuals with early-stage FL should have a unilateral bone marrow biopsy (stages I and II). However, it can be omitted in patients with advanced disease (stage III and IV) as it provides no extra information in such a scenario [19, 20]. For assessment of organ functions and prognostic information, baseline complete blood count, renal and hepatic functions, serology for hepatitis B and C, β2-microglobulin, and LDH are necessary. Patients planned for anthracycline-based therapy should have their cardiac function evaluated by 2D-ECHO or a MUGA scan. Fertility preservation should be discussed with all patients of reproductive age [21].

5. Histologic transformation

Histological transformation of FL to high-grade lymphoma during the natural history of disease is a well-known entity. 15–20% patients demonstrating transformation at 5 years of follow up [22, 23]. Risk of transformation is about 1–3 percent per year. Histological examination reveals loss of follicular architecture and replacement by large-sized cells with a high proliferation index. FL most commonly transforms to diffuse large B cell lymphoma (DLBCL), but other histology like Burkitt's lymphoma, lymphoblastic lymphoma, and Hodgkin's disease have also been reported [24]. Rapidly progressing lymphadenopathy, unusual extra-nodal involvement, constitutional symptoms, elevated lactate dehydrogenase (LDH) and hypercalcemia are clinical pointers of histological transformation. Diagnosis is confirmed by guided biopsy of the highest metabolically active lesion in case of high clinical suspicion [25, 26].

6. Prognostic factors

Age, stage, nodal burden, LDH, hemoglobin, and β2-microglobulin have been recognized as important prognostic factors. Various prognostic models have been developed based on these factors (**Table 2**), including FLIPI (follicular lymphoma international prognostic index), FLIPI 2, and PRIMA-PI (Primary Rituximab and Maintenance study prognostic index). FLIPI is a widely used tool

Prognostic model and risk factors	Risk stratification
FLIPI 1. Age: >60 years 2. Ann Arbor Stage: III–IV 3. Hb concentration: <12 g/dL 4. Number of nodal sites: >4 5. Serum LDH: >ULN	Low: 0–1 risk factors→5-year OS: 92%; Intermediate: 2 risk factors→5-year OS: 78% High: 3–5 risk factors→5-year OS: 52%
FLIPI 2 1. Age: >60 years 2. Bone marrow involvement 3. Hb concentration: <12 g/dL 4. Greatest diameter of largest involved node: >6 cm 5. Serum beta 2 microglobulin concentration: >ULN	Low: 0–1 risk factors→ 3-year OS: 99% Intermediate: 2 risk factors→ 3-year OS: 96% High: 3–5 risk factors→ 3-year OS: 84%
PRIMA-PI 1. Serum beta 2 microglobulin >3 g/L 2. Bone marrow involvement	Low: 0 risk factors→5-year PFS: 69% Intermediate: 1 risk factor→5-year PFS: 55% High: 2 risk factors→5-year PFS: 37%
POD 24 (Progression of disease within 24 months of chemoimmunotherapy)	POD >24 months→ 5-year OS 90% POD <24 months→ 5-year OS 50%

ECOG, Eastern Cooperative Oncology Group; FLIPI, follicular lymphoma international prognostic index; Hb, hemoglobin; LDH, lactate dehydrogenase; OS, overall survival; PFS, progression-free survival; POD, Progression of disease; PRIMA-PI, Primary Rituximab and Maintenance study prognostic index; PS, performance status; ULN, upper limit of normal.

Table 2.
Prognostics tools in follicular lymphoma.

developed in the pre-rituximab era, but it has been validated in several prospective trials in patients receiving rituximab [27–29]. PRIMA-PI incorporates only two parameters, serum 2-microglobulin levels, and bone marrow involvement, however it has not been prospectively validated [30]. POD24 (progression within 24 months of therapy) has recently been found as a key prognostic and predictive marker [31, 32]. It may be used method for predicting relapse and aid in therapy selection.

7. Management

Management of FL is based on the stage at presentation, tumor grade, and burden of disease. Early-stage local diseases are treated with curative intent, while in advanced diseases aim is to reduce symptom burden, increase survival, and enhance the quality of life.

7.1 Limited stage FL

Early-stage (stage I and II) patients have an excellent prognosis with median survival approaching 20 years [33–35]. There are several management options available, including radiation, single-agent rituximab, chemo-immunotherapy, and observation. The recommended radiation dosage is involved site radiotherapy (ISRT) with 24 Gy (Gray) administered in 12 fractions [36]. Higher dose does not provide any survival advantage and is associated with greater toxicity [37]. When compared to observation alone, patients who receive RT have better disease-specific survival as well as overall survival [38, 39]. PFS benefit was observed by adding rituximab or chemotherapy to the radiotherapy, however, there was no difference in overall survival [40, 41]. Patients unwilling for treatment may also be considered for observation [42]. High grade (grade 3B) FL patients are managed on the lines of other high-grade NHL like DLBCL (diffuse large B cell lymphoma). Combination chemo-immunotherapy R-CHOP (rituximab, cyclophosphamide, vincristine, doxorubicin, prednisone) is preferred in such cases. If involved sites cannot be encompassed in a single radiation field, patients should be treated as advanced FL.

7.2 Advanced stage FL

Advanced stage FL is a very diverse group, with some patients having an indolent course and long-term survival and others having a more aggressive course, with frequent relapses. Although the majority of patients respond to currently available therapies, relapses are common. The treatment of advanced FL is determined by the histologic grade and disease load [43]. For assessing disease load in advanced FL, Groupe d'Etude des Lymphomes Folliculaires (GELF) criteria are widely employed (**Table 3**). Patient with any of the GELF feature is categorized as high tumor load disease [44].

Patients who do not fulfill any of the GELF features are considered to have a low disease load and can be initially observed. This is based on the results of a randomized trial, which showed no difference in cause-specific survival and overall survival between observation and active treatment with chlorambucil [44]. Another approach is to use single-agent rituximab followed by maintenance. In a randomized trial comparing observation, single-agent rituximab and rituximab followed by maintenance rituximab for 2 years, PFS and time to start of new treatment was better with rituximab treatment. However, there is no survival benefit with

GELF criteria
1. Nodal or extra nodal tumor size: any site >7 cm or ≥ 3 sites >3 cm
2. Presence of B symptoms*
3. Presence of compressive symptoms
4. Palpable spleen below umbilicus
5. Presence of ascites or pleural effusions
6. Presence of leukemic phase (circulating malignant cells >5 × 10^9/L)
7. Presence of cytopenia due to disease: neutropenia (<1 × 10^9/L) or thrombocytopenia (<100 × 10^9/L)

**B symptoms are defined as recurrent unexplained fever >38°C, or recurrent night sweats or unexplained ≥10% loss of bodyweight in last 6 months. GELF Groupe d-Etude des Lymphomes Folliculaires.*
High tumor load is defined if any one or more risk factors are present.

Table 3.
GELF criteria for assessment of tumor load in follicular lymphoma [43, 44].

rituximab [45]. Similarly, no survival benefit was observed with rituximab maintenance in the RESORT study. In this study, patients received four cycles of weekly rituximab followed by randomization to maintenance rituximab or retreatment on progression [46]. Due to lack of any overall survival advantage with upfront treatment over observation, low burden FL may be kept on close follow-up.

FL with a high disease load warrants immediate treatment with chemo-immunotherapy. Various chemo-immunotherapy induction regimens available for patients with FL are R-CVP (rituximab, cyclophosphamide, vincristine, and prednisone), R-CHOP (rituximab, cyclophosphamide, adriamycin, vincristine, and prednisone), and BR (bendamustine and rituximab). Patients who have a partial or complete remission with the above therapies are further treated with rituximab maintenance. Choice of chemo-immunotherapy regimen is based on patients performance status, pre-existing comorbidities, and side effect profile of drugs as no overall survival advantage has been shown for any regimen above other in a randomized trial. R-CVP has lower response rates and progression-free survival compared to R-CHOP. BR is associated with better progression-free survival and lower rates of neutropenia, infections, neuropathy, and alopecia. However, there was no difference concerning overall survival over R-CHOP and R-CVP [47–49]. Use of newer anti-CD20 agent obinutuzumab has shown improvement in progression-free survival but no overall survival benefit and is associated with higher infusion reactions, neutropenia, and infections [50]. Use of chemotherapy-free regimens using lenalidomide and rituximab (R2) has similar survival with a different toxicity profile compared to chemo-immunotherapy regimens [51].

The role of maintenance rituximab in patients with either complete or partial remission after initial chemo-immunotherapy has not been proven beyond doubt. In the PRIMA (Primary Rituximab And Maintenance) trial, patients were randomized to rituximab maintenance (every 8 weeks for 2 years) or a placebo after initial chemo-immunotherapy. Rituximab arm had higher progression-free survival but at the cost of higher adverse effects (infusion reaction, neutropenia, and infections). However, initial chemo-immunotherapy regimens did not include a bendamustine-based regimen, which is most commonly used in the current era [52]. So these results could not be extrapolated after initial bendamustine-based therapy in absence of prospective evidence. Similarly, there was no survival benefit with rituximab maintenance in patients aged 60–75 years [53].

8. Relapse or refractory follicular lymphoma

FL has a protracted course with multiple remissions and relapses. About 20% of patients do not respond to initial therapy and another 20% of patients relapse within 24 months of initial therapy [54]. Interval between initial treatment and relapse is the most important prognostic and predictive factor for relapsed FL. Those who relapse after 24 months of initial therapy have good long-term outcomes, while those relapsing within 24 months have a dismal prognosis. There is no set consensus on the management of relapsed patients. Multiple options are available including chemo-immunotherapy, novel agents, and stem cell transplant. Choice of therapy depends upon the disease burden, prior therapy, response to prior therapies, duration of previous remission, performance status, comorbidities, and adverse effect profile of the drugs. The goal of therapy is improvement in symptoms, increase survival, and a better quality of life.

Patients who relapse more than 24 months after initial chemoimmunotherapy are considered late relapses. These late relapses have an indolent course and survivals rates can approximate that of the general population [55]. Patients who do not meet GELF criteria have no immediate requirement to initiate treatment and may be observed. An alternate approach is to use single-agent rituximab. Symptomatic FL patients with high disease load may be managed with single-agent rituximab, chemoimmunotherapy, lenalidomide plus rituximab (R2), or novel agents. Single-agent rituximab is preferred in patients with comorbidities and poor performance status [56]. Relapsed FL with good performance status can be treated with anti CD20 monoclonal antibody in combination with chemotherapy or lenalidomide. If the patient has previously received BR-based therapy, R-CHOP, R-CVP, or R2 may be used at the time of relapse. Similarly, if the patient has received R-CHOP-based therapy, he may be considered for BR or R2. If the patient has relapsed during anti-CD20 monoclonal antibody maintenance, it is preferable to use an alternate anti-CD20 agent like obinutuzumab [57, 58]. Radio-immunoconjugates have been used for management of FL in patients with good bone marrow reserve but because of the associated high risk of secondary malignancies and difficult administration have not gained much acceptance [59].

Patients who have progression of disease within 24 months (POD 24) of initial chemo-immunotherapy are considered early relapses and have poor outcomes. 5-year overall survival in this group is 50% compared to 90% for patients who do not progress in 2 years [54]. Histological transformation should be ruled out in these patients with a repeat biopsy. The patient's further therapy is determined by whether he or she is transplant eligible or not. Transplant eligible patients are managed by chemo-immunotherapy followed by autologous hematopoietic stem cell transplant (HSCT). Autologous HSCT in early relapse has shown 20% improvement in 5-year overall survival. There is no survival benefit of allogenic over autologous HSCT [60, 61]. For patients with late relapse autologous HSCT may be deferred for later relapses. Allogenic stem cell transplant may be reserved for fit patients who have persistent marrow involvement, poor mobilizers stem cells for autologous HSCT and failure of autologous HSCT.

Newer drugs in the arena of follicular lymphoma management are PI3K inhibitors (idelalisib, copanlisib, duvelisib, umbralisib). EZH2 (enhancer of zeste homolog 2) mutations are observed in up to 20% of cases of relapsed FL and predict a favorable outcome. EZH2 inhibitor tazemetostat is an oral drug approved in relapsed FL patients in the first relapse in presence of EZH2 mutations and post two lines irrespective of EZH2 mutation status. Responses are observed in approximately 70% of patients with EZH2 mutations and 35% without EZH2 mutations. Adverse effects are mild and include hematotoxicity, hepatotoxicity, and elevation in serum creatinine [51]. Phosphatidylinositol-3- kinase (PI3K) inhibitors are approved in relapsed FL post multiple lines of therapy. Overall response rates range from 40 to 60%, most of which are partial responses. Common toxicities include fatigue, gastrointestinal toxicity (diarrhea, colitis), hepatotoxicity, pneumonitis, opportunistic infections, and metabolic derangements (hypertriglyceridemia, hyperglycemia). Idelalisib is an oral inhibitor of PI3K delta isoform. Copanlisib is an intravenous drug inhibiting PI3K alpha and delta isoforms. Duvelisib is an oral drug, is a dual inhibitor of delta and gamma isoforms of PI3K. Umbralisib is an oral multikinase inhibitor, acting on PI3K delta and casein kinase [62–65].

Two chimeric antigen receptor T (CART) therapy products have been approved for relapsed/refractory FL post two or more lines of therapy are tisagenlecleucel and axicabtagene ciloleucelis [66, 67]. Response are seen in about 90% of patients with the majority achieving complete remission. Characteristic adverse effects include cytokine release syndrome (CRS), neurotoxicity, cytopenia, infections, and hypogammaglobulinemia.

9. Future directions

Multiple newer therapies are currently under trial in patients with relapsed follicular lymphoma including checkpoint inhibitors, monoclonal antibodies, immunomodulatory drugs, vaccines, and chimeric antigen receptor T cell therapy. Future research should focus on identifying the predictive and prognostic biomarkers to identify patients at risk of early relapse and the role of therapy intensification in such cases.

Author details

Gopila Gupta[1] and Vikas Garg[2*]

1 Department of Hematology and Bone Marrow Transplant, Fortis Hospital, New Delhi, India

2 Department of Medical Oncology, Dr. B. R. Ambedkar Institute Rotary Cancer Hospital, All India Institute of Medical Sciences, New Delhi, India

*Address all correspondence to: vg18007@gmail.com

References

[1] SH S, E C, NL H, ES J, SA P, H S, et al. WHO Classification of Tumours of Haematopoietic and Lymphoid Tissues [Internet]. [cited 2020 Aug 9]. Available from: https://publications.iarc.fr/Book-And-Report-Series/Who-Classification-Of-Tumours/WHO-Classification-Of-Tumours-Of-Haematopoietic-And-Lymphoid-Tissues-2017

[2] Morton LM, Wang SS, Devesa SS, Hartge P, Weisenburger DD, Linet MS. Lymphoma incidence patterns by WHO subtype in the United States, 1992-2001. Blood. 2006;**107**(1):265-276

[3] Biagi JJ, Seymour JF. Insights into the molecular pathogenesis of follicular lymphoma arising from analysis of geographic variation. Blood. 2002;**99**(12):4265-4275

[4] Sandhu DS, Sharma A, Kumar L. Non-Hodgkin's lymphoma in Northern India: An analysis of clinical features of 241 cases. Indian Journal of Medical and Paediatric Oncology. 2018;**39**(1):42

[5] Morton LM, Slager SL, Cerhan JR, Wang SS, Vajdic CM, Skibola CF, et al. Etiologic heterogeneity among non-Hodgkin lymphoma subtypes: The InterLymph Non-Hodgkin lymphoma subtypes Project. Journal of the National Cancer Institute. Monographs. 2014;**2014**(48):130-144

[6] Chan WC, Armitage JO, Gascoyne R, Connors J, et al. A clinical evaluation of the International Lymphoma Study Group classification of non-Hodgkin's lymphoma. The Non-Hodgkin's Lymphoma Classification Project. Blood. 1997;**89**(11):3909-3918

[7] Gogia A, Raina V, Kumar L, Sharma A, Sharma MC, Mallick SR. Follicular lymphoma: An Institutional Analysis. The Asian Pacific Journal of Cancer Prevention (APJCP). 2017;**18**(3):681-685

[8] Anderson T, Chabner BA, Young RC, Berard CW, Garvin AJ, Simon RM, et al. Malignant lymphoma. 1. The histology and staging of 473 patients at the National Cancer Institute. Cancer. 1982;**50**(12):2699-2707

[9] Hehn ST, Grogan TM, Miller TP. Utility of fine-needle aspiration as a diagnostic technique in lymphoma. Journal of Clinical Oncology: Official Journal of the American Society of Clinical Oncology. 2004;**22**(15):3046-3052

[10] Cheson BD, Fisher RI, Barrington SF, Cavalli F, Schwartz LH, Zucca E, et al. Recommendations for initial evaluation, staging, and response assessment of hodgkin and non-hodgkin lymphoma: The lugano classification. Journal of Clinical Oncology. 2014;**32**(27):3059-3067

[11] Swerdlow SH, Campo E, Pileri SA, Harris NL, Stein H, Siebert R, et al. The 2016 revision of the World Health Organization classification of lymphoid neoplasms. Blood. 2016;**127**(20):2375-2390

[12] Hellmuth JC, Louissaint A, Szczepanowski M, Haebe S, Pastore A, Alig S, et al. Duodenal-type and nodal follicular lymphomas differ by their immune microenvironment rather than their mutation profiles. Blood. 2018;**132**(16):1695-1702

[13] Okosun J, Bödör C, Wang J, Araf S, Yang C-Y, Pan C, et al. Integrated genomic analysis identifies recurrent mutations and evolution patterns driving the initiation and progression of follicular lymphoma. Nature Genetics. 2014;**46**(2):176-181

[14] Green MR, Gentles AJ, Nair RV, Irish JM, Kihira S, Liu CL, et al. Hierarchy in somatic mutations arising

during genomic evolution and progression of follicular lymphoma. Blood. 2013;**121**(9):1604-1611

[15] Meda BA, Buss DH, Woodruff RD, Cappellari JO, Rainer RO, Powell BL, et al. Diagnosis and subclassification of primary and recurrent lymphoma. The usefulness and limitations of combined fine-needle aspiration cytomorphology and flow cytometry. American Journal of Clinical Pathology. 2000;**113**(5): 688-699

[16] Smith SD, Redman M, Dunleavy K. FDG PET-CT in follicular lymphoma: a case-based evidence review. Blood. 2015;**125**(7):1078-1082

[17] Batlevi CL, Sha F, Alperovich A, Ni A, Smith K, Ying Z, et al. Positron-emission tomography-based staging reduces the prognostic impact of early disease progression in patients with follicular lymphoma. European Journal of Cancer (Oxford, England: 1990). 2020;**126**:78-90

[18] Weiler-Sagie M, Bushelev O, Epelbaum R, Dann EJ, Haim N, Avivi I, et al. 18F-FDG avidity in lymphoma readdressed: A study of 766 patients. Journal of Nuclear Medicine. 2010;**51**(1):25-30

[19] Nakajima R, Moskowitz AJ, Michaud L, Mauguen A, Batlevi CL, Dogan A, et al. Baseline FDG-PET/CT detects bone marrow involvement in follicular lymphoma and provides relevant prognostic information. Blood Advances. 2020;**4**(8):1812-1823

[20] Luminari S, Biasoli I, Versari A, Rattotti S, Bottelli C, Rusconi C, et al. The prognostic role of post-induction FDG-PET in patients with follicular lymphoma: a subset analysis from the FOLL05 trial of the Fondazione Italiana Linfomi (FIL). Annals of Oncology. Official Journal of the European Society for Medical Oncology. 2014;**25**(2): 442-447

[21] Howell SJ, Shalet SM. Fertility preservation and management of gonadal failure associated with lymphoma therapy. Current Oncology Reports. 2002;**4**(5):443-452

[22] Sarkozy C, Trneny M, Xerri L, Wickham N, Feugier P, Leppa S, et al. Risk factors and outcomes for patients with follicular lymphoma who had histologic transformation after response to first-line immunochemotherapy in the PRIMA trial. Journal of Clinical Oncology: Official Journal of the American Society of Clinical Oncology. 2016;**34**(22):2575-2582

[23] Al-Tourah AJ, Gill KK, Chhanabhai M, Hoskins PJ, Klasa RJ, Savage KJ, et al. Population-based analysis of incidence and outcome of transformed non-Hodgkin's lymphoma. Journal of Clinical Oncology: Official Journal of the American Society of Clinical Oncology. 2008;**26**(32): 5165-5169

[24] Bischin AM, Dorer R, Aboulafia DM. Transformation of follicular lymphoma to a high-grade B-Cell lymphoma with MYC and BCL2 translocations and overlapping features of Burkitt lymphoma and acute lymphoblastic leukemia: A case report and literature review. Clinical Medicine Insights: Blood Disorders. 2017;**10**:1-8. [cited 2020 Aug 15];10. Available from: https://www.ncbi.nlm.nih.gov/pmc/articles/PMC5428247/

[25] Lossos IS, Gascoyne RD. Transformation of Follicular Lymphoma. Best Practice & Research. Clinical Haematology. 2011;**24**(2): 147-163

[26] Link BK, Maurer MJ, Nowakowski GS, Ansell SM, Macon WR, Syrbu SI, et al. Rates and outcomes of follicular lymphoma transformation in the immunochemotherapy era: A report from the University of Iowa/MayoClinic Specialized Program of Research

Excellence Molecular Epidemiology Resource. Journal of Clinical Oncology: Official Journal of the American Society of Clinical Oncology. 2013;**31**(26):3272-3278

[27] Buske C, Hoster E, Dreyling M, Hasford J, Unterhalt M, Hiddemann W. The Follicular Lymphoma International Prognostic Index (FLIPI) separates high-risk from intermediate- or low-risk patients with advanced-stage follicular lymphoma treated front-line with rituximab and the combination of cyclophosphamide, doxorubicin, vincristine, and prednisone (R-CHOP) with respect to treatment outcome. Blood. 2006;**108**(5):1504-1508

[28] Nooka AK, Nabhan C, Zhou X, Taylor MD, Byrtek M, Miller TP, et al. Examination of the follicular lymphoma international prognostic index (FLIPI) in the National LymphoCare study (NLCS): A prospective US patient cohort treated predominantly in community practices. Annals of Oncology. Official Journal of the European Society for Medical Oncology. 2013;**24**(2):441-448

[29] Federico M, Bellei M, Marcheselli L, Luminari S, Lopez-Guillermo A, Vitolo U, et al. Follicular lymphoma international prognostic index 2: A new prognostic index for follicular lymphoma developed by the international follicular lymphoma prognostic factor project. Journal of Clinical Oncology: Official Journal of the American Society of Clinical Oncology. 2009;**27**(27):4555-4562

[30] Bachy E, Maurer MJ, Habermann TM, Gelas-Dore B, Maucort-Boulch D, Estell JA, et al. A simplified scoring system in de novo follicular lymphoma treated initially with immunochemotherapy. Blood. 2018;**132**(1):49-58

[31] Casulo C, Byrtek M, Dawson KL, Zhou X, Farber CM, Flowers CR, et al. Early relapse of follicular lymphoma after rituximab plus cyclophosphamide, doxorubicin, vincristine, and prednisone defines patients at high risk for death: An analysis from the national lymphocare study. Journal of Clinical Oncology. 2015;**33**(23): 2516-2522

[32] Maurer MJ, Bachy E, Ghesquières H, Ansell SM, Nowakowski GS, Thompson CA, et al. Early event status informs subsequent outcome in newly diagnosed follicular lymphoma. American Journal of Hematology. 2016;**91**(11):1096-1101

[33] Friedberg JW, Taylor MD, Cerhan JR, Flowers CR, Dillon H, Farber CM, et al. Follicular lymphoma in the United States: First report of the national lymphocare study. Journal of Clinical Oncology. 2009;**27**(8): 1202-1208

[34] Guadagnolo BA, Li S, Neuberg D, Ng A, Hua L, Silver B, et al. Long-term outcome and mortality trends in early-stage, Grade 1-2 follicular lymphoma treated with radiation therapy. International Journal of Radiation Oncology, Biology, Physics. 2006;**64**(3):928-934

[35] Seymour JF, Pro B, Fuller LM, Manning JT, Hagemeister FB, Romaguera J, et al. Long-term follow-up of a prospective study of combined modality therapy for stage I-II indolent non-Hodgkin's lymphoma. Journal of Clinical Oncology: Official Journal of the American Society of Clinical Oncology. 2003;**21**(11):2115-2122

[36] Wirth A, Mikhaeel NG, Aleman BMP, Pinnix CC, Constine LS, Ricardi U, et al. Involved site radiation therapy in adult lymphomas: An overview of international lymphoma radiation oncology group guidelines. International Journal of Radiation Oncology, Biology, Physics. 2020;**107**(5):909-933

[37] Lowry L, Smith P, Qian W, Falk S, Benstead K, Illidge T, et al. Reduced dose radiotherapy for local control in non-Hodgkin lymphoma: A randomised phase III trial. Radiotherapy and Oncology: Journal of the European Society for Therapeutic Radiology and Oncology. 2011;**100**(1):86-92

[38] Pugh TJ, Ballonoff A, Newman F, Rabinovitch R. Improved survival in patients with early stage low-grade follicular lymphoma treated with radiation: A Surveillance, Epidemiology, and End Results database analysis. Cancer. 2010;**116**(16):3843-3851

[39] Vargo JA, Gill BS, Balasubramani GK, Beriwal S. What is the optimal management of early-stage low-grade follicular lymphoma in the modern era? Cancer. 2015;**121**(18):3325-3334

[40] MacManus M, Fisher R, Roos D, O'Brien P, Macann A, Davis S, et al. Randomized trial of systemic therapy after involved-field radiotherapy in patients with early-stage follicular lymphoma: TROG 99.03. Journal of Clinical Oncology. 2018;**36**(29): 2918-2925

[41] Friedberg JW, Byrtek M, Link BK, Flowers C, Taylor M, Hainsworth J, et al. Effectiveness of first-line management strategies for stage I follicular lymphoma: analysis of the National LymphoCare Study. Journal of Clinical Oncology: Official Journal of the American Society of Clinical Oncology. 2012;**30**(27):3368-3375

[42] Advani R, Rosenberg SA, Horning SJ. Stage I and II follicular non-Hodgkin's lymphoma: long-term follow-up of no initial therapy. Journal of Clinical Oncology: Official Journal of the American Society of Clinical Oncology. 2004;**22**(8):1454-1459

[43] Brice P, Bastion Y, Lepage E, Brousse N, Haïoun C, Moreau P, et al. Comparison in low-tumor-burden follicular lymphomas between an initial no-treatment policy, prednimustine, or interferon alfa: a randomized study from the Groupe d'Etude des Lymphomes Folliculaires. Groupe d'Etude des Lymphomes de l'Adulte. Journal of Clinical Oncology: Official Journal of the American Society of Clinical Oncology. 1997;**15**(3):1110-1117

[44] Ardeshna KM, Smith P, Norton A, Hancock BW, Hoskin PJ, MacLennan KA, et al. Long-term effect of a watch and wait policy versus immediate systemic treatment for asymptomatic advanced-stage non-Hodgkin lymphoma: a randomised controlled trial. Lancet (London, England). 2003;**362**(9383):516-522

[45] Ardeshna KM, Qian W, Smith P, Braganca N, Lowry L, Patrick P, et al. Rituximab versus a watch-and-wait approach in patients with advanced-stage, asymptomatic, non-bulky follicular lymphoma: an open-label randomised phase 3 trial. The Lancet Oncology. 2014;**15**(4):424-435

[46] Kahl BS, Hong F, Williams ME, Gascoyne RD, Wagner LI, Krauss JC, et al. Rituximab extended schedule or re-treatment trial for low–tumor burden follicular lymphoma: Eastern cooperative oncology group protocol E4402. Journal of Clinical Oncology. 2014;**32**(28):3096-3102

[47] Federico M, Luminari S, Dondi A, Tucci A, Vitolo U, Rigacci L, et al. R-CVP versus R-CHOP versus R-FM for the initial treatment of patients with advanced-stage follicular lymphoma: Results of the FOLL05 trial conducted by the Fondazione Italiana Linfomi. Journal of Clinical Oncology: Official Journal of the American Society of Clinical Oncology. 2013;**31**(12):1506-1513

[48] Rummel MJ, Niederle N, Maschmeyer G, Banat GA, von Grünhagen U, Losem C, et al. Bendamustine plus rituximab versus

CHOP plus rituximab as first-line treatment for patients with indolent and mantle-cell lymphomas: an open-label, multicentre, randomised, phase 3 non-inferiority trial. Lancet (London, England). 2013;**381**(9873):1203-1210

[49] Flinn IW, van der Jagt R, Kahl BS, Wood P, Hawkins TE, Macdonald D, et al. Randomized trial of bendamustine-rituximab or R-CHOP/R-CVP in first-line treatment of indolent NHL or MCL: The BRIGHT study. Blood. 2014;**123**(19):2944-2952

[50] Marcus R, Davies A, Ando K, Klapper W, Opat S, Owen C, et al. Obinutuzumab for the first-line treatment of follicular lymphoma. The New England Journal of Medicine. 2017;**377**(14):1331-1344

[51] Morschhauser F, Fowler NH, Feugier P, Bouabdallah R, Tilly H, Palomba ML, et al. Rituximab plus lenalidomide in advanced untreated follicular lymphoma. The New England Journal of Medicine. 2018;**379**(10): 934-947

[52] Salles G, Seymour JF, Offner F, López-Guillermo A, Belada D, Xerri L, et al. Rituximab maintenance for 2 years in patients with high tumour burden follicular lymphoma responding to rituximab plus chemotherapy (PRIMA): A phase 3, randomised controlled trial. Lancet (London, England). 2011;**377**(9759):42-51

[53] Vitolo U, Ladetto M, Boccomini C, Baldini L, De Angelis F, Tucci A, et al. Rituximab maintenance compared with observation after brief first-line R-FND chemoimmunotherapy with rituximab consolidation in patients age older than 60 years with advanced follicular lymphoma: a phase III randomized study by the Fondazione Italiana Linfomi. Journal of Clinical Oncology: Official Journal of the American Society of Clinical Oncology. 2013;**31**(27): 3351-3359

[54] Casulo C, Byrtek M, Dawson KL, Zhou X, Farber CM, Flowers CR, et al. Early relapse of follicular lymphoma after rituximab plus cyclophosphamide, doxorubicin, vincristine, and prednisone defines patients at high risk for death: An analysis from the national lymphocare study. Journal of Clinical Oncology: Official Journal of the American Society of Clinical Oncology. 2015;**33**(23):2516-2522

[55] Maurer MJ, Bachy E, Ghesquières H, Ansell SM, Nowakowski GS, Thompson CA, et al. Early event status informs subsequent outcome in newly diagnosed follicular lymphoma. American Journal of Hematology. 2016;**91**(11):1096-1101

[56] Maloney DG, Ogura M, Fukuhara N, Davis J, Lasher J, Izquierdo M, et al. A phase 3 randomized study (HOMER) of ofatumumab vs rituximab in iNHL relapsed after rituximab-containing therapy. Blood Advances. 2020;**4**(16): 3886-3893

[57] Salles GA, Morschhauser F, Solal-Céligny P, Thieblemont C, Lamy T, Tilly H, et al. Obinutuzumab (GA101) in patients with relapsed/refractory indolent non-Hodgkin lymphoma: results from the phase II GAUGUIN study. Journal of Clinical Oncology: Official Journal of the American Society of Clinical Oncology. 2013;**31**(23): 2920-2926

[58] Radford J, Davies A, Cartron G, Morschhauser F, Salles G, Marcus R, et al. Obinutuzumab (GA101) plus CHOP or FC in relapsed/refractory follicular lymphoma: results of the GAUDI study (BO21000). Blood. 2013;**122**(7):1137-1143

[59] Witzig TE, Gordon LI, Cabanillas F, Czuczman MS, Emmanouilides C, Joyce R, et al. Randomized controlled trial of yttrium-90-labeled ibritumomab tiuxetan radioimmunotherapy versus

rituximab immunotherapy for patients with relapsed or refractory low-grade, follicular, or transformed B-cell non-Hodgkin's lymphoma. Journal of Clinical Oncology: Official Journal of the American Society of Clinical Oncology. 2002;**20**(10):2453-2463

[60] Schouten HC, Qian W, Kvaloy S, Porcellini A, Hagberg H, Johnsen HE, et al. High-dose therapy improves progression-free survival and survival in relapsed follicular non-Hodgkin's lymphoma: results from the randomized European CUP trial. Journal of Clinical Oncology: Official Journal of the American Society of Clinical Oncology. 2003;**21**(21):3918-3927

[61] Smith SM, Godfrey J, Ahn KW, DiGilio A, Ahmed S, Agrawal V, et al. Autologous versus allogeneic transplantation in follicular lymphoma patients experiencing early treatment failure. Cancer. 2018;**124**(12):2541-2551

[62] Fowler NH, Samaniego F, Jurczak W, Ghosh N, Derenzini E, Reeves JA, et al. Umbralisib, a dual PI3Kδ/CK1ε inhibitor in patients with relapsed or refractory indolent lymphoma. Journal of Clinical Oncology: Official Journal of the American Society of Clinical Oncology. 2021;**39**(15):1609-1618

[63] Gopal AK, Kahl BS, de Vos S, Wagner-Johnston ND, Schuster SJ, Jurczak WJ, et al. PI3Kδ inhibition by idelalisib in patients with relapsed indolent lymphoma. The New England Journal of Medicine. 2014;**370**(11):1008-1018

[64] Matasar MJ, Capra M, Özcan M, Lv F, Li W, Yañez E, et al. Copanlisib plus rituximab versus placebo plus rituximab in patients with relapsed indolent non-Hodgkin lymphoma (CHRONOS-3): a double-blind, randomised, placebo-controlled, phase 3 trial. The Lancet Oncology. 2021;**22**(5):678-689

[65] Flinn IW, Miller CB, Ardeshna KM, Tetreault S, Assouline SE, Mayer J, et al. DYNAMO: A phase II study of duvelisib (IPI-145) in patients with refractory indolent non-hodgkin lymphoma. Journal of Clinical Oncology: Official Journal of the American Society of Clinical Oncology. 2019;**37**(11):912-922

[66] Schuster SJ, Svoboda J, Chong EA, Nasta SD, Mato AR, Anak Ö, et al. Chimeric antigen receptor T cells in refractory B-cell lymphomas. The New England Journal of Medicine. 2017;**377**(26):2545-2554

[67] Hirayama AV, Gauthier J, Hay KA, Voutsinas JM, Wu Q, Pender BS, et al. High rate of durable complete remission in follicular lymphoma after CD19 CAR-T cell immunotherapy. Blood. 2019;**134**(7):636-640

Chapter 3

Primary Gastrointestinal Lymphoma

Ramiz Bayramov and Ramila Abdullayeva

Abstract

The gastrointestinal tract (GIT) is the most common (30–40%) extranodal site involved in lymphoma. Although primary gastrointestinal lymphoma (PGIL) is a rare disease, comprising only 1–4% of gastrointestinal (GI) malignant tumors, its incidence is increasing. Different regions of the GIT are involved in different subtypes of PGIL with a various frequency that reflects the diversity of the causative agents and predisposing factors for each site and subtype of PGIL. Even though these malignant diseases are categorized under the common term of "lymphoma" they represent a heterogeneous group of malignant neoplasms which are different entities in terms of etiologic factors, predisposing conditions, pathogenesis, immunohistochemical profile, treatment strategy and prognosis. In this chapter the epidemiology of all subtypes of PGIL, factors and disorders contributing to the development of them, non-inherited and inherited conditions associated with a higher risk of them, diagnostic difficulties and pitfalls, and novel treatment strategies were comprehensively and concisely illuminated.

Keywords: gastrointestinal lymphoma, gastric lymphoma, intestinal lymphoma, extranodal lymphoma, non-Hodgkin lymphoma

1. Introduction

The incidence of lymphoma, especially extranodal lymphoma, such as non-Hodgkin lymphoma (NHL) of the central nervous system (CNS), GI and cutaneous lymphomas has been increasing over the last decades [1–3].

The definition of PGIL has differed among different authors but typically refers to a lymphoma that develops in any part of the gastrointestinal tract (GIT) from the oropharynx to the anal canal. PGIL is the most common type of extranodal lymphoma comprising 25–40% of the latter depending on geographic regions [4, 5]. PGIL, however, is a rare malignancy, accounting for 1% to 4% of the malignant lesions in GIT [3, 6]. GIT several times more frequently is involved secondarily from nodal lymphoma [4].

Dawson's criteria that were suggested 6 decades ago are used for the definition of PGIL, that include (1) absence of peripheral lymphadenopathy at the time of presentation; (2) lack of enlarged mediastinal lymph nodes (LNs); (3) normal total and differential white blood cell count; (4) predominance of bowel lesion at the time of laparotomy with only LNs affected in the immediate vicinity (LNs which are confined to the drainage area of the primary tumor site); and (5) no involvement of liver and spleen [7].

Histopathologically, almost 90% of the PGILs are of B-cell lineage, and T-cell lymphomas (TCLs) and Hodgkin lymphoma (HL) are rarely encountered in GIT [4, 8, 9]. Some histological subtypes of lymphoma have a relative propensity to develop in specific sites as mucosa-associated lymphoid tissue (MALT) lymphoma in the stomach, follicular lymphoma (FL) in the duodenum, enteropathy-associated T-cell lymphoma (EATL) in the jejunum, mantle cell lymphoma (MCL) in the terminal ileum and colon [10].

Due to the rarity of PGIL, opinions upon some aspects of this neoplasm are still controversial. The increasing incidence of this malignancy, makes it necessary for clinicians to understand the characteristic clinical manifestation, diagnostic properties, treatment and prognosis of PGIL more comprehensively [11].

In the last decades, a great achievement has been reached in the diagnosis, staging and management of PGIL attributed to a better understanding of its etiology and molecular aspect including signaling pathways [4]. The therapeutic approach to the cure of PGIL has completely changed over the last decade, including innovative conservative options to reduce the complication rate following treatment [11]. Nevertheless, the prognostic and diagnostic significance of mutational analysis in daily practice and its role in novel targeted therapy remains and requires to be determined [12].

2. Epidemiological properties

PGIL, as mentioned above, is a rare malignancy, constituting 1% to 4% of the GIT cancer [4, 6]. Although theoretically lymphoma can arise from any region of the GIT stomach is the most frequently involved site (60–75%) followed by the small intestine [20–30%], ileocecal region (7%) and colon (6–12%). More than one gastrointestinal (GI) site is involved in 6–13% of the cases [4, 6, 13–15].

Primary esophageal lymphoma (PEL) is extremely rare comprising <1% of all PGILs. Less than 30 cases of PEL have been reported in the literature [4]. Primary gastric lymphoma (PGL) accounts for up to 5% of all malignancies of the stomach [16]. Primary small intestinal lymphoma (PSIL) constitutes 15–20% of all small bowel neoplasms [4]. Primary colorectal lymphoma (PCRL) comprises only 0.2% of all malignancies arising from the colorectum with caecum, ascending colon and rectum more frequently involved in decreasing order [14].

PGIL approximately 2–3 times more frequently is seen in men compared to women [4, 8, 11]. This ratio can be varied depending on the sites of PGIL and pathological subtypes. For example, DLBCL is seen in males 1.2–2 times more [17, 18], and FL affects males and females equally [19] or demonstrates a clear female predominance [20].

The age of the patients with PGIL can range from 19 to >90 years with a median age of 55 years [4, 8, 21]. The age range (and median age) depends on involved sites and pathological subtypes of PGIL. The median age of patients with TCL is usually by 10–14 years younger compared to B-cell lymphoma (BCL) [8, 22].

Different entities of the PGILs of B-cell lineage can demonstrate different peak ages. MALT lymphoma and MCL are most commonly detected between the age of 50 and 60 years [23]. On the contrary immunoproliferative small intestine disease (IPSID) is mainly seen in adolescents and younger adults [24, 25] and endemic Burkitt's lymphoma (BL) is mainly detected in children [26].

Some forms of PGIL have a tendency to increase in its incidence in younger age group of people, the other ones tend to be encountered among some ethnics or have different geographical distribution. It has been observed that the incidence of MALT lymphoma has increased significantly in people older than 40 years [27].

Monomorphic epitheliotropic intestinal TCL (MEITL) is more common in people of Hispanic descent and is the most frequent primary intestinal TCL being detected in Asia [28]. PGL is the most common extranodal site of lymphoma in the USA. The predominant part of this neoplasm is either extranodal marginal zone lymphoma (MZL) of MALT or DLBCL. PSIL, while uncommon in Western countries, comprises up to 75% of PGIL in the Middle East, North and South Africa, and Mediterranean basin, because of that is commonly called "Mediterranean type lymphoma". Endemic BL, the most common type of BL, has a geographical distribution identical to that of *Plasmodium falciparum* [29]. That is why the incidence of BL in Africa is nearly 50-fold higher than that in the USA [11, 24].

3. Predisposing factors and disorders

Certain risk factors and disorders can be involved in the pathogenesis of PGIL including *Helicobacter pylori*, *Campylobacter jejuni*, human immunodeficiency virus (HIV), Epstein-Barr virus (EBV), hepatitis B virus (HBV), human T-cell lymphotropic virus-1 (HTLV-1), celiac disease, inflammatory bowel disease (IBD) and immunosuppression [4, 30].

Chronic gastritis related to *H. pylori* infection has been considered a major predisposing factor for the development of MALT lymphoma [11] and the latter is strongly associated with *H. pylori* infection. This pathogen is the most common infectious agent related to global malignancy (5.5% of total cancers) [31]. The prevalence of *H. pylori*-related gastritis is dependent on geographical regions, socio-economic status, education level, living environment, occupation and age [32]. Patients with *H. pylori* gastritis have a great risk for the development of gastric MALT lymphoma, and the development of this neoplasm requires some circumstances or co-factors [33]. Studies demonstrated that only 1 of the 13 different tested *H. pylori* strains was capable of inducing B-cell proliferation and making T-cells produce IL-2 [25]. However, unlike gastric MALT lymphoma, esophageal MALT lymphoma is not associated with *H. pylori* infection [4].

MALT lymphoma can be divided into *H. pylori*-positive or negative based on association with *H. pylori* infection. Typically, gastric MALT lymphoma is a low-grade (LG) neoplasm, but it can be transformed into a high-grade (HG) lymphoma. In the last years, it has been discovered that *H. pylori* infection plays a role in the development of gastric DLBCL as well [34] and few studies have shown complete remission of that after eradication therapy alone [35]. Recent studies detected that CagA-positive strains of *H. pylori* are more frequent in DLBCL than in LG MALT lymphoma of the stomach [36]. It should be noted that although "LG MALT lymphoma" is widely used in the literature despite its official name is "extranodal MZL of MALT" in the 2016 revision of WHO classification (for comprehensive explanation see subsection 5). However, following the commonly used by most of the authors terminology "LG MALT lymphoma" will be employed in this chapter keeping the original style of spelling of the authors.

The role of *H. pylori* in the pathogenesis of PCRL has not been fully clarified. Niino et al. reported that in five of the eight cases (63%) endoscopic examination showed that the rectal MALT lymphoma had disappeared following antibiotic therapy which was confirmed histologically [37]. These results indirectly discover the role of unknown infection, which is a target for antibiotics in the development of rectal MALT lymphoma.

IPSID, also recognized as an alpha-chain disease, is considered as a variant of MALT lymphoma related to *C. jejuni* (sometimes to *Campylobacter coli*) infection that prevalently involves the proximal part of the small intestine. The disease is characterized by a lymphoid infiltrate of mucosa composed of plasma cells and lymphocytes with centrocyte features. The plasma cells secrete truncated immunoglobulin, consisting of the heavy chains without associating light chains [24].

Pathogenesis of primary PGIL can also be associated with other infectious agents like EBV, HIV, HBV and HTLV-1 [11]. The role of EBV-infection in the pathogenesis of B-cell NHL has been established [38]. Hui et al. reported 11 cases of PGL that harbor the EBV encoded small messenger RNA, EBER-1, detected by fluorescence in situ hybridization (FISH). The cases comprised 18% of 61 consecutive PGL. Nine of the 11 (81.8%) EBER-1-positive PGL cases were DLBCL-type without LG components. None of the EBER-1-positive gastric BCLs showed histological features characteristic of LG lymphoma of MALT-type being common in Western countries. Of the two patients with TCL, one had a pleomorphic TCL and the other had an angiocentric lymphoma. They concluded that a significant proportion of PGL in Hong Kong Chinese are EBV-related and that they show histological features more similar to conventional nodal lymphomas than to MALT-type lymphomas [39].

BL has three recognized clinical variants: endemic form, sporadic variant and immunodeficiency-associated BL. There is clear evidence regarding the role of EBV and *P. falciparum* as a co-factor in the pathogenesis of endemic BL. It demonstrates an association with HIV-1 as well, but the data is insufficient to support the role of those factors in sporadic cases, where the association with EBV is observed in only 20–30% of the patients [29, 40].

EBV infection is also associated with the EBV-positive DLBCL, recently recognized as a definite entity. The term "elderly" in the 2008 WHO classification has been substituted by NOS (not otherwise specified) because this lymphoma can be encountered in younger patients as well [12].

A recently recognized entity, EBV-positive mucocutaneous ulcer (MCU) is characteristically associated with iatrogenic immunosuppression (for autoimmune or inflammatory conditions and solid organ transplantation), HIV-infection and age-related immunosenescence that leads to inadequate immune surveillance for EBV. It is characterized by the propagation of EBV-positive atypical large B-cells affecting the skin or mucous sites, presumably related to local trauma or inflammation [41, 42]. Most cases of EBV-positive MCU are detected in the elderly (due to predisposing age-associated immunosenescence in half of the patients), but the patients with iatrogenic immunosuppression usually have a younger age. Patients treated by immunosuppressive therapy for IBD may be all the more vulnerable due to the presence of local tissue injury related to the mentioned disease [19].

NK/T cell neoplasms are invariably associated with EBV infection and are mostly aggressive; thus, differentiation from a benign NK-cell enteropathy is paramount [15]. BL is associated with EBV and HIV/AIDS, and most commonly affects children [26].

GI lesions as the most frequent extranodal manifestation of HIV-associated NHL lymphoma (occurs in 5–10% of individuals with HIV-infection), are late events of HIV-infection with severe immunosuppression and are mostly diagnosed in advanced stages of the disease. They are characterized by HG B-cell histology, frequently multifocal location in the GIT, high rates of life-threatening complications (bleeding, perforation or obstruction) [43, 44]. NHL is the second most common type of malignancy in HIV-patients following Kaposi sarcoma [45]. The high incidence of GI NHL prompted Powitz et al. to commence a prospective survey on 93 of 341 HIV-infected patients with GI symptoms who were examined by endoscopy, some selected patients by endoscopic ultrasound (EUS). NHL of the GIT was detected in seven of 93 endoscopically examined patients (7.5%) [44].

Nearly 70–90% of AIDS-related lymphomas are highly aggressive and are almost exclusively BL and an immunoblastic variant of DLBCL. Compared to the general population, the relative risk for highly aggressive lymphomas is higher >400-fold overall [46], and 260-fold and 650-fold for BL and DLBCL, respectively among HIV-infected people [47]. BL can be one of the diseases associated with the initial manifestation of AIDS [48]. The indolent lymphomas are less common, comprising <10% of AIDS-related lymphomas. Compared to the general population, the relative risk is increased nearly 15-fold for indolent lymphomas and TCLs in the HIV-positive population [46, 47, 49]. However, TCLs are less common in HIV-infected people as well despite the increased relative risk. Of note, 40–50% of cases of HIV-associated BL are positive for EBV [48].

The epidemiologic association between HBV-infection and NHL, notably DLBCL is well established. Most studies concerning this association have been conducted in endemic areas. Some researchers report up to 2.5 times higher risk of NHL in HBV-infected people. Deng et al. studied HBV-infection status and clinicopathologic features of 587 patients with DLBCL in HBV-endemic China. Eighty-one (13.8%) patients were HBsAg-positive, 20 of which (25%) had DLBCL in GIT. Compared to HBsAg-negative DLBCL, HBsAg-positive DLBCL demonstrated a younger median onset age by 10 years, more advanced stages of the disease and significantly worse outcome [50].

PGL with a T-cell phenotype is very rare, comprising only 7% of PGLs in endemic areas of HTLV-1 infection. Primary gastric TCL without HTLV-1 infection is extremely rare, and sporadic cases have been occasionally reported [51].

PGIL is one of the major and serious complications of different diseases and conditions presenting with immunodepression, both congenital (Wiskott-Aldrich syndrome, ataxia-telangiectasia, X-linked agammaglobulinemia) and acquired immunodeficiency (HIV-infection, iatrogenic immunosuppression). Lymphomas developed in the setting of the diseases associated with immunodepression are pathologically and clinically heterogeneous, but share some hallmarks such as frequent involvement of extranodal sites, association with EBV-infection, B-cell lineage genesis, and aggressive behavior. Although PGIL associated with congenital immunodeficient conditions seems to be an infrequent occasion despite the higher prevalence of post-transplantation lymphoproliferative disorders GIT is one of the most involved sites of lymphoma [43]. It should be noted that PEL in an immunocompetent patient is very rare [52].

The three most common systemic autoimmune diseases—rheumatoid arthritis, primary Sjögren's syndrome (PSS) and systemic lupus erythematosus, are characterized by an increased risk of lymphoma. Of these diseases, the highest risk of lymphoma is associated with PSS [53]. The development of the NHL is the most serious complication of PSS. Up to 25% of NHL associated with PSS is PGL that predominantly demonstrates MALT lymphoma. NHLs complicated PSS are not associated with viral agents known to be present in other types of lymphoma [54].

TCL of the small bowel comprises 10–25% of all primary intestinal lymphomas (PIL) primarily occurring as EATL, and most of them are often associated with Crohn's disease [55, 56]. Intestinal EATL, type I in particular, usually occurs in the setting of celiac disease [15]. T-cell gene rearrangement confirms clonality [57]. MEITL was formerly known as type II EATL. Even in this older classification, it had been recognized that the "type II" form of the disease had rarely demonstrated (if demonstrated) association with underlying gluten-sensitive enteropathy [19].

4. Pathogenesis

Although the stomach is devoid of lymphoid tissue, it is the organ most commonly involved of MALT lymphoma, especially the antrum and distal body.

Lymphoid cells are attracted and transformed into gastric MALT tissue by a chronic *H. pylori* infection. Lymphoid follicles develop in the setting of chronic inflammation (gastritis) associated with *H. pylori* infection. It is evidenced by the fact that the rate of *H. pylori* infection prevalence is >90% in patients with MALT lymphoma. These lymphoid follicles resemble LN tissue and are composed of activated plasma cells, B-cells and reactive T-cells. When these cells are continuously stimulated by *H. pylori*, the B-cells undergo clonal expansion [57, 58]. Overtime, B-cell clones that still depend on antigens for growth and survival, acquiring unknown genetic mutations, will give rise to MALT lymphoma. At this stage, the proliferation is monoclonal but not yet able to spread beyond the site of inflammation. With the acquisition of additional mutations, including chromosomal abnormalities, the tumor becomes antigen-independent and capable of systemic spread [11]. In addition to B-cells, T-cells and macrophages play an important role in MALT lymphomagenesis [57, 58].

The association of gastric MALT lymphoma with *H. pylori* is undeniable. *E. coli* and *C. jejuni* were also tested, two Gram-negative intestinal bacteria which share different antigens with *H. pylori*, and they failed to induce B-cell proliferation in culture, so *H. pylori* strains have a specific role [25]. In addition, *H. pylori* can translocate the CagA protein directly into B-cells resulting in extracellular signal-regulated kinase activation and *BCL2* expression up-regulation, leading to apoptosis inhibition [59].

In normal B and T-cells signals produced by the interaction of antigen with antigen receptors on the cell surface cause the protein bcl-10 (B-cell leukemia/lymphoma 10) to bind to the protein MALT1 (lymphoma-associated translocation protein 1) [60]. During *H. pylori* infection, normal B-cells are transformed into malignant clones via three chromosomal translocations—t(14;18)(q32;q21), t(1;14)(p22;q32) and t(11;18)(q21;q21), which produces activation of nuclear factor kappa B (NF-kB), a transcription factor that promotes cell survival and plays a role in immunity, inflammation, and apoptosis [61, 62]. These events result in enhancing the survival of extranodal lymphoma cells [63].

The t(14;18)(q32;q21) fuses the *IGH* gene on chromosome 14 with the *MLT/MALT1* gene on chromosome 18. The rare t(1;14)(p22;q32) translocation fuses the coding sequence of *BCL10* gene on chromosome 1 to the *IGH* promoter/enhancer elements [11, 64]. These all lead to overexpression of the *BCL10* gene, which causes cellular transformation [65] and guarantees a survival advantage to the neoplastic B-cells. Nuclear expression of bcl-10 or NF-kB in gastric MALT lymphoma is characterized by resistance of those cases to the *H. pylori* eradication therapy, even in the cases without the t(11;18)(q21;q21) translocation [66]. The t(3;14)(p13;q32) translocation fuses the *FOXP1* gene on chromosome 3 to the *IGH* gene and leads to upregulation of the FOXP1 transcription factor [67]. MALT lymphoma cases with *FOXP1* rearrangement appear to grow into DLBCL more frequently compared with those with t(11;18)(q21;q21) translocation the mechanism of that is unclear [68].

In *H. pylori*-negative gastric MALT lymphomas, the theory suggesting that infection leads to lymphomagenesis loses validity. Today, many propose that there are various mechanisms by which pathogenesis occurs in the development of *H. pylori*-negative gastric MALT lymphoma, including the relationship between genetic alterations and other activation pathways [11]. Recently, the t(11;18) (q21;q21) translocation is associated with LG MALT lymphoma, extranodal MZL [69]. The t(11;18) rearrangement fuses the apoptosis inhibitor gene *API2* (apoptosis inhibitor 2 gene) on chromosome 11 with the novel *MLT/MALT1* gene, a human paracaspase, on chromosome 18 [70, 71]. According to the data in literature, *H. pylori*-negative MALT lymphoma tends to have a high positive rate for t(11;18)(q21;q21) translocation than *H. pylori*-positive MALT lymphoma [69]. Studies show that t(11;18) (q21;q21) was found to be more prevalent in patients with CagA-positive *H. pylori* strains compared to CagA-negative *H. pylori*-infection [72]. Some authors reported this translocation to be closely associated with *H. pylori*-negative gastric MALT lymphoma [73]. It should be noted that the t(11;18)(q21;q21) has mainly been observed in LG MALT lymphomas of the GIT. Recent studies have also demonstrated that the t(11;18)(q21;q21) translocation presents important biological characteristics since this translocation is associated with resistance to antibiotic treatment in cases of *H. pylori*-positive gastric MALT lymphoma and with a more aggressive clinical behavior in cases of *H. pylori*-negative gastric MALT lymphoma [69, 74, 75]. The publications have also reported that t(11;18)(q21;q21) is never seen in early gastric MALT lymphomas that regressed after *H. pylori* eradication treatment [74]. In gastric LG MALT lymphomas, the reported frequency of t(11;18)(q21;q21) ranges from 0% to 48% (mean, 30%). It should be noted that the t(11;18)(q21;q21) translocation or the *API2–MLT/MALT1* fusion transcript has been detected in some percentage of patients with extranodal MZL of MALT (LG MALT lymphoma), but not in cases of DLBCL (HG lymphoma). Results of some studies indicate that t(11;18)(q21;q21) may be closely associated with colonic MALT lymphoma, but not with gastric MALT lymphoma [69]. Niino et al. (2010) reported that of the 8 cases of rectal MALT lymphoma analyzed with FISH for *MALT1* translocation, two demonstrated *MALT1* genetic abnormality. These cases were resistant to antibiotic treatment [37].

In specific subtypes of non-Hodgkin's BCL particular oncogene rearrangements related to chromosomal translocations have been determined. The t(11;14)(q13;q32) translocation is one of such fusions specific for MCL, which involves the *BCL1/cyclin D1* gene on chromosome 11. The t(14;18)(q32;q21) translocation that leads to overexpression of the *BCL2* gene has been found in 80–90% of FL cases. The *c-MYC* gene (8q24.1) is known to be rearranged in BL, in association with t(8;14)(q32;q32) translocation. In addition, the t(3;14)(q27;q32) is the most common translocation involving the *BCL6* gene (3q27.3) which results in deregulation of *BCL6* and is predominantly associated with DLBCL, rarely with FL [69].

Nakamura et al. (2000) believe that gastric MALT lymphoma can be rationally subdivided into 3 subtypes, MALT-A, MALT-B, and MALT-C. They suppose that MALT-A may represent a dysplasia or incipient neoplasm, MALT-B a neoplasm promoted by antigenic stimulation of *H. pylori*, and MALT-C a lymphoma independent of *H. pylori* infection. Polypoid lesions in MALT-C were associated with *c-IAP2-MALT1/MLT* gene alteration resulting from t(11;18)(q21;q21) translocation [73].

Data of Wang et al. show that identification of a t(11;18)(q21;q21) by reverse transcription real-time PCR is highly specific for extranodal MZL of MALT and helps in the diagnosis of this type of lymphoma. This translocation correlates with morphological features of gastric extranodal MZL of MALT and frequently shows monocytoid morphology, less often small lymphocytic morphology and not purely plasmacytoid morphology [76].

Proto-oncogene *BCL6* encodes a transcriptional repressor necessary for the development of germinal centers (GCs) and is directly implicated in lymphomagenesis. Post-GC development of B-cells requires *BCL6* down-regulation, while its constitutive expression caused by chromosomal translocations leads to the development of DLBCL [77]. The *BCL6* gene, which functions as a transcription repressor, is the target of multiple chromosomal translocations in NHL. These translocations occur in the nontranslated region of the *BCL6* gene; the BCL6 promoter region is thought to deregulate *BCL6* gene expression [78]. BCL6 promoter region can also be altered as a result of somatic mutations [79]. Most B-cell NHL, including DLBCL and FL, arise from GC B-cells; a stage at which B cells undergo rounds of proliferation and edit their immunoglobulins [80]. Therefore, *BCL6* is frequently overexpressed in the majority of extranodal HG lymphomas caused by chromosomal translocation leading to the development of lymphoma in various ways [79, 81]. Chromosomal translocations and mutations of the BCL6 promoter region are associated with ~40% of DLBCL and ~10% of FL [77]. The levels of expression of the *BCL6* gene and protein have been shown to predict the clinical outcome of DLBCLs [78, 79]. It has remained unclear whether DLBCL (gastric DLBCL is sometimes called HG gastric lymphoma) arises *de novo* or it transforms from LG gastric MALT lymphoma [82].

C. jejuni is considered an agent promoting lymphoid cell proliferation in the wall of the small intestine. *C. jejuni* has been revealed to persist in Peyer's patches and mesenteric LNs, and is capable of inducing a strong mucosal response in the small intestine as a B-cell proliferation that results in the production of IgA of the same type seen in IPSID [25].

MCL as a rule has been known to be an aggressive and incurable small BCL that is derived from naïve B-cells of the pregerminal center. Two types of clinically indolent variants are now identified reflecting that MCL might develop along 2 very different pathways [12]. Classical MCL is consisting of *IGH*-unmutated (in 20–30% of the cases) or minimally/borderline mutated (in 40–50% of the cases) B-cells that usually express SOX11 and characteristically involves LNs and extranodal sites. Acquisition of additional cytogenetic abnormalities targeting different oncogenic pathways can lead to the development of more aggressive variants (pleomorphic or blastoid) of MCL. Other MCLs are derived from *IGH*-mutated SOX11-negative B-cells which leads to leukemic non-nodal MCL, which commonly involves the peripheral blood, bone marrow and spleen [83]. These cases are commonly clinically indolent; however, secondary alterations involving *TP53* (17p13.1) may happen and subsequently result in the development of very aggressive disease [12, 83]. Therefore, *IGH*-mutational status can identify clinically distinct subtypes of MCL which are characterized by different biological behavior.

Genetics plays an essential role in the development of PGL. Patients with MALT lymphomas have a high prevalence of HLA-DQA1*0103, HLA-DQB1*0601 and R702W mutation in the *NOD2*/*CARD15* gene (16q12.1) [84, 85]. Cases of LG lymphoma are associated with the presence of TNF-857 T allele [59] probably due to fact that tumor necrosis factor-α (TNF-α) plays a crucial role in *H. pylori*-associated inflammation. Positive associations have been found also between variant alleles in *TNF*-308G > A and *IL10*-3575 T > A genes and risk of DLBCL. In the genetic susceptibility of PGL plays a substantial role the rare allele (TLR4 Asp299Gly) of the Toll-like receptor 4 [86] which belongs to the family of pattern recognition receptors and recognizes conserved microbial components. According to the results of some studies genetics associated with homozygous haplotypes for the rare allele G (rs12969413) of SNP3 (single nucleotide polymorphism) covering the *MALT1* locus protect the people against gastric HG lymphomas, but not of LG [87].

It should be noted that the list of genetic aberrations that are present in NHL and that are useful either for diagnosis or for understanding the pathogenesis of different diseases has been growing continuously [12].

5. Pathological characteristics

Although lymphoma can involve any part of the GIT, the most frequent sites in order of its occurrence are the stomach followed by the small intestine and the ileocaecal region as mentioned earlier. Visually PGIL appears as a polyp, mass, ulcer or infiltration depending on the pathological subtypes of lymphoma and the involved sites. Sometimes PGIL can be multifocal. Multifocality has been reported particularly in MALT lymphoma and FL [4]. Multiple lymphomatous polyposis (MLP) is a rare and particular clinical type of GI lymphoma characterized by the development of multiple polyps. Polypoid lesions of MLP are commonly encountered in several sites of the GIT including the esophagus, stomach, duodenum, and bowel. This is classified as B-cell centrocytic NHL; most of the cases of MLP pathohistologically tend to be classified as MCL, rarely as MALT lymphoma [23] and a few cases of FL or TCL have been reported [88, 89].

According to 2016 revised WHO classification there are around 40 different subtypes of NHL, each with characteristics and peculiar clinical behavior. Although the goals of the WHO classification are to identify well-defined entities and to facilitate the recognition of uncommon subtypes that require further clarification, as they move forward some challenges in the classification continue. The borders between some of the disease entities remain ill-defined for example nodular lymphocyte predominant HL with diffuse growth pattern versus T-cell/histiocyte rich large BCL [12].

Some discoveries have been rapidly incorporated into daily diagnostic practice such as IHC for SOX11 or BRAF used to help in the diagnosis of MCL or hairy cell leukemia (HCL), respectively. Molecular detection of the recurrent *MYD88* (3p22.2) and *RHOA* (3p21.31) or *IDH2* (15q26.1) mutations are helping to delineate the morphological spectrum of lymphoplasmocytic lymphoma and angioimmunoblastic T-cell lymphoma, respectively [12].

Theoretically, with the possible exception of a few subtypes, any lymphoma entities listed in the last WHO classification of lymphoid malignancies may arise in the GIT. There are various inflammatory and reactive conditions in the GIT that can give rise to, mimic, or mask lymphomas. As mentioned earlier, the GIT is home to various lymphoid neoplasms, most of which are of B-cell lineage, including the most common DLBCL subtype. Not frequently TCLs also are encountered in GIT, however, some of them are related to underlying GI disorders or treatment. Some subtypes of GI lymphoma are characterized by aggressive clinical behavior, but others are indolent and may not require treatment. Identifying these entities can provide adequate treatment and, equally importantly, avoiding of overtreatment when aggressive therapy is not needed. The 2016 revised WHO classification has introduced some important changes to the schema used to categorize lymphomas that affect the GIT, and several TCL and NK-cell lymphomas have been reclassified and/or introduced [90].

DLBCL is the most common pathological type of lymphomas in essentially all sites of the GIT, although recently the frequency of other forms has also increased in certain regions of the world. Histopathologically, almost 90% of the PGIL are of B-cell lineage with very few TCLs and HL [4, 8].

The majority of PELs are the DLBCL type of NHL. Only a few cases of MALT lymphoma, MCL, TCL involving the esophagus have been reported [91–93]. HL of the esophagus is extremely rare. FL affecting the esophagus is a part of the multifocal presentation in the GIT [4].

PGL is the most common extranodal NHL and represents a wide spectrum of diseases, ranging from indolent extranodal MZL of MALT to aggressive DLBCL [11]. Although all histological types of nodal lymphoma can arise from the stomach, the majority of them are of B-cell origin, and MALT lymphoma and DLBCL account for over 90%. Gastric DLBCL occurs in 59% while the extranodal MZL of the MALT occurs in 38% of the PGL cases. Approximately one-fourth of the cases of DLBCL is encountered with the MALT component. MCL is seen in 1% of the cases, FL in 0.5%. Peripheral TCL accounts for 1.5% of PGL [94]. It should be noted that small BCLs are composed mainly of small lymphocytes and are often referred to as "LG" BCLs. The WHO classification intentionally does not divide lymphomas by grade, and because they ("LG" BCLs) are not surely indolent, the preferred name used is "small BCLs". They include MALT lymphoma, FL, MCL, etc. In the literature, most of the authors use the terms "HG MALT lymphoma" and "LG MALT lymphoma" without reference to the official name in the classification. The use of such terminology is confusing, because, this leads to some tangles. So, the "MALT" descriptor implies that there is only one type of lymphoma with various grades that develops in organs with mucosa. In terms of biological behavior, however, there are two common subtypes of lymphoma that arise in mucosal locations, one indolent and the other aggressive. Therefore, the term "MALT" would comprise both subtypes and blur the border between them. This was the main ground why WHO classification chose the term "extranodal MZL" for the indolent entity—to distinguish it from DLBCL, the aggressive entity. The acronym "MALT" is fine for shorthand but should not be used without reference to the official name for the indolent neoplasm "extranodal MZL" [83] as it is specified in the 2008 WHO classification and 2016 revised WHO classification [95, 96].

PSIL that are more heterogeneous than those in the stomach includes MALT lymphoma, DLBCL, MCL, EATL, FL, IPSID [97], a variant of extranodal MZL of MALT, and BL. IPSID and EATL are the main histological subtypes of PSIL. TCL of the small intestine accounts for approximately 10–25% of all PILs primarily occurring as EATL [55, 56]. Lymphocytic lymphoma (chronic lymphocytic leukemia) rarely arises primarily from GIT [4].

PCRL is mostly (>90%) of the B-cell lineage as other sites of the GIT [37, 97]. The most common histological subtype of PCRL is DLBCL. Other histological subtypes include FL, BL, MALT lymphoma, MCL [60, 98] and TCL. MALT lymphoma is less common in the large bowel than in the small intestine (0.5–1% vs. 1–2% of total cases, respectively). MCL in the colorectum presents commonly in the setting of diffuse systemic diseases. Peripheral TCL is rare in Western countries but has an increasing incidence in many Asian countries, and is more aggressive than the other types of lymphoma. Perforation is a common feature of TCL, and its prognosis is poor [22, 98].

As mentioned earlier DLBCL is the most common histological subtype (up to 58%) of all PGILs [99] and is encountered in all sites of GIT more than 50% being seen in the stomach followed by the small intestine [18]. It originates from GC B-cells or post-germinal B-cells [100]. DLBCL is characterized by large lymphoid cells, with nuclei greater than twice the size of a small lymphocyte, and frequently larger than nuclei of tissue macrophage. The tumor cells contain round, oval, or slightly irregular nuclei with vesicular nuclear chromatin, prominent nucleoli, and ample amount of basophilic cytoplasm and have a diffuse growth pattern [15, 100, 101]. In most cases, the predominant cells resemble either large centroblasts or immunoblasts; nonetheless, a mixture of these two cell types is also commonly encountered. So cytologically, DLBCL is diverse and can be divided into the following morphologic variants: centroblastic, immunoblastic, T-cell/histiocyte rich and anaplastic. Histologically, there is an intense cellular infiltration of the lamina propria [15]. The tumor cells are CD45 positive and express the pan-B antigens (CD19, CD20, CD22 and CD79a) [4, 100, 101]. Variability has been observed in CD5 and CD10 expression [102]. CD10 is expressed in 30 to 60% of cases though CD5 is generally negative and only seen in *de novo* cases. MUM1/IRF4 is present in 35–65% of cases. Nuclear PAX-5 immunoreactivity is seen almost in all DLBCL cases and 70% of tumor cells may express bcl-6 protein [101]. CD10 expression is considered a marker of follicular-derived DLBCL. Immunohistochemical evaluation shows a moderate to high proliferative index with a Ki-67 [15, 100]. The most commonly seen translocations as mentioned earlier include t(14;18)(q32;q21), t(3;14)(p27;q32) and t(8;14)(q24;q32) with *BCL2*, *BCL6* and *MYC* rearrangement, respectively [4].

2008 WHO classification recognized GC B-cell-like (GCB) and activated B-cell-like (ABC) molecular "subgroups" of DLBCL based on gene expression profiling

(GEP). The GCB and ABC subgroups are distinct biologic entities and differed in their chromosomal alterations, activation of signaling pathways, and clinical outcome. The identification of the molecular characteristics of these 2 subgroups, however, has led to the investigation of more adequate treatment strategies to improve the worse outcome of the cases with ABC/non-GCB type DLBCL [83].

MALT lymphoma mainly involves the stomach and also can rarely be encountered in the small intestine and colorectum [103]. Gastric MALT lymphoma can involve any part of the organ, but more frequently it affects the antrum [32]. It is typically an LG neoplasm, characterized by a dense lymphoid infiltration that invades and destroys gastric glands and results in the so-called "lymphoepithelial lesion" which is pathognomonic for lymphoma [103]. It has been postulated that MALT lymphoma arises from post-germinal center memory B-cells with the capacity to differentiate into marginal zone cells and plasma cells [104]. MALT lymphomas do not have a specific antigenic profile, the B-cells share the immunophenotype with marginal zone B-cells present in the spleen, Peyer's patches and LNs [4, 33]. So, the tumor B-cells can express the surface immunoglobulins (often IgM, not frequently IgA and IgG, rarely IgD) and pan-B antigens (CD19, CD20, CD22 and CD79a), the marginal zone-associated antigens (CD35 and CD21, and lack CD5, CD10, CD23) [4]. Therefore, gastric MALT lymphoma is CD20+, rarely CD5+; CD10-, CD23- and cyclin D1- [15, 32, 33]. *H. pylori*-negative MALT lymphoma tends to have a high positive rate for t(11;18)(q21;q21) translocation than *H. pylori*-positive MALT lymphoma [69]. The PCR for *IGH* gene rearrangement should be performed only when there is a lymphoid infiltrate morphologically suspicious of lymphoma, and MALT lymphoma should not be diagnosed in the absence of clear histological evidence [105].

B lymphocytes of the extranodal marginal zone are the lineage of MALT lymphoma and are characterized by the heterogeneous cellular population which is prevalently composed of small (monocytoid) lymphocytes and large cells (immunoblasts and centroblasts) [106]. The increase in the proportion of large cells in MALT lymphoma can lead pathologists to confusion, suggesting a conversion into DLBCL which is characterized by the presence of solid aggregates or sheet-like proliferation of large cells [107].

The question about whether all cases of primary gastric DLBCL are derived from previous LG MALT lymphomas or they develop *de novo* remains unsolved. It should be noted that the cytogenetic alterations observed in gastric MALT lymphomas are different from those of typical primary gastric DLBCL. Therefore, cytogenetics can differentiate the two variants in some cases [11]. MALT lymphomas have a nonspecific antigenic profile that can differentiate them from primary DLBCL which is characterized by different immunophenotypes, especially about CD45, CD5, and CD10 expression [102]. Moreover, both transformed MALT lymphomas and *de novo* DLBCLs show bcl-6 positivity; however, DLBCLs with a GC-like phenotype is frequently CD10 and bcl-2 positive, whereas transformed MALT lymphomas are CD10 and bcl-2 negative [108].

IPSID or alpha heavy chain disease (αHCD) is an extranodal BCL and represents a variant of MALT lymphoma, which involves mainly the proximal small intestine [24, 25]. This disorder is morphologically characterized by small bowel infiltration by a uniform population of lymphoplasmacytic cells associating with atypical lymphoid propagation to DLBCL. The centrocyte-like lymphocytes express CD20, and both atypical lymphocytic and plasmacytic populations will strongly stain with IgA heavy chain, with lack of light chain staining [25]. IPSID lymphomas reveal excessive plasma cell differentiation and produce truncated alpha heavy chain proteins lacking the light chains as well as the first constant domain. Cytogenetic studies demonstrated clonal rearrangements involving predominantly the heavy and light chain genes, including t(9;14)(p13;q32) translocation with the involvement of the *PAX5* gene [24].

BL, a type of non-Hodgkin BCL, displays a diffuse, monotonous infiltrate of medium-sized neoplastic lymphoid cells with round nuclei and little cytoplasm showing finely clumped and dispersed, with multiple basophilic nucleoli, presenting pathologically with a "starry sky" pattern [15, 29, 109]. It is most often found in the abdomen and the jaw, however, localization in the abdomen other than the ileocecal area is very rare [15, 109]. Mutations in the transcription factor 3 gene, *TCF3* (19p13.3) or in its negative regulator *ID3* (1p36.12) take place in about 70% of sporadic and immunodeficiency-related BL and less frequently (40%) in endemic cases. TCF3 supports the proliferation and survival of lymphoid cells by activating the B-cell receptor/phosphatidylinositol 3-kinase signaling pathways and modulating the expression of *CCND3* (*cyclin D3*, 6p21.1), which also undergoes mutation in 30% of BL cases. One of the questions not fully settled is whether genuine BL without *MYC* arrangement exists in reality. A subset of lymphomas that resemble BL morphologically, to a great extent phenotypically and by GEP, surprisingly lack *MYC* rearrangements. Instead, they have an alteration in chromosome 11q which is characterized by telomeric losses and proximal gains. Compared with BL, these lymphomas have more complex karyotypes, weak *MYC* expression, a certain degree of cytological pleomorphism, sometimes a follicular pattern, and frequently a nodal presentation. Although the clinical course seems to be similar to BL this subtype of BL was classified as a new provisional entity designated as Burkitt-like lymphoma with 11q aberration in the 2016 revised WHO classification. In literature, the number of reported cases of this entity is still limited and more studies are needed to resolve the controversial issues [83]. Tumor cells express membrane immunoglobulins (IgM, Ig light chain), B-cell antigens (CD19, CD20, CD22), CD10, bcl-6, c-MYC while expressing negative results for CD5, CD23, and bcl-2. The most common cytogenetic change is t(8;14)(q24;q32) and t(8;22)(q24;q11) translocations that are characterized by overexpression of *c-MYC* oncogene and can be detected in 90% of cases by classical karyotyping or FISH. The proliferation index Ki-67 of BL is very high, usually over 95%, so it is not surprising because BL is the fastest growing human cancer [29, 109]. Cytogenetic analysis is recommended to allow a clear distinction between BL and other *c-MYC*-driven B-cell NHL, especially DLBCL [29].

The morphological distinction between BL and DLBCL has been problematic for pathologists [12, 109]. Distinguishing between these two lymphomas, however, is critical, especially in adults (BL is rare in adults and rarely found in the stomach and colon), as the two diseases are treated differently [109]. GEP studies have demonstrated that BL has a specific signature but that there are cases that resemble DLBCL and aggressive BCLs, and have a molecular signature similar to BL, hence fall into an intermediate category. 2008 WHO classification recognized this issue and added a provisional entity of BCL, unclassifiable, with characteristics intermediate between DLBCL and BL (BCLU) [12, 29].

MCL originates from small to medium-sized lymphocytes located in the mantle zone (inner layer) of follicular tissue. Extra nodal involvement is present in the majority of cases, with a peculiar tendency to invade the GIT in the form of MLP. MLP is one of the most common primary GI presentations of MCL and accounts for approximately about 9% of PGIL [110]. MLP most commonly occurs in the ascending colon and the small bowel (particularly in the ileum and ileocecal region) and gastric involvement are next common [110, 111]. Occasionally, however, numerous polyps are present throughout the entire GIT. Polyps may be sessile, polypoid or both. They range in size from 0.1 to 4–5 cm and present with ulceration [110]. MCL is now recognized as an aggressive BCL with various growth patterns (mantle zone, nodular, or diffuse) and a broad range of cytological features [112, 113].

The prototype MCL is positive for pan B-cell antigens, although few cases of CD5-negative MCL have been reported [24]. Most cases of MCL exhibit a characteristic phenotype (CD20+, CD5+, CD43+, CD3-, CD10-, CD23-) and have the t(11;14)(q13;q32) translocation with overexpression of the *CCND1* (*cyclin D1*) gene on chromosome 11q13 [112]. Neuronal transcription factor SOX11 nuclear expression is also characteristic of MCL and can help distinguish MCL from other BCLs. The current WHO guidelines for the diagnosis of MCL rely on morphologic examination and immunophenotyping, with the demonstration of cyclin D1 protein overexpression and/or the t(11; 14)(q13;q32) for confirmation [114]. Few cases of cyclin D1-negative MCL, however, have been reported with up-regulated cyclin D2 or D3 [112]. The existence of cyclin D1 negative MCL has been controversial and difficult to substantiate since cyclin D1 overexpression is believed to be essential in the pathogenesis of MCL [112].

Duodenal-type FL, formerly known as primary intestinal FL, is a variant of FL sharing many morphological and immunohistochemical characteristics with nodal FL [19] but is a distinct entity from nodal FL in terms of clinicopathological and molecular standpoints [115] and demonstrates almost universally LG cytology. Morphologically, the mucosa and submucosa are infiltrated with well-circumscribed round neoplastic follicles which form small nodules and polyps corresponding to the endoscopic manifestation. The neoplastic follicles are similar to those seen in nodal FL and are composed of monotypic centrocytes and rare centroblasts. Although the disease is not graded in the same manner as nodal FL, it corresponds to LG (grades 1–2) lymphoma. The lymphoma cells often infiltrate into the surrounding lamina propria [19]. The immunoprofile of the lymphoma cells demonstrate similarity to that of nodal FL, with the expression of CD20, CD10, bcl-2, and bcl-6. The proliferation marker Ki-67 demonstrates a low rate. In contrast with systemic FL, duodenal-type FL is not characterized by the expression of activation-induced cytidine deaminase (AID) [116]. The indolent biological behavior of duodenal-type FL may bring its neoplastic nature into question. But it harbors the same t(14;18)(q32;q21) translocation with *IGH/BCL2* rearrangement observed in conventional FL. Furthermore, the duodenal-type entity seems to have rarer additional genetic aberrations than conventional FL. In addition, some evidence suggest that its gene expression profile overlaps with that of extranodal MZLs of MALT [19]. Although FL is very rare, it expresses surface immunoglobulin (often IgM) and pan B-cell antigens. CD10 and bcl-2 are expressed in almost 90% of the cases. Duodenal-type FL does not express CD5 and cyclin D1 thereby can be differentiated from MCL. *IGH/BCL2* rearrangement related to t(14;18)(q32;q21) translocation can be found by FISH or PCR analysis in most of the cases [117].

MEITL differs from the "classic" form of EATL by characteristic morphologic and immunophenotypic features [19]. Recognizing these distinctions, 2016 revised WHO classification formally separated these 2 entities and now defines MEITL as a primary intestinal TCL not associated with celiac disease [118]. It is a rare and aggressive peripheral TCL deriving from intestinal intraepithelial T lymphocytes. The small intestine is affected most frequently, with rare cases involving the stomach and colon. The spreading pattern of MEITL is in contrast with EATL as well; the former often spreads diffusely within the intestinal mucosa with or without tumefactive lesions, since the latter is frequently associated with large and ulcerative tumors that may perforate the intestine. Ulceration may occur in cases of MEITL, and mesenteric LNs involvement is common [28]. No background villous atrophy in small intestinal mucosa associates the tumor. MEITL cells are positive for CD3, CD8, CD56, and MATK in most of the cases, but negative for CD4, CD5, CD30. Nearly 20% of the cases demonstrate aberrant expression of CD20, a feature that can potentially lead to diagnostic confusion with B-cell entities, such as DLBCL or BL. By contrast, classic EATL is usually negative for CD8, CD56, and MATK, with CD4 negativity and variable CD30 positivity [19].

Intestinal TCL, not otherwise specified, does not represent a specific disease entity; it is a term used to denote a heterogenous group of TCLs developing in the GIT with insufficient evidence to be diagnosed as EATL or MEITL, due to incomplete clinical information, scarce biopsy specimens, or insufficient immunophenotypic data. Furthermore, a part of the cases may be peripheral TCL, not otherwise specified, with GI involvement [19]. No reported cases of this TCL subset with a history of celiac disease at initial diagnosis [119]. The morphologic and immunohistochemical characteristics are heterogenous, because this term likely encompasses multiple disease entities [19]. This subset of lymphoma has an aggressive clinical course, with several reported cases demonstrating widespread disease at initial diagnosis [119].

The EBV-positive MCU has been added as a newly recognized entity and is characterized by limited growth despite the aggressive morphological features, and good outcome with a conservative approach [12]. In the involved mucosal surfaces of GIT is encountered superficial ulceration with underlying dense infiltrate of atypical lymphoid cells, necrotic debris, and a rim of reactive T-cells around B-cell areas. Plasma cells are present to a varying degree; they may be prominent and maybe light chain-restricted. The background inflammatory infiltrate can contain histiocytes, eosinophils as well. A significant number of large atypical lymphocytes are found within the necrosis, sometimes in dense sheets. The atypical lymphocytes are large and various in appearance and can resemble those seen in DLBCL or classic HL. They have large pleomorphic nuclei and prominent nucleoli with often Hodgkin and Reed-Sternberg (HRS) cytology. In the setting of iatrogenic immunosuppression for a solid organ transplant, this is a type of post-transplantation lymphoproliferative disorder [120]. The distinction between DLBCL and EBV-positive MCU is important in the post-transplantation setting because EBV-positive MCU has an indolent course. The lesions are typically well-circumscribed at the base and surrounded by a rim of reactive lymphocytes, which are mainly T-cells [115]. The large, atypical lymphocytes are positive for PAX-5, OCT2, MUM1, CD30, EBER and LMP1, and negative for CD10. BOB1 and bcl-6 are frequently positive, with variable expression of CD15, CD20, CD45 and CD79a [42]. T-cells in the inflammatory background are EBER-negative and express normal pan-T-cell markers, including CD3 and CD8. It is particularly important to distinguish these cases from classical HL, which is extremely rare in the GIT [19].

Indolent T-cell lymphoproliferative disorder (ITLPD) of the GIT is a provisional entity in the updated WHO classification and is a nonaggressive, largely nonepitheliotropic small, mature T-cell disorder of the GIT with evidence of clonality by T-cell receptor gene rearrangement studies [19, 121, 122]. This disease is encountered in adulthood (it occurs in children occasionally) and can involve any part of the GIT with the small intestine and colon being the most commonly involved sites. However, because many of the histologic features may overlap with IBD, it is uncertain whether these patients truly have to precede IBD, or whether the lymphoproliferative disorder itself has been initially misdiagnosed as IBD. No cases have been reported in association with celiac disease [121]. Moreover, GI ITLPD may be misdiagnosed as EATL or MEITL and lead to aggressive therapy since the latter lymphoma subtypes are rare but aggressive lymphomas of the GIT. Microscopically, the lamina propria is expanded by a dense and monotonous lymphoid infiltrate. The mucosal crypts or glands are displaced and often distorted, but not destroyed. Cryptitis and crypt abscesses are absent, but granulomas may be focally present, potentially mimicking those seen in Crohn's disease. The lymphoid infiltrate is composed of small, mature lymphocytes with round nuclei and regular nuclear contours [19, 121, 122]. The lymphoma cells are mature T-cells that express

CD2, CD3, CD4, CD5, or CD8, and variably CD7. The absence of CD56 expression is particularly important for diagnosis, distinguishing this entity from MEITL. All reported cases have demonstrated TCRβ expression, with no cases showing TCRγ expression. The proliferation marker Ki-67 rate is low (<10%) [121, 122]. Clonal rearrangements of TCR (either γ or β) have been observed in all cases, and all have been negative for EBV (EBER) by FISH, distinguishing this entity from extranodal NK/TCL of nasal type, which can involve the GIT [19].

5.1. Staging of PGIL

Accurate diagnosis and staging of PGIL are essential for the stratification of treatment in this heterogeneous group of malignancies [4]. In other words, tumor stage is one of the most important guidelines in the choice of local (surgery, radiotherapy) and systemic (chemotherapy—ChTh) management modalities. There is a lack of consensus regarding the best staging system for PGIL. Different subtypes of PGIL have a different dissemination pattern from their nodal counterparts, which limits the use of the conventional Ann Arbor staging system [101]. The Ann Arbor staging system, developed for and routinely used in nodal NHL, is not optimal for documentation of the specific relevant features of primary extranodal lymphoma in the GIT [123]. Various modifications have been proposed to aid the staging of PGILs, including those of Musshoff, Blackledge and the Lugano Workshop [101, 123, 124].

TNM staging for tumors of epithelial origin has also been proposed as an alternative in PGIL to describe to what extent the disease is localized or spread. The "T" part of this system pertains to the anatomical structure of the organs and sufficiently fulfills the requirements for the staging of the local extent of the disease. The European Gastro-Intestinal Lymphoma Study (EGILS) Group proposed a modified TNM staging system, named after the first venue of the group in Paris. The modified staging system adjusted to the PGIL, considering histopathological characteristics of extranodal B and T-cell lymphomas, and accordingly enroll: (1) depth of tumor infiltration along with the thickness of GIT; (2) extent of nodal involvement; (3) lymphoma spreading [123]. Paris staging system is valid for lymphomas originating from the gastro-esophageal junction to the anus [123] and has increasingly gained its significance [4].

Paris staging system classifies PGIL as follows:

TX—lymphoma extent not specified

T0—no evidence of lymphoma

T1—lymphoma confined to the mucosa/submucosa

T1m—lymphoma confined to mucosa

T1sm—lymphoma confined to submucosa

T2—lymphoma infiltrates muscularis propria or subserosa

T3—lymphoma penetrates serosa (visceral peritoneum) without invasion of adjacent structures

T4—lymphoma invades adjacent structures or organs

NX—involvement of LNs not assessed

N0—no evidence of LN involvement

N1—involvement of regional LNs

N2—involvement of intra-abdominal LNs beyond the regional area

N3—spread to extra-abdominal LNs

MX—dissemination of lymphoma not assessed

M0—no evidence of extranodal dissemination

M1—non-continuous involvement of separate site in GIT (e.g., stomach and rectum)

M2—non-continuous involvement of other tissues (e.g., peritoneum, pleura) or organs (e.g., tonsils, ocular adnexa, lung, liver, spleen, breast, etc.)

BX—involvement of bone marrow not assessed

B0—no evidence of bone marrow involvement

B1—lymphomatous infiltration of bone marrow

TNM—clinical staging: status of tumor, node, metastasis, bone marrow

pTNMB—histopathological staging: status of the tumor, node metastasis, bone marrow

pN—the histological examination will ordinarily include six or more LNs

According to the site of the PGIL "regional" LNs implies: (a) stomach: perigastric LNs and those located along the branches of the coeliac artery (left gastric artery, common hepatic artery, and splenic artery); (b) duodenum: pancreatoduodenal, suprapyloric and infrapyloric, hepatic LNs, and those located along superior mesenteric artery; (c) small intestine: mesenteric LNs; the ileocolic as well as the posterior caecal LNs for the terminal ileum only; (d) colorectum: pericolic and perirectal LNs and those located along the ileocolic, right, middle, and left colic, inferior mesenteric, superior rectal, and internal iliac arteries [123].

6. Clinical characteristics

PGIL is a relatively rare cancer that is easily misdiagnosed and indistinguishable from other benign and malignant conditions due to its unspecific symptoms attributable to the site of involvement [4, 11]. The clinical manifestation of PGIL is dependent on the involved site, pathological subtype and the stage of the tumor. The age of presentation varies with the histological subtypes of lymphoma [97].

Although PEL is often asymptomatic, the common symptoms of symptomatic patients include dysphagia, odynophagia, weight loss, chest pain or symptoms developed as a result of complications such as hemorrhage, obstruction or perforation [4, 125, 126]. Constitutional B symptoms (fever, night sweats) are not typically present and are seen rarely [4]. Some researchers suppose that the diagnosis of GI lymphoma, including PEL (despite its rare incidence) should be considered in any HIV-infected patient presenting with unexplained GI symptoms [44, 93].

Clinical manifestation of PGL is nonspecific and indistinguishable from other benign and malignant conditions. The most common complaints of patients with PGL are epigastric pain, nausea and vomiting (due to pyloric stenosis or reflex), iron-deficiency anemia due to chronic gastric bleeding, and weight loss. Occasionally, an abdominal mass is palpable. Severe complications such as perforation and life-threatening haemorrhage are seen rarely (4%) [127]. Lymphadenopathy is rare and such patients often have no physical signs [4]. Unlike nodal lymphoma, B constitutional symptoms are not common. Gastric MALT lymphoma is often an indolent, multifocal disease and in 10% of the cases, it can have synchronous involvement of intestinal and extraintestinal sites [128] with appropriate clinical signs.

The clinical presentation of PSIL is nonspecific and the patients have symptoms, such as colicky abdominal pain, nausea, vomiting, weight loss and rarely acute obstructive symptoms, intussusceptions, perforation or diarrhea [97]. However, the typical clinical features of IPSID, a subtype of MALT lymphoma, are different because the dominant region for IPSID is the duodenum and upper jejunum, and present diarrhea, malabsorption syndrome or protein-losing enteropathy [23, 24]. Intussusception is a common clinical finding in ileocecal lymphomas, occurring mainly in patients with the fungating type of the lesion [129]. In general, the most commonly affected region with PSIL is the ileum followed by the jejunum and duodenum (6–8%) [100].

PCRL presents with abdominal pain, altered bowel habit, palpable abdominal mass, lower GI bleeding and weight loss [22, 101, 130, 131]. Obstruction and perforation are relatively rare in patients with PCRL [131]. Primary colorectal TCLs are characterized by multifocal ulcerative lesions in relatively young patients and a high rate of hematochezia, fever or perforation, and aggressive clinical course even for cases of localized disease [22]. The caecum is the most common site of involvement because of the abundance of lymphatic tissue [101].

Some features of some PILs should be peculiarly noted. MCL, FL and MALT lymphoma of the small intestine rarely present with multiple polyps called MLP [20, 110, 132]. In one-third of the cases, MLP is due to MCL. MLP can present with symptoms such as abdominal pain, diarrhea, bleeding, and less frequently, protein losing enteropathy, intestinal malabsorption, intestinal obstruction or chylous ascites. MLP polyps usually occur in the ileocecal region and one-third of cases present as a mass [110].

7. Diagnostics

During diagnostics, the clinician verifies the lymphoma, determines its site and stage, and detects possible relationship of some lymphoma subtypes with some infections and disorders, and inherited conditions. Comprehensive history taking and physical examination may provide a very important clues for reaching the goal promptly. The first objective examination tool depends on the patient's complaints and the result of the physical examination.

Endoscopy is the firstly used diagnostic modality for visualization of the lesion and for getting biopsy samples depending on the involved site. The histological examination of biopsy samples taken during endoscopy is the "gold standard" for the diagnosis of PGIL. The endoscopy by itself cannot identify lymphoma or differ it from the more common GI carcinomas [127]. The injury patterns of PGIL (ulceration, diffuse infiltration, polypoid mass, etc.) are characteristic also of GI carcinomas. However, the most common endoscopic appearances of PGIL are ulcerative and massive [8]. One of the main difficulties for accurate visual diagnosis of PGIL is the variation in endoscopic abnormalities, which varies from minimal mucosal irregularities to bigger ulcerations [18].

Endoscopic findings in PEL vary greatly and are nonspecific, which poses diagnostic challenges when it is differentiated from other benign and malignant lesions. The morphological features of PEL seen at endoscopy are nodular, polypoid, ulcerated or stenotic [92]. Multiple biopsies should be obtained from the stomach, gastroesophageal junction, duodenum, and from lesions in cases of PGL since gastroduodenal lymphomas (MALT lymphoma, duodenal-type FL, etc.) can occasionally present as a multifocal disease with involvement of tissue that appears to be unaffected on endoscopic visualization [133]. Endoscopic findings may vary from subtle mucosal changes (mucosal edema, friability, patchy redness, irregular patchy gray or whitish granularity, contact bleeding, superficial irregular erosions and ulcerations) to gross lesions (ulceration, diffuse infiltration, and a polypoid mass) [124] that are characteristic also for early gastric carcinoma and gastric carcinoma respectively and are not diagnostic (**Figure 1A**). The extension of a gastric lesion across the pylorus into the duodenum is highly suggestive of lymphoma, not of carcinoma, but is not pathognomonic. Endoscopy, however, is an indispensable tool for the initial diagnosis, for obtaining biopsy samples and as well as for follow-up of the cases. Conventional pinch biopsy results may be false-negative (up to 8%) owing to submucosal localization [127] without involving the mucosa. Repeated endoscopic biopsies are mandatory in case of clinical suspicion and negative or

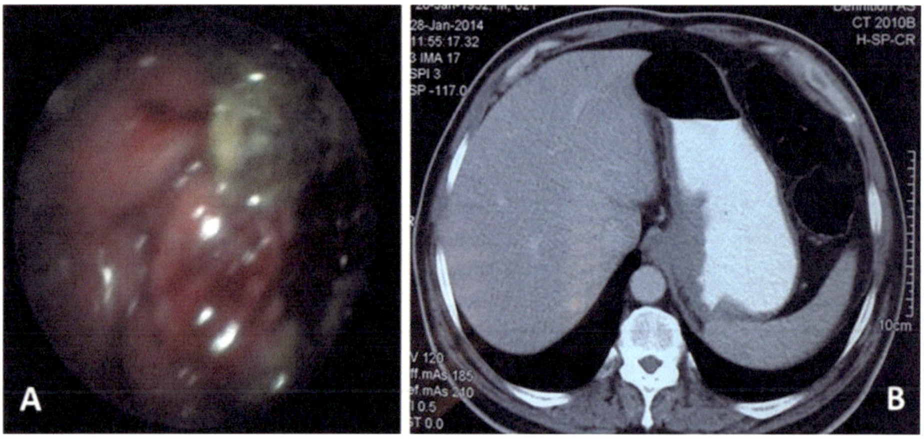

Figure 1.
Endoscopic (A) and CT (B) views of gastric DLBCL in H. pylori-positive 63-year-old man who complained of anorexia, epigastral discomphort and vomiting. The diagnosis of DLBCL was confirmed pathohistologically and immunohistochemically. The lesion involved the proximal third of the stomach. Perigastric, regional, paraaortic and mesenteric LNs were enlarged on CT.

inconclusive histology [124] EUS-guided fine-needle aspiration biopsy can help to increase the yield in some cases. The presence of *H. pylori* in tissue samples obtained by esophagogastroscopy must also be tested in all cases through immunohistochemistry (IHC) [11]. In the last years, magnifying endoscopy has improved endoscopic diagnosis of PGL by detection of destructed gastric pits, irregular pit size or distribution [62].

The duodenum and the terminal ileum can be investigated by conventional endoscopy which is home to special subtypes of PGIL. Detection and assessment of PSIL have been revolutionized since the introduction of capsule endoscopy and double-balloon enteroscopy (push-and-pull enteroscopy) which is capable of providing biopsy samples, thereby limiting major surgical interventions. PSIL is presented as a polyp, bulky lesion, or ulcer on capsule endoscopy which cannot be visually differentiated from other lesions [134]. Unlike the other endoscopic approaches, capsule endoscopy does not permit tissue sampling. Primary ileocolonic lymphoma and PCRL can be classified endoscopically into fungating, ulcerative, infiltrative and mixed types. Among these, fungating and ulcerofungating are the most frequent [129]. Total colonoscopy with tissue sampling is crucial for accurate diagnosis in cases of suspicion of PCRL.

As mentioned earlier MCL, FL and MALT lymphoma of the small intestine rarely present with multiple polyps called MLP [20, 110, 132]. Upper GI endoscopy, enteroscopy and colonoscopy are important tools in diagnosing MLP to assess the locations of the polyps and obtain tissue biopsies. Differentiating MLP from adenomatous or hamartomatous polyposis by endoscopic or radiological evaluation alone is impossible and tissue diagnosis is required [110].

MALT lymphoma of the large intestine is manifested as multiple mucosal nodularities [22, 135]. IPSID tends to affect proximally with a disseminated nodular pattern leading to mucosal fold thickening, irregularity and speculation [136]. Extranodal BL is frequently seen but GIT involvement varies among the three clinical subtypes, with the sporadic variant usually presenting as a bulky mass, commonly in the terminal ileum and caecum [15, 29].

About 10% of all FL is of GI origin and the GIT is the most frequently involved site [115]. Primary FL of the GIT is very rare and constitute <7% of all GI NHL lymphomas [20]. Many cases (43–77%) of GI FL are asymptomatic and sometimes accidentally found by endoscopic examination [115]. Cases of GI FL often present as an incidental whitish polypoid lesion described as small polypoid nodules, multiple polypoid lesions, multiple small polyps, multiple nodules, or multiple granules in patients undergoing upper endoscopy for other unrelated reasons, such as dyspepsia or suspected gastroesophageal reflux [19, 137]. Other macroscopic features are infrequent, but they can present as erosions or ulcers [137]. The disease is usually found in the proximal part of the small intestine [19, 20, 115, 137–139] most often with duodenal involvement in the second portion [19, 115, 137]. Gastric and colorectal FL have been occasionally reported [137]. Multiple sites of small intestinal involvement are seen in 56–80% of cases [20, 139]. The most reliable way to distinguish primary GI FL from GI involvement of conventional FL, is to rule out intestinal involvement by mesenteric/retroperitoneal disease and/or systemic diseases by imaging and bone marrow biopsy [19].

PTCL preferentially involves the jejunum with an increased tendency to perforate [130]. EATL, usually proximal or diffuse, shows nodules, ulcers or strictures [136]. PTCL of the large intestine presents as a diffuse or focal segmental lesion with extensive mucosal ulceration similar to that observed in granulomatous conditions as Crohn's disease or tuberculosis [22, 135]. The GIT EBV-positive MCU usually presents with sharply circumscribed ulcers in the oral mucosa, esophagus, colon, rectum, and/or perianal area. It is usually a localized (albeit potentially locally aggressive) process, and lymphadenopathy, bone marrow involvement, and disseminated disease are exceedingly rare [41, 42]. In cases of ITLPD, the affected GI mucosa (the disease most often localizes in the small intestine and colon; however, all sites in the GIT may be involved) is viewed thickened with prominent folds, nodularity, and/or polyps. The surface can be hyperemic with superficial erosions [121].

It is recommended that biopsy specimens should undergo histological, immunohistochemical and genotyping studies to make the diagnosis [124]. It should be noted that on histological examination Reed-Sternberg-like cells can be seen in LG BCLs [140] including extranodal MZL, FL, IPSID that can be confused with HL. Histological assessment is currently considered the "gold standard" also for the assessment of treatment response in gastric lymphoma [5].

The different procedures employed for the pre-treatment staging include computed tomography (CT), magnetic resonance imaging (MRI), EUS, 18F-fluorodeoxyglucose positron emission tomography (FDG-PET). Contrast-enhanced techniques and functional imaging such as perfusion CT can also help the monitoring, assessment, and prediction of response [4, 11].

Radiographic patterns of PEL, described in the literature, are nonspecific and not diagnostic and include thickening of the wall mimicking other tumors, stricture, ulcerated mass, multiple submucosal nodules, varicoid pattern, achalasia-like pattern, progressive aneurysmal dilatation, and tracheoesophageal fistula formation, and none of them is specific and diagnostic [91, 141]. CT, however, is valuable for the evaluation of the mediastinal extension of PEL, fistula formation, and status of LNs, thus playing a role in staging disease, assisting in stratification of available treatment modalities, evaluating treatment responses, monitoring disease progression, and detecting relapses [141]. CT scan of the chest, abdomen and pelvis is should be employed to stage PGIL irrespective of the involved site.

Radiographic patterns of PGL observed in double-contrast upper GI studies include ulcers, thickened fold, polypoid mass, mucosal nodularities or infiltrating lesions, which are not conclusive, thus posing a diagnostic challenge while differentiating from other malignant and benign lesions, hence requiring pathological confirmation [142]. The radiological findings usually do not correlate to its pathological subtypes [4]. Conservation of pliability and distensibility of the gastric wall despite the substantial gastric fold thickening and extensive infiltration of the gastric wall is a finding very suggestive of lymphoma. Gastric wall thickening is much more severe in HG lymphoma compared to LG lymphoma on CT images, and abdominal lymphadenopathy is more common in cases of HG lymphoma (**Figure 1B**) [142]. The patterns of gastric involvement can be as localized polypoid mass or segmental/diffuse infiltrative lesion. Tumor infiltration is usually homogeneous, however, areas of low attenuation may be observed in larger tumors. Segmental infiltration and diffuse infiltration involving more than 50% of the stomach are the most common hallmarks of gastric NHL on CT images [143]. Preservation of the fat plane which is an indirect sign that there is no invasion into surrounding anatomical structures may be suggestive of lymphoma as well, however, it is nonspecific. Transpyloric extension of the PGL with involvement of the duodenal wall and presence of bulky LNs, notably below the renal hilum is more suggestive of lymphoma than carcinoma [142].

The radiologic appearances of PCRL are variable and significantly overlapped with other benign and malignant conditions of the colorectal region. The imaging findings during double-contrast barium enema can be divided into focal and diffuse lesions. The observed focal lesions include mucosal nodularity, mucosal fold thickening, polypoid mass, circumferential infiltration with smooth mucosal surface or extensive ulceration, cavitary mass. Diffuse lesions encompass diffuse ulcerative and nodular lesions [22, 135].

The MRI characteristics of PGIL include exophytic tumor mass, irregularly thickened mucosal folds with submucosal infiltration, a circular infiltrating lesion which narrows the lumen, mesenteric or/and retroperitoneal lymphadenopathy. The lymphomas are mostly homogeneous on T1-weighted images and have intermediate signal intensity. Heterogeneously increased signal intensities are observed on T2-weighted images. The enhancement is commonly mild-moderate after intravenous administration of gadolinium-based contrast agents [144].

In routine clinical practice, EUS is being employed widely for assessment of the primary lesion and clinical staging because it is able accurately to depict the neoplastic disease in the wall of the GIT organs, extent of the lesion and depth of invasion. EUS findings, however, are not pathognomonic, because PGILs can be presented as anechoic, hypoechoic or even rarely hyperechoic masses [5, 93, 127]. Infiltrative carcinoma tends to grow vertically along the gastric wall, while PGL demonstrates mostly horizontal growth. Moreover, the involvement of perigastric LNs is most common in PGL cases [5]. EUS is highly accurate in detecting the depth of infiltration of tumor and the presence of perigastric LNs, which are essential for adequate treatment planning. It should be noted that EUS can provide significant information to distinguish lymphoma from carcinoma regardless of the stage of the mentioned tumors [124].

EUS has become an integral tool in the diagnosis, locoregional staging, and monitoring response of PGIL to treatment. EUS is superior to CT scan for the T- and N-staging by providing vivid details for any invasion within and beyond the gastric wall. The significance of EUS and CT, however, is a matter of debate in the follow-up of patients, since it has been well studied that histological remission is confirmed earlier than the disappearance of the wall changes in cases of PGIL. It eliminates the necessity for endoscopic biopsy follow-up in the relevant patients. Gastric MALT lymphoma, often requires a more meticulous staging procedure despite its indolent clinical behavior since it is not infrequently multifocal, can be transformed into DLBCL, and is difficult to diagnose due to normal endoscopic appearance in many cases. Therefore, endoscopic biopsy samples should be taken from multiple sites of the stomach and duodenum encompassing the areas with normal and abnormal appearance [145]. Some authors suppose that EUS seems sufficient for the routine follow-up of patients with PGL without using gastroscopy with biopsy [5].

Recently, the incorporation of PET-CT has emerged as an indispensable tool in staging the disease and following up the patients with extranodal involvement of HL and NHL, with increased sensitivity and specificity. The intensity of FDG uptake in lymphoma is influenced by various intrinsic tumor factors such as histological features and grade, as well as various extrinsic factors [144]. Application of 18F-FDG PET-CT in the diagnosis of PGL is challenging due to the physiologic FDG activity in the stomach and variability in the degree of uptake in various histologic subtypes [146]. FDG-PET has a significant advantage in the staging of DLBCL independent of the affected anatomic site, and MCL, although it has no added benefit for MALT lymphomas due to their indolent behavior [11, 147]. PET-scanning has no sufficient sensitivity (<50%) and is not reliable to diagnose the intestinal FL [137]. Currently, for PGL, PET CT is a standard initial imaging study in DLBCL histology but not recommended in cases of gastric MALT lymphoma [11] and intestinal FL because aggressive PGILs have more intense uptake than LG MALT lymphoma and GI FL [137, 146]. GI DLBCL is manifested as circumferential thickening of the wall, with diffuse increased FDG uptake. FDG PET-CT can also detect indolent lesions that are undetectable on conventional cross-sectional imaging [147]. New promising techniques using recent PET tracers like 18F-fluoro-thymidine may significantly benefit the overall management of lymphomas [4].

In some cases, the diagnosis of PGIL cannot be made by traditional methods and novel diagnostic methods and surgery is needed. Chen et al. report that 48.4% (201/415) of their patients with PGIL were diagnosed by surgery. Reasons for that surgery became a method of diagnosis were as follows: (1) the lesions of PGIL mainly locate submucosally, which increase the difficulty of diagnosis through endoscopic biopsy; (2) when the diagnosis of a visualized malignant lesion after repeating endoscopic biopsy still cannot be confirmed, surgery can be the choice; (3) part of PGIL patients came to the hospital because of acute abdomen, especially patients of TCL and in those cases diagnosis could only be verified after an emergency operation. They report that in their study, 37 (18.4%) of the 201 patients diagnosed by surgery underwent emergency operations. It makes suggests that surgery is an essential way for diagnosis of PGIL, particularly in the cases of TCL because of their high frequency of acute abdomen [8].

The other laboratory analyses conducted encompass a complete haemogram, hepatic and renal function panels, measurement of blood glucose, serum lactate dehydrogenase, uric acid, potassium, calcium, and phosphorus levels. Bone marrow aspirate with a biopsy is fulfilled for assessment of lymphoma dissemination and monitoring of treatment response. In certain types of lymphoma serum protein electrophoresis and identification of paraproteins can be performed as well. For recognition of etiological factors, appropriate serological tests are frequently conducted in various types of lymphoma [145].

8. Treatment strategies

The optimal treatment of PGIL is a matter of debate. The treatment strategy of PGİL depends on multiple factors; involved site, pathological variants, stage of the tumor, the existence of bacterial or viral associations and chromosomal translocations. Accurate staging is necessary for the important therapeutic implications. If the disease affects beyond the organ and regional nodes, treatment strategies can no longer be focused on local control and systemic aggressive ChTh must be the mandatory option.

Surgery was the main treatment modality in the past, but now, in uncomplicated cases, it is replaced by the combination of anthracycline-containing ChTh and rituximab, a chimeric monoclonal antibody against the protein CD20 [13]. Treatment of PGIL is largely ChTh based, augmented with surgical and radiation therapy in many cases. The length and type of chemotherapeutic interventions depend on the extent of the disease but generally systemic therapy, as well as intrathecal delivery of agents, is required to prevent or treat involvement in the cerebrospinal fluid. Surgical resection is controversial and generally considered when complete resection is possible rather than debulking unless indicated by obstruction or perforation. Consolidation therapy with radiation is recommended in patients with localized disease [18]. So, the global therapeutic approach to the cure of primary GI NHL has completely changed over the last 10 years: innovative, conservative options to reduce treatment toxicity, therefore preventing systemic relapses, have made their appearance and are on the rise [16].

The discovery of a causative link between *H. pylori* and the development of gastric MALT lymphoma has revolutionized treatment options [5]. The literature has reported that approximately 60–100% of *H. pylori*-positive localized gastric MALT lymphoma without t(11;18)(q21;q21) chromosomal translocation obtain complete remission after the eradication of this bacteria [4]. Based on this recently, treatment to eradicate *H. pylori* has become standard management for primary gastric MALT lymphoma [148, 149]. Histological evaluation of tumor response to treatment, however, requires serial follow-up and needs standardization. The GELA histological evaluation system of residual disease in gastric biopsy samples following treatment is commonly used at certain centers. It has been reported that monoclonal B-cells persist in up to 50% of the cases with confirmed endoscopic and histological remission following treatment with antibiotics [150]. Patients with negative *H. pylori* infection and those with failure to eradication therapy should benefit from alternative therapeutic regimens that include radiation therapy or ChTh [32]. Gastric MALT lymphoma-specific chromosomal translocation t(11;18)(q21;q21) has been discovered to be a negative predictive parameter for regression following *H. pylori* eradication [73].

No definite guidelines have been advocated for the treatment of advanced or *H. pylori*-negative gastric MALT lymphoma. Although surgery has been used as its initial treatment, recent studies showed that moderate-dose radiotherapy alone can achieve a remission rate of 93–100%. Before antibiotic therapy, radiotherapy was the first-line therapy for gastric MALT lymphomas [32]. Thus, "involved-field" (stomach and perigastric LNs) irradiation at the total dose of 30 Gy for over 4 weeks has become the treatment of choice for stages I and II MALT lymphoma without *H. pylori* or with persistent lymphoma following therapy. Surgery is, at present, no longer a curative first-line treatment for gastric MALT lymphoma and reserved only for refractory cases to nonsurgical approaches and for those with complications such as perforation, hemorrhage or obstruction that cannot be treated with other alternative therapies [11, 151]. Systemic therapy must be taken into consideration in patients with advanced stages [151]. Patients with localized disease, who did not respond to antibiotic therapy or radiation therapy, should be considered for systemic ChTh [59]. Treatment options include ChTh and the use of monoclonal antibodies. ChTh using the CHOP (cyclophosphamide, vincristine, doxorubicin, and prednisone) regimen is highly effective in the treatment of patients with localized primary HG PGL [18]. Thus ChTh and rituximab immunotherapy could be used in all stages of gastric MALT lymphoma alone or combination of both [11, 32].

Surgery traditionally was the standard procedure or an indispensable component of combined treatment strategy in primary GI DLBCL. The arguments in favor of the surgery include removal of the primary tumor, availability of precise histological assessment and tumor staging, as well as avoidance of life-threatening complications (perforation, hemorrhage) that may emerge during radiotherapy and ChTh. In recent decades, opinions have increasingly shifted away toward conservative treatment even for patients with the resectable disease [152]. Gastric DLBCL is treated with aggressive poly-ChTh, which is usually combined with rituximab. Thus, gastric DLBCL should be treated with the front-line ChTh (CHOP) or chemoimmunotherapy with R-CHOP (CHOP with rituximab). Frontline chemoimmunotherapy with 3–4 cycles of standard R-CHOP followed by "involved-field" radiotherapy could be considered as a standard option for localized stages. Complete remission can be achieved in advanced gastric DLBCL patients after 6–8 cycles of R-CHOP as their nodal counterparts [4, 11, 16, 152]. In other words in the case of gastric DLBCL, either arising *de novo* or the following transformation from MALT lymphoma, conservative approaches demonstrate excellent results, as gastric DLBCL appears to be a highly chemosensitive disease [151]. A higher cost of rituximab was the prohibitive factor for cure in these patients [18]. Therefore, radical intent surgery might be proposed for the patients unfit for rituximab treatment [152] as rituximab use has raised concerns about a higher incidence of neutropenic infections [100].

If the patient has the progressive disease (according to PET CT), the consideration for second-line treatment (salvage ChTh) for DLBCL with a regimen, such as rituximab, ifosfamide, carboplatin, and etoposide or Gemcitabine, dexamethasone, cisplatin and rituximab, followed by autologous stem cell transplantation (SCT) should be considered [11].

Various recent studies have demonstrated a significant rate (50%) of complete regression (analogous to MALT lymphomas) in localized gastric DLBCL following anti-*H. pylori* therapy. These results exhibit that eradication, keeping chemoradiotherapy for unresponsive patients, is a fair strategy for patients with limited-stage gastric DLBCL [153]. This suggests that a subset of gastric DLBCL might still contain an antigenic drive, though antibiotics could be paired with ChTh at the clinician's discretion (**Figure 2**). Nevertheless, these results need to be valid in larger prospective studies before broad usage [11].

Lymphomas originating from the duodenal bulbs might have similar characteristics with gastric MALT lymphomas. Unfortunately, the lesions observed over the descending portion might be less associated with *H. pylori* infection, indicating that *H. pylori* eradication therapy cannot be expected to be effective [23]. Nevertheless, various reports are showing that the eradication of *H. pylori* is effective for duodenal and even rectal MALT lymphomas [37, 154].

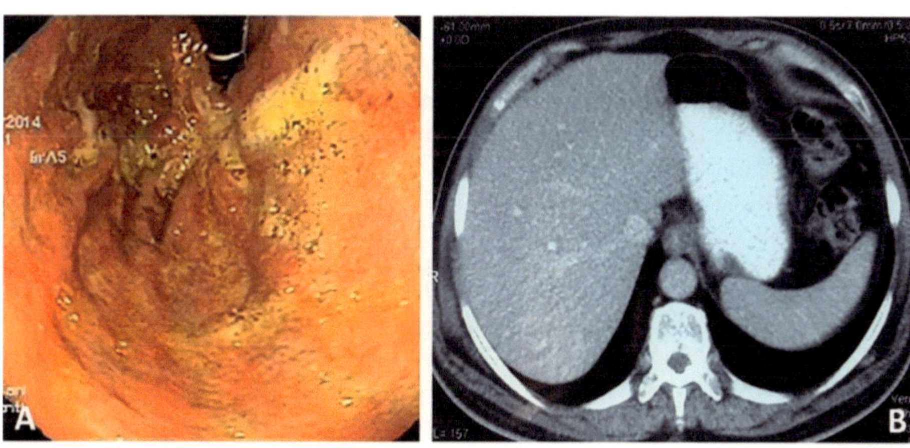

Figure 2.
*Endoscopic (A) and CT (B) views of the patient with a history of gastric DLBCL (described in **Figure 1**) following H. Pylori eradication therapy and 6 cycles of ChTh with CHOP regimen. According to gastroscopy and CT scan, a complete response was achieved after treatment. The patient lived 6 years without the signs of recurrence confirmed by regular endoscopy and CT scan performed annually and died of unrelated disease.*

The treatment outcome of PIL is relatively poorer than that of PGL depending on their histological subtypes. Lymphoma primarily located in the small bowel usually warrants laparotomy with the affected segment removed both for its diagnosis and its treatment. LG BCL of the small intestine (stage IE) only requires surgical resection. A multi-agent chemotherapeutic strategy is warranted for advanced stage PIL with multifocal cases of lymphoma. Systemic treatment with anthracycline-based ChTh followed by radiotherapy is proposed for advanced PIL which cannot be removed [4]. No guidelines exist for the treatment of small intestinal DLBCL. Historically, in HIV patients ChTh combined with antiretroviral therapy remains the first step in the management of aggressive lymphomas [100].

IPSID in the early stage responds to antibiotics such as tetracycline or combined metronidazole and ampicillin, with remission occurring within 6–12 months. Patients without substantial regression following a 6-month course of antibiotic therapy or complete remission within 12 months should be administered ChTh with CHOP. ChTh is also recommended up-front combined with antibiotics for patients with intermediate or advanced stage of the disease at initial diagnosis. Surgery plays a limited role in the majority of cases due to diffuse involvement, although it may be required for accurate diagnosis [4, 24]. Most untreated IPSID patients progress to lymphoplasmacytic and immunoblastic lymphoma invading the intestinal wall and mesenteric LNs, and may metastasize to a distant organ [24].

No optimized therapeutic guideline is available for BL which usually requires an aggressive approach. High-intensity chemotherapeutic agents for a short duration, such as cyclophosphamide, vincristine, doxorubicin, methotrexate and cytarabine, can significantly improve the treatment outcome [4]. The risks of emerging tumor lysis syndrome (TLS) and CNS dissemination of the disease are also important issues that should be taken into consideration at the first presentation of patients with BL. To reduce the risk of TLS, many regimens use relatively low doses of ChTh drugs (especially cyclophosphamide) and administration of prednisone. High-dose intravenous (as well as intrathecal) methotrexate and cytarabine, both of which have CNS penetration, are commonly administered to reduce CNS dissemination of the disease [155].

CODOX-M/IVAC, Magrath regimen (CODOX-M, cyclophosphamide, vincristine, doxorubicin, methotrexate; /IVAC, ifosfamide, cytarabine, and etoposide) is commonly used for the treatment of BL. Hyper-CVAD (hyperfractionated cyclophosphamide, vincristine, doxorubicin, and dexamethasone) alternating with methotrexate and cytarabine is another effective strategy in BL. Most adults with BL can favor the Magrath or modified Magrath regimens (depending on risk group) with the addition of rituximab. The benefit of administering rituximab in front-line BL therapy has been demonstrated in both adults and children, and it is a standard treatment in both cases. Dose-adjusted EPOCH-R (etoposide, prednisone, vincristine, cyclophosphamide, doxorubicin, and rituximab) is an intermediate-intensity strategy, which was tested in BL because of its high efficacy in DLBCL and its hypothetical ability to overcome high tumor proliferation. Studies testing this strategy in patients with sporadic and immunodeficiency-associated BL demonstrated a progression-free rate > 90%, with low toxicity and low rates of TLS. A randomized trial comparing DA-EPOCH-R (dose-adjusted EPOCH-R) with R-CODOX-M/RIVAC (CODOX-M/IVAC with rituximab) is currently being conducted in several European countries for its comparative effect [155]. Rituximab exhibits sufficient promising results to recommend its adjunction to ChTh and it may even erase the prognostic difference between young and elderly patients. However, its administration is avoided during the debulking phase given the high risk of TLS [29].

Involved-field radiotherapy should not be considered in BL, except for patients with CNS involvement. In case of initial CNS invasion, the number of intrathecal

ChTh administrations is increased. SCT should not be recommended for patients with complete responses. This approach must be employed for cases of partial response or patients with chemosensitive recurrence. Due to the high proliferative ability of BL, graft-versus-tumor effects that appeared following allogeneic SCT are too sluggish to be manifested. Therefore, this type of transplant should not be employed [29]. It should be noted that because modern ChTh may be curative for the majority of BL patients and up to 90% of adolescents and young adults, the interest in hematopoietic cell transplantation has now considerably diminished [156].

MCL is an aggressive and incurable type of B-cell NHL [110, 113]. Conventional therapeutic regimens are not effective in MCL cases and are associated with poor survival [4, 110]. Current combinations of multi-drug ChTh and monoclonal antibodies have conferred significant improvement in response rates of MCL. Overall response rates comprise 80–95% and complete response rates of 30–50% are not being achieved. Other ChTh regimens such as R-Hyper-CVAD (Rituximab with hyperfractionated cyclophosphamide, vincristine, doxorubicin, and dexamethasone alternating with high-dose methotrexate and cytarabine) have demonstrated good results. However, it is a more aggressive regimen associated with increased toxicity. The R-CHOP regimen can be used in patients with poor performance status as a less toxic regimen [110]. Those who are eligible for grafting are previously induced with R-CHOP. ChTh regimen, consisting of rituximab alone or purine nucleoside analogs with rituximab, can be applied to those ineligibles for SCT [4, 157].

Compared with nodal FL, GI FL usually presents with localized disease [115] and shows indolent clinical course [4, 20, 117, 158, 159], with excellent long-term survival, even when the disease recurs in the intestine until they are symptomatic or show evidence of its progression [4, 117, 158, 159]. A small subset of patients (<10%) progress to nodal disease [158, 159]. Surgical resection might be curative for patients with GI FL who, after thorough evaluation, are considered to have disease confined to one segment of the bowel. However, given the multifocal nature of GI FL, the role of surgery is generally limited to establishing a diagnosis and treating actual or imminent complications [139]. Therefore, there is no consensus in the management strategy and some clinical problems are yet to be solved [115]. A variety of therapies have been used, but treatment is not likely to be necessary for most patients and a "watch-and-wait" approach is reasonable [4, 115] because unlike nodal FL, GI FL is known to be indolent [115]. Symptomatic cases, or advanced disease of FL necessitates surgery and ChTh (CHOP). Although rituximab is beneficial for FL, its true value has not been well ascertained [4].

No guidelines are available for the management of EATL although anthracyclin-based ChTh is a mainstay treatment modality. ChTh as the first-line therapy is more effective in GI BCL when compared with the T-cell subtype. In cases of serious comorbidities and complications attributed to ChTh, such as perforation, and profuse bleeding multimodal approaches including debulking or radical intent surgery should be performed to remove the gross EATL before ChTh, if the patients can tolerate it. It was reported that two-thirds of the patients with EATL undergone surgical resection followed by combination ChTh and autologous SCT can obtain a sustained complete response [4].

Most patients with EBV-positive MCU have a favorable clinical course, with nearly all reported cases showing resolution following a reduction of immunosuppressive therapy [41, 42]. Other interventions, such as local radiation or ChTh, may be necessary for those patients in whom the immunosuppression cannot be reversed, such as in the elderly [19].

GI ITLPD usually presents as an indolent neoplasm with no progression to aggressive TCLs. These cases are often misdiagnosed as TCL with little or no response to

ChTh. Radiotherapy may be a more effective option compared with ChTh. But there are not enough clinical observations to confirm it [160].

Since the introduction of highly active antiretroviral therapy (HAART) in the treatment of AIDS patients, a decrease in the incidence of GI lymphoma among AIDS patients and improved survival rates for relevant lymphoma patients have been achieved. Therefore, therapeutic strategies including ChTh, immunotherapy and HAART can be able to demonstrate promising results in response and survival rates [43].

9. Prognosis

The clinical course and prognosis of PGİL are dependent on histopathological subtype and stage at the time of initial diagnosis [11]. The best overall survival (OS) and progression-free survival (PFS) were observed in MALT lymphoma and FL, followed by DLBCL, and the poorest in EATL and other lymphomas of T-cell lineage [8]. Overall survival rates remain poor also in MCL [110].

Gastric MALT lymphoma is commonly an indolent, multifocal disease and because of that, it has a high rate of relapse after surgery. In 10% of cases, it can have synchronous involvement of intestinal and extraintestinal sites [91]. In the early stages, the disease may completely resolve following antibiotic therapy; however, transformation to DLBCL is not uncommon [25].

There are many prognostic systems for prognostication of DLBCL of which the International Prognostic Index (IPI) is the most valuable and main clinical tool widely employed [101]. GEP is a new evolving approach to diagnose, classify and prognosticate DLBCL. According to GEP two prognostically significant types of DLBCL have been identified [12, 83, 101, 161]. The molecular subgroups include GCB and ABC, which are associated with different chromosomal aberrations. GCB group has a better prognosis than the ACB group [101]. GEP is considered the "gold standard" to identify the molecular subtypes of DLBCL, however, is not available in routine diagnostics due to its cost-ineffectiveness. Several studies have attempted to define the molecular subtypes (GCB and non-GCB) by IHC using a limited panel of available antibodies [12]. The Hans algorithm which used antibodies to CD10, BCL6, and IRF4/MUM1 has been the most widely used in clinical trials [83] with nearly 80% concordance with the GEP [161]. According to the results of most of the relevant studies, IHC algorithms can predict the prognosis in DLBCL, however, all researchers believe that these methods cannot perfectly substitute GEP. Taking into consideration of the possible prognostic significance of cell lineage and the incremental efforts to adjust the treatment strategy based on molecular characteristics, 2016 revised WHO classification recommends distinguishing the above-mentioned molecular subtypes of DLBCL. Therefore, the application of IHC algorithms is now considered an acceptable and effective tool by many experts [12].

BL, a type of non-Hodgkin BCL, is a substantially aggressive mature B cell neoplasm and the fastest growing human cancer that is seen mainly in children and young adults [15, 109]. Despite very aggressive biology most of the cases of BL can be cured by modern ChTh [156]. BL comprises up to 20% of HIV-associated lymphomas and is usually associated with higher median CD4 counts when compared with many other lymphoma types. In a recently presented multicenter study, there were no differences in survival between HIV-negative and HIV-positive counterparts [155].

Primary GI MCL is highly aggressive and survival is poor compared to nodal MCL involving the GIT. Patients respond poorly to CHOP chemotherapy [157].

Despite the improved response rate of ChTh for MCL, current overall survival rates remain poor because of the advanced stage in most of the cases and the early relapse. Median survival with standard treatment for MCL patients remains between 1.5 and 4 years [110, 113]. For risk prediction, the MCL International Prognostic Index (MIPI) that include also pretreatment Ki-67 proliferation rate, an important determinant of risk, is employed [157]. MIPI might be helpful to allow individualized, risk-adapted treatment decisions in patients with MCL.

GI FL has poorer outcomes than previously suggested [138]. Anatomical location within the GIT may have prognostic implications, with primary duodenal and small intestinal disease having a significantly higher progression-free survival rate than non-duodenal presentations [138, 139]. For risk stratification of FL patients, FLIPI (FL International Prognostic Index) and FLIPI2 have been developed as prognostic indexes. Despite the usefulness of these risk assessment criteria in nodal cases, no studies have been conducted on intestinal FL patients [115, 137]. Most of the GI FL cases are assessed as low risk or intermediate risk, but it is not confirmed by larger studies if these criteria are suitable for GI cases [115].

MLP may be one of the GI lymphomas with a poor prognosis, even though several regimens of systemic ChTh have been adapted for its treatment [23].

EATL and MEITL is clinically aggressive disease, with frequent early dissemination and a median survival of several months [28, 162].

EBV-positive MCU has an indolent clinical course and may spontaneously regress in some cases [41, 42].

ITLPD is a nonaggressive disease and its clinical course is chronic and relapsing, with rarely reported disseminated disease, including bone marrow and peripheral blood involvement, usually after many years [121, 122].

10. Summary and conclusions

GIT is the most common extranodal site involved in lymphoma. Histopathologically, almost 90% of PGILs are of B-cell lineage. PGILs represent a heterogeneous group of malignant neoplasms which are different entities in terms of cancerogenesis, cell lineage, pathological characteristics, immunoprofile, biological behavior, response to modern treatment approaches and prognosis. In most cases, pathogenesis of primary PGIL is associated with infectious agents such as *H. pylori*, *C. jejuni*, EBV, HIV, HBV and HTLV-1. Immunodepressive (congenital and acquired) and autoimmune conditions are the second most significant disorders associated with PGIL. Regardless of the etiologic factors in the pathogenesis of PGIL play a great role in chromosomal translocation that lead to overexpression or down-expression of some genes that promote uncontrolled lymphoid cell proliferation. Some specific gene rearrangements take place in the pathogenesis of different subtypes of PGIL. After the introduction of GEP some lymphoma subtypes, such as DLBCL and BL were further subdivided into distinct entities, hence some new provisional entities were added in the 2008 WHO classification and revised 2016 WHO classifications. Pathologically and immunohistochemically distinct subtypes of PGIL represent different entities that have characteristic hallmarks and molecular signatures. The distinction is also observed in the predominance of involved sites for different subtypes of lymphoma. The clinical course can range from indolence to very aggressive behavior depending on the lymphoma subtypes and concomitant gene rearrangements. In most cases, diagnosis of PGIL can be made endoscopically, however, few cases of intestinal lymphoma are being detected during surgery performed for its complications. Treatment of PGIL is largely ChTh based and anthracycline-containing ChTh and rituximab is the mainstay treatment modality. Despite this, some PGIL subtypes (especially MCL) remain to be resistant to modern therapeutic approaches and associated with poor survival rates.

Conflict of interest

The authors declare no conflict of interest.

Author details

Ramiz Bayramov* and Ramila Abdullayeva
Department of Oncology, Azerbaijan Medical University, Baku, Azerbaijan

*Address all correspondence to: ramizbayramov@gmail.com

References

[1] Groves F, Linet M, Travis L, Devesa S. Cancer surveillance series: Non-Hodgkin's lymphoma incidence by histologic subtype in the united states from 1978 through 1995. Journal of the National Cancer Institute. 2000;**92**(15):1240-1251. DOI: 10.1093/jnci/92.15.1240

[2] Chiu B, Weisenburger D. An update of the epidemiology of non-Hodgkin's lymphoma. Clinical Lymphoma. 2003;**4**(3):161-168. DOI: 10.3816/clm.2003.n.025

[3] Devesa S, Fears T. Non-Hodgkin's lymphoma time trends: United States and international data. Cancer Research. 1992;**52**(Suppl. 19):5432s-5440s

[4] Ghimire P, Wu G-Y, Zhu L. Primary gastrointestinal lymphoma. World Journal of Gastroenterology. 2011;**17**(6): 697-707. DOI: 10.3748/wjg.v17.i6.697

[5] Püspök A, Raderer M, Chott A, et al. Endoscopic ultrasound in the follow up and response assessment of patients with primary gastric lymphoma. Gut. 2002;**51**:691-694. DOI: 10.1136/gut.51.5.691

[6] Nakamura S, Matsumoto T. Gastrointestinal lymphoma: Recent advances in diagnosis and treatment. Digestion. 2013;**87**:182-188. DOI: 10.1159/000350051

[7] Dawson IM, Cornes JS, Morson BC. Primary malignant lymphoid tumours of the intestinal tract. Report of 37 cases with a study of factors influencing prognosis. The British Journal of Surgery. 1961;**49**:80-89. DOI: 10.1002/bjs.18004921319

[8] Chen Y, Chen Y, Chen S, et al. Primary gastrointestinal lymphoma: Aretrospective multicenter clinical study of 415 cases in Chinese province of Guangdong and a systematic review containing 5075 Chinese patients. Medicine (Baltimore). 2015; **94**(47):e2119. DOI: 10.1097/MD.0000000000002119

[9] Herrmann R, Panahon AM, Barcos MP, et al. Gastrointestinal involvement in non-Hodgkin's lymphoma. Cancer. 1980;**46**(1): 215-222. DOI: 10.1002/1097-0142(19800701)46:1<215::aid-cncr2820460136>3.0.co;2-6

[10] Rizvi MA, Evens AM, Tallman MS, et al. T-cell non-Hodgkin lymphoma. Blood. 2006;**107**:1255-1264. DOI: 10.1182/blood-2005-03-1306

[11] Juárez-Salcedo LM, Sokol L, Chavez JC, Dalia S. Primary gastric lymphoma, epidemiology, clinical diagnosis, and treatment. Cancer Control. 2018;**25**(1):1-12. DOI: 10.1177/1073274818778256

[12] Quintanilla-Martinez L. The 2016 updated WHO classification of lymphoid neoplasias. Hematol Oncology. 2017;**35**(S1):37-45. DOI: 10.1002/hon.2399

[13] Papaxoinis G, Papageorgiou S, Rontogianni D, et al. Primary gastrointestinal non-Hodgkin's lymphoma: A clinicopathologic study of 128 cases in Greece. A Hellenic Cooperative Oncology Group study (HeCOG). Leukemia & Lymphoma. 2006;**47**(10):2140-2146. DOI: 10.1080/10428190600709226

[14] Dionigi G, Annoni M, Rovera F, et al. Primary colorectal lymphomas: Review of the literature. Surgical Oncology. 2007;**16**(Suppl. 1):S169-S171. DOI: 10.1016/j.suronc.2007.10.021

[15] Bautista-Quach MA, Ake CD, Chen M, Wang J. Gastrointestinal lymphomas: Morphology, immunophenotype and molecular features. Journal of Gastrointestinal

Oncology. 2012;**3**(3):209-225. DOI: 10.3978/j.issn.2078-6891.2012.024

[16] Ferrucci PF, Zucca E. Primary gastric lymphoma pathogenesis and treatment: What has changed over the past 10 years? British Journal of Haematology. 2007;**136**:521-538. DOI: 10.1111/j.1365-2141.2006.06444.x

[17] Morton LM, Wang SS, Devesa SS, et al. Lymphoma incidence patterns by WHO subtype in the United States, 1992-2001. Blood. 2006;**107**(1):265-276. DOI: 10.1182/blood-2005-06-2508

[18] Suresh B, Asati V, Lakshmaiah KC, et al. Primary gastrointestinal diffuse large B-cell lymphoma: A prospective study from South India. South Asian Journal of Cancer. 2019;**8**(1):57-59. DOI: 10.4103/sajc.sajc_52_18

[19] Weindorf SC, Smith LB, Owens SR. Update on gastrointestinal lymphomas. Archives of Pathology & Laboratory Medicine. 2018;**142**:1347-1351. DOI: 10.5858/arpa.2018-0275-RA

[20] Damaj G, Verkarre V, Delmer A, et al. Primary follicular lymphoma of the gastrointestinal tract: A study of 25 cases and a literature review. Annals of Oncology. 2003;**14**(4):623-629. DOI: 10.1093/annonc/mdg168

[21] Kitamura K, Yamaguchi T, Okamoto K, et al. Early gastric lymphoma: A clinicopathologic study of ten patients, literature review, and comparison with early gastric adenocarcinoma. Cancer. 1996;**77**(5): 850-857. DOI: 10.1002/(sici)1097-0142 (19960301)77:5<850::aid-cncr7>3.0.co;2-i

[22] Kim YH, Lee JH, Yang SK, et al. Primary colon lymphoma in Korea: A KASID (Korean Association for the Study of Intestinal Diseases) study. Digestive Diseases and Sciences. 2005;**50**:2243-2247. DOI: 10.1007/s10620-005-3041-7

[23] Hirata N, Tominaga K, Ohta K, et al. A case of mucosa-associated lymphoid tissue lymphoma forming multiple lymphomatous polyposis in the small intestine. World Journal of Gastroenterology. 2007;**13**:1453-1457. DOI: 10.3748/wjg.v13.i9.1453

[24] Al-Saleem T, Al-Mondhiry H. Immunoproliferative small intestinal disease (IPSID): A model for mature B-cell neoplasms. Blood. 2005;**105**(6): 2274-2280. DOI: 10.1182/blood-2004-07-2755

[25] Lecuit M, Abachin E, Martin A, et al. Immunoproliferative Small Intestinal Disease Associated with Campylobacter jejuni. The New England Journal of Medicine. 2004;**350**(3):239-248. DOI: 10.1056/nejmoa031887

[26] Biko DM, Anupindi SA, Hernandez A, et al. Childhood Burkitt lymphoma: Abdominal and pelvic imaging findings. American Journal of Roentgenology. 2009;**192**(5):1304-1315. DOI: 10.2214/AJR.08.1476

[27] Ge Z, Liu Z, Hu X. Anatomic distribution, clinical features, and survival data of 87 cases primary gastrointestinal lymphoma. World Journal of Surgical Oncology. 2016;**14**(1):1-7. DOI: 10.1186/s12957-016-0821-9

[28] Tse E, Gill H, Loong F, et al. Type II enteropathy-associated T-cell lymphoma: A multicenter analysis from the Asia Lymphoma Study Group. American Journal of Hematology. 2012;**87**(7): 663-668. DOI: 10.1002/ajh.23213

[29] Bonnet C, Janssens A, Wu KL, et al. BHS Guidelines for the treatment of Burkitt's lymphoma. Belgian Journal of Hematology. 2015;**6**(2):61-69

[30] Engels EA. Infectious agents as causes of non-Hodgkin lymphoma. Cancer Epidemiology, Biomarkers & Prevention. 2007;**16**(3):401-404. DOI: 10.1158/1055-9965.epi-06-1056

[31] Wang F, Meng W, Wang B, Qiao L. Helicobacter pylori-induced gastric

inflammation and gastric cancer. Cancer Letters. 2014;**345**(2):196-202. DOI: 10.1016/j.canlet.2013.08.016

[32] Filip PV, Cuciureanu D, Diaconu LS, et al. MALT lymphoma: Epidemiology, clinical diagnosis and treatment. Journal of Medicine and Life. 2018;**11**(3):187-193. DOI: 10.25122/jml-2018-0035

[33] Zullo A, Cerro P, Chios A, et al. A very unusual cause of dysphagia: Mantle cell lymphoma. Annals of Gastroenterology. 2016;**29**(3):383-385

[34] Mulalic E, Delibegovic S. An Aggressive Form of MALT Lymphoma of the Stomach with Pancreas Infiltration. Medical Archives. 2016;**70**(3):235-237. DOI: 10.5455/medarh.2016.70.235-237

[35] Hussell T, Isaacson PG, Crabtree JE, Spencer J. Helicobacter pylori-specific tumour-infiltrating T cells provide contact dependent help for the growth of malignant B cells in low-grade gastric lymphoma of mucosa-associated lymphoid tissue. The Journal of Pathology. 1996;**178**:122-127. DOI: 10.1002/(SICI)1096-9896(199602)178:2<122::AID-PATH486>3.0.CO;2-D

[36] Tsai HF, Hsu PN. Interplay between Helicobacter pylori and immune cells in immune pathogenesis of gastric inflammation and mucosal pathology. Cellular & Molecular Immunology. 2010;7(4):255-259. DOI: 10.1038/cmi.2010.2

[37] Niino D, Yamamoto K, Tsuruta O, et al. Regression of rectal mucosa-associated lymphoid tissue (MALT) lymphoma after antibiotic treatments. Pathology International. 2010;**60**:438-442. DOI: 10.1111/j.1440-1827.2010.02538.x

[38] Wang F, Xu RH, Han B, et al. High incidence of hepatitis B virus infection in B-cell subtype non-Hodgkin lymphoma compared with other cancers. Cancer. 2007;**109**:1360-1364. DOI: 10.1002/cncr.22549

[39] Hui PK, Tokunaga M, Chan WY, et al. Epstein-Barr virus-associated gastric lymphoma in Hong Kong Chinese. Human Pathology. 1994;**25**(9):947-952. DOI: 10.1016/0046-8177(94)90017-5

[40] Stefan DC, Lutchman R. Burkitt lymphoma: Epidemiological features and survival in a South African centre. Infectious Agents and Cancer. 2014;**9**:19. DOI: 10.1186/1750-9378-9-19

[41] Bunn B, van Heerden W. EBV-positive mucocutaneous ulcer of the oral cavity associated with HIV/AIDS. Oral Surgery, Oral Medicine, Oral Pathology, Oral Radiology. 2015;**120**(6):725-732. DOI: 10.1016/j.oooo.2015.06.02

[42] Dojcinov SD, Venkataraman G, Raffel M, et al. EBV-positive mucocutaneous ulcer—A study of 26 cases associated with various sources of immunosuppression. The American Journal of Surgical Pathology. 2010;**34**(3):405-417. DOI: 10.1097/pas.0b013e3181cf8622

[43] Heise W. GI-lymphomas in immunosuppressed patients (organ transplantation; HIV). Best Practice & Research. Clinical Gastroenterology. 2010;**24**(1):57-69. DOI: 10.1016/j.bpg.2010.01.001

[44] Powitz F, Bogner JR, Sandor P, et al. Gastrointestinal lymphomas in patients with AIDS. Zeitschrift für Gastroenterologie. 1997;**35**(3):179-185

[45] Andhavarapu S, Tolentino AM, Jha C, et al. Diffuse large B-cell lymphoma presenting as multiple lymphomatous polyposis of the gastrointestinal tract. Clinical Lymphoma & Myeloma. 2008;**8**:179-183. DOI: 10.3816/CLM.2008.n.023

[46] Dal Maso L, Franceschi S. Epidemiology of non-Hodgkin lymphomas and other haemolymphopoietic neoplasms in

people with AIDS. The Lancet Oncology. 2003;**4**(2):110-119. DOI: 10.1016/s1470-2045(03)00983-5

[47] Coté TR, Biggar RJ, Rosenberg PS, et al. Non-Hodgkin's lymphoma among people with AIDS: Incidence, presentation and public health burden. AIDS/Cancer Study Group. International Journal of Cancer. 1997;**73**(5):645-650. DOI: 10.1002/(sici)1097-0215(19971127)73:5<645::aid-ijc6>3.0.co;2-x

[48] Omar FE. Childhood lymphomas—A brief overview. CME. 2010;**27**(7):332-336

[49] Biggar RJ, Engels EA, Frisch M, et al. Risk of T-cell lymphomas in persons with AIDS. Journal of Acquired Immune Deficiency Syndromes. 2001;**26**(4):371-376. DOI: 10.1097/00042560-200104010-00015

[50] Deng L, Song Y, Young KH, et al. Hepatitis B virus-associated diffuse large B-cell lymphoma: Unique clinical features, poor outcome, and hepatitis B surface antigen-driven origin. Oncotarget. 2015;**6**(28):25061-25073. DOI: 10.18632/oncotarget.4677

[51] Sugita S, Iijima T, Furuya S, et al. Gastric T-cell lymphoma with cytotoxic phenotype. Pathology International. 2007;**57**:108-114. DOI: 10.1111/j.1440-1827.2006.02065.x

[52] Weeratunge CN, Bolivar HH, Anstead GM, Lu DH. Primary esophageal lymphoma: A diagnostic challenge in acquired immunodeficiency syndrome--two case reports and review. Southern Medical Journal. 2004;**97**:383-387. DOI: 10.1097/01.SMJ.0000100120.49153.3F

[53] Zintzaras E, Voulgarelis M, Moutsopoulos HM. The risk of lymphoma development in autoimmune diseases: A meta-analysis. Archives of Internal Medicine. 2005;**165**(20):2337-2344. DOI: 10.1001/archinte.165.20.2337

[54] Royer B, Cazals-Hatem D, Sibilia J, et al. Lymphomas in patients with Sjögren'ssyndrome are marginal zone B-cell neoplasms, arise in diverse extranodal and nodal sites, and are not associated with viruses. Blood. 1997;**90**(2):766-775. DOI: 10.1182/blood.V90.2.766

[55] Garrido A, Luque A, Vázquez A, et al. Primary small bowel neoplasms as a complication of celiac disease. Gastroenterología y Hepatología. 2009;**32**:618-621. DOI: 10.1016/j.gastrohep.2009.05.003

[56] Ko YH, Karnan S, Kim KM, et al. Enteropathy-associated T-cell lymphoma--a clinicopathologic and array comparative genomic hybridization study. Human Pathology. 2010;**41**(9):1231-1237. DOI: 10.1016/j.humpath.2009.11.020

[57] Craig VJ, Arnold I, Gerke C, et al. Gastric MALT lymphoma B cells express polyreactive, somatically mutated immunoglobulins. Blood. 2010;**115**(3):581-591. DOI: 10.1182/blood-2009-06-228015

[58] Greiner A, Knörr C, Qin Y, et al. Low-grade B cell lymphomas of mucosa-associated lymphoid tissue (MALT-type) require CD40-mediated signaling and Th2-type cytokines for in vitro growth and differentiation. The American Journal of Pathology. 1997;**150**(5):1583-1593

[59] Kuo SH, Yeh KH, et al. Helicobacter pylori-related diffuse large B-cell lymphoma of the stomach: A distinct entity with lower aggressiveness and higher chemosensitivity. Blood Cancer Journal. 2014;**4**(6):e220. DOI: 10.1038/bcj.2014.40

[60] Ruland J, Duncan GS, Elia A, et al. Bcl10 is a positive regulator of antigen receptor-induced activation of

NF-kappaB and neural tube closure. Cell. 2001;**104**(1):33-42. DOI: 10.1016/s0092-8674(01)00189-1

[61] Ruskoné-Fourmestraux A, Fischbach W, Aleman BMP, et al. EGILS consensus report. Gastric extranodal marginal zone B-cell lymphoma of MALT. Gut. 2011;**60**(6):747-758. DOI: 10.1136/gut.2010.224949

[62] Zullo A, Hassan C, et al. Gastric MALT lymphoma: Old and new insights. Annals of Gastroenterology. 2014;**27**(1): 27-33

[63] Sagaert X, De Wolf-Peeters C, Noels H, Baens M. The pathogenesis of MALT lymphomas: Where do we stand? Leukemia. 2007;**21**(3):389-396. DOI: 10.1038/sj.leu.2404517

[64] Zhang Q, Siebert R, Yan M, et al. Inactivating mutations and overexpression of BCL10, a caspase recruitment domain containing gene, in MALT lymphoma with t(1,14)(p22;q32). Nature Genetics. 1999;**22**(1):63-68. DOI: 10.1038/8767

[65] Willis TG, Jadayel DM, Du MQ, et al. Bcl10 is involved in t(1, 14) (p22;q32) of MALT B cell lymphoma and mutated in multiple tumor types. Cell. 1999;**96**(1):35-45. DOI: 10.1016/s0092-8674(00)80957-5

[66] Yeh KH, Kuo SH, Chen LT, et al. Nuclear expression of BCL10 or nuclear factor kappa B helps predict Helicobacter pylori-independent status of low-grade gastric mucosa-associated lymphoid tissue lymphomas with or without t(11,18) (q21;q21). Blood. 2005;**106**(3):1037-1041. DOI: 10.1182/blood-2005-01-0004

[67] Wlodarska I, Veyt E, De Paepe P, et al. FOXP1, a gene highly expressed in a subset of diffuse large B-cell lymphoma, is recurrently targeted by genomic aberrations. Leukemia. 2005;**19**(8):1299-1305. DOI: 10.1038/sj.leu.2403813

[68] Sagaert X, de Paepe P, Libbrecht L, et al. Forkhead box protein P1 expression in mucosa-associated lymphoid tissue lymphomas predicts poor prognosis and transformation to diffuse large B-cell lymphoma. Journal of Clinical Oncology. 2006;**24**(16):2490-2497. DOI: 10.1200/jco.2006.05.6150

[69] Nakamura S, Matsumoto T, Nakamura S, et al. Chromosomal translocation t(11,18)(q21;q21) in gastrointestinal mucosa associated lymphoid tissue lymphoma. Journal of Clinical Pathology. 2003;**56**:36-42. DOI: 10.1136/jcp.56.1.36

[70] Dierlamm J, Baens M, Wlodarska I, et al. The apoptosis inhibitor gene API2 and a novel 18q gene, MLT, are recurrently rearranged in the t(11,18) (q21;q21) associated with mucosa-associated lymphoid tissue lymphomas. Blood. 1999;**93**(11):3601-3609. DOI: 10.1182/blood.v93.11.3601

[71] Yonezumi M, Suzuki R, Suzuki H, et al. Detection of AP12-MALT1 chimaeric gene in extranodal and nodal marginal zone B-cell lymphoma by reverse transcription polymerase chain reaction (PCR) and genomic long and accurate PCR analyses. British Journal of Haematology. 2001;**115**(3):588-594. DOI: 10.1046/j.1365-2141.2001.03158.x

[72] Streubel B, Seitz G, et al. MALT lymphoma associated genetic aberrations occur at different frequencies in primary and secondary intestinal MALT lymphomas. Gut. 2006;**55**(11):1581-1585. DOI: 10.1136/gut.2005.090076

[73] Nakamura T, Nakamura S, Yonezumi M, et al. Helicobacter pylori and the t(11,18)(q21;q21) translocation in gastric low-grade B-cell lymphoma of mucosa-associated lymphoid tissue type. Japanese Journal of Cancer Research.

2000;**91**:301-309. DOI: 10.1111/j. 1349-7006.2000.tb00945.x

[74] Liu H, Ye H, Ruskone-Fourmestraux A, et al. t(11,18) is a marker for all stage gastric MALT lymphomas that will not respond to H. pylori eradication. Gastroenterology. 2002;**122**:1286-1294. DOI: 10.1053/gast.2002.33047

[75] Ye H, Liu H, Raderer M, et al. High incidence of t(11,18)(q21;q21) in Helicobacter pylori-negative gastric MALT lymphomas. Blood. 2003;**101**(7): 2547-2550. DOI: 10.1182/blood-2002-10-3167

[76] Wang G, Auerbach A, Wei M, et al. t(11,18)(q21;q21) in extranodal marginal zone B-cell lymphoma of mucosa-associated lymphoid tissue in stomach: A study of 48 cases. Modern Pathology. 2009;**22**:79-86. DOI: 10.1038/modpathol.2008.155

[77] Saito M, Gao J, Basso K, et al. Signaling Pathway mediating downregulation of BCL6 in germinal center B cells is blocked by BCL6 gene alterations in B cell lymphoma. Cancer Cell. 2007;**12**(3):280-292. DOI: 10.1016/j.ccr.2007.08.011

[78] Lossos I, Akasaka T, Martinez-Climent J, et al. The BCL6 gene in B-cell lymphomas with 3q27 translocations is expressed mainly from the rearranged allele irrespective of the partner gene. Leukemia. 2003;**17**:1390-1397. DOI: 10.1038/sj.leu.2402997

[79] Offit K, Lococo F, Louie DC, et al. Rearrangement of the bcl-6 gene as prognostic marker in diffuse large cell lymphoma. The New England Journal of Medicine. 1994;**331**(2):74-80. DOI: 10.1056/nejm199407143310202

[80] Yang H, Green MR. Epigenetic Programing of B-Cell Lymphoma by BCL6 and Its Genetic Deregulation. Frontiers in Cell and Development Biology. 2019;**7**:272. DOI: 10.3389/fcell.2019.00272

[81] Davis RE, Ngo VN, Lenz G, et al. Chronic active B-cell-receptor signalling in diffuse large B-cell lymphoma. Nature. 2010;**463**:88-92. DOI: 10.1038/nature08638

[82] Foster LH, Portell CA. The role of infectious agents, antibiotics, and antiviral therapy in the treatment of extranodal marginal zone lymphoma and other low-grade lymphomas. Current Treatment Options in Oncology. 2015;**16**(6):28. DOI: 10.1007/s11864-015-0344-6

[83] Swerdlow SH, Campo E, Pileri SA, et al. The 2016 revision of the World Health Organization classification of lymphoid neoplasms. Blood. 2016; **127**(20):2375-2390. DOI: 10.1182/blood-2016- 01-643569

[84] Zullo A, Hassan C, et al. Effects of Helicobacter pylori eradication on early stage gastric mucosa-associated lymphoid tissue lymphoma. Clinical Gastroenterology and Hepatology. 2010;**8**(2):105-110. DOI: 10.1016/j.cgh.2009.07.017

[85] Rosenstiel P, Hellmig S, Hampe J, et al. Influence of polymorphisms in the NOD1/CARD4 and NOD2/CARD15 genes on the clinical outcome of Helicobacter pylori infection. Cellular Microbiology. 2006;**8**(7):1188-1198. DOI: 10.1111/j.1462-5822.2006.00701.x

[86] Ronchi A, Montella M, Panarese I, et al. Malt gastric lymphoma:an pathogenetic features. WCRJ. 2016;**3**(2):e715

[87] Hellmig S, Bartscht T, Fischbach W, et al. Germline variations of the MALT1 gene as risk factors in the development of primary gastric B-cell lymphoma. European Journal of Cancer. 2009;**45**(10): 1865-1870. DOI: 10.1016/j.ejca.2009.03.010

[88] Tomita S, Kojima M, Imura J, et al. Extranodal diffuse follicular center

lymphoma mimicking mantle cell lymphoma of the intestine. American Journal of Hematology. 2003;**74**(4): 287-289. DOI: 10.1002/ajh.10437

[89] Isomoto H, Maeda T, Akashi T, et al. Multiple lymphomatous polyposis of the colon originating from T-cells: A case report. Digestive and Liver Disease. 2004;**36**(3):218-221. DOI: 10.1016/j.dld.2003.09.019

[90] Swerdlow SH, Campo E, Harris NL, et al. 2017 Revised WHO Classification of Tumors of Haematopoietic and Lymphoid Tissues. Lyon, France: IARC Press; 2017

[91] Coppens E, El Nakadi I, Nagy N, Zalcman M. Primary Hodgkin's lymphoma of the esophagus. American Journal of Roentgenology. 2003;**180**: 1335-1337. DOI: 10.2214/ajr.180.5.1801335

[92] Zhu Q, Xu B, Xu K, et al. Primary non-Hodgkin's lymphoma in the esophagus. Journal of Digestive Diseases. 2008;**9**:241-244. DOI: 10.1111/j.1751-2980.2008.00354.x

[93] Kalogeropoulos IV, Chalazonitis AN, Tsolaki S, et al. A case of primary isolated non-Hodgkin's lymphoma of the esophagus in an immunocompetent patient. World Journal of Gastroenterology. 2009;**15**:1901-1903. DOI: 10.3748/wjg.15.1901

[94] Koch P. Treatment results in localized primary gastric lymphoma: Data of patients registered within the German multicenter study (GIT NHL 02/96). Journal of Clinical Oncology. 2005;**23**(28):7050-7059. DOI: 10.1200/jco.2005.04.031

[95] Ely S. Distinction between "high grade MALT" and diffuse large B cell lymphoma. Gut. 2002;**51**(6):893-894. DOI: 10.1136/gut.51.6.893

[96] Jaffe ES. The 2008 WHO classification of lymphomas: Implications for clinical practice and translational research. Hematology. American Society of Hematology. Education Program. 2009;**1**:523-531. DOI: 10.1182/asheducation-2009.1.523

[97] Li B, Shi YK, He XH, et al. Primary non-Hodgkin lymphomas in the small and large intestine: Clinicopathological characteristics and management of 40 patients. International Journal of Hematology. 2008;**87**:375-381. DOI: 10.1007/s12185-008-0068-5

[98] Said J, Pinter-Brown L. Clinical and pathological diagnosis of peripheral T-cell lymphoma and emerging treatment options: A case-based discussion. Clinical Advances in Hematology & Oncology. 2009;7(11):S1. S4-13, quiz S15

[99] Ding W, Zhao S, Wang J, et al. Gastrointestinal lymphoma in Southwest China: Subtype distribution of1,010 cases using the WHO (2008) classification in a single institution. Acta Haematologica. 2016;**135**:21-28. DOI: 10.1159/000437130

[100] Lodhi HT, Sadat I, Qulsoom H, et al. Primary small bowel diffuse large B-cell lymphoma: Excellent endoscopic appearance. The American Journal of Gastroenterology. 2018;**113**:S1422-S1423. DOI: 10.14309/00000434-201810001-02554

[101] Barbaryan A, Ali AM, Kwatra SG, et al. Primary diffuse large B-cell lymphoma of the ascending colon. Rare Tumors. 2013;**5**(2):85-88. DOI: 10.4081/rt.2013.e23

[102] Ponzoni M, Ferreri AJ, Pruneri G, et al. Prognostic value of bcl-6, CD10 and CD38 immunoreactivity in stage I-II gastric lymphomas: Identification of a subset of CD10+ large B-cell lymphomas with a favorable outcome. International Journal of Cancer. 2003;**106**:288-291. DOI: 10.1002/ijc.11179

[103] Foon KA, Lichtman MA. General Considerations of Lymphoma:

Epidemiology, Etiology, Heterogeneity, and Primary Extranodal Disease. In: Kaushansky K, Lichtman MA, Beutler E et al., editors. Williams Hematology 8th ed. McGraw-Hill; 2010. pp. 1-39

[104] Novak U, Basso K, Pasqualucci L, et al. Genomic analysis of non-splenic marginal zone lymphomas (MZL) indicates similarities between nodal and extranodal MZL and supports their derivation from memory B-cells. British Journal of Haematology. 2011;**155**(3): 362-365. DOI: 10.1111/j.1365-2141.2011.08841.x

[105] Bacon CM, Du MQ, Dogan A. Mucosa-associated lymphoid tissue (MALT) lymphoma: A practical guide for pathologists. Journal of Clinical Pathology. 2007;**60**(4):361-372. DOI: 10.1136/jcp.2005.031146

[106] Zucca E, Roggero E, Pileri S. B-cell lymphoma of MALT type: A review with special emphasis on diagnostic and management problems of low-grade gastric tumours. British Journal of Haematology. 1998;**100**(1):3-14. DOI: 10.1046/j.1365-2141.1998.00513.x

[107] Isaacson P, Muller-Hermelink H, Piris M, et al. Extranodal marginal zone B-cell lymphoma of mucosa-associated lymphoid tissue (MALT lymphoma). In: Jaffe ES, Harris NL, Stein H, Vardiman JW, editors. Pathology and Genetics of Tumours of Haematopoietic and Lymphoid Tissues. World Health Organization Classification of Tumours. Lyon, France: IARC Press; 2001. pp. 157-160

[108] Ferreri AJ, Montalbán C. Primary diffuse large B-cell lymphoma of the stomach. Critical Reviews in Oncology/Hematology. 2007;**63**(1):65-71. DOI: 10.1016/j.critrevonc.2007.01.003

[109] Čubranić A, Golčić M, Fučkar-Čupić D, et al. Burkitt lymphoma in gastrointestinal tract: A report of two cases. Acta Clinica Croatica. 2019;**58**:386-390. DOI: 10.20471/acc.2019.58.02.25

[110] Kella VKN, Constantine R, Parikh NS, et al. Mantle cell lymphoma of the gastrointestinal tract presenting with multiple intussusceptions—Case report and review of literature. World Journal of Surgical Oncology. 2009;7:60. DOI: 10.1186/1477-7819-7-60

[111] Bajpai S, Narang J, Narang S, et al. Mantle Cell Lymphoma: Incidence of gastrointestinal involvement and correlation with overall response-retrospective review of multiple multicenter trials. Blood. 2020;**136** (Suppl. 1):33-34. DOI: 10.1182/blood-2020-137657

[112] Fu K, Weisenburger DD, Greiner TC, et al. Cyclin D1-negative mantle cell lymphoma: A clinicopathologic study based on gene expression profiling. Blood. 2005; **106**(13):4315-4321. DOI: 10.1182/blood-2005-04-1753

[113] Vose JM. Mantle cell lymphoma: 2012 update on diagnosis, risk-stratification, and clinical management. American Journal of Hematology. 2012;**87**(6):604-609. DOI: 10.1002/ajh.23176

[114] Jaffe ES, Harris NL, Stein H, Vardiman JW, editors. World Health Organization Classification of Tumors: Pathology and Genetics of Tumors of Haematopoietic and Lymphoid Tissues. Lyon, France: IARC Press; 2001

[115] Takata K, Miyata-Takata T, Sato Y, et al. Gastrointestinal follicular lymphoma: Current knowledge and future challenges. Pathol Intl. 2018;**68**(1):1-6. DOI: 10.1111/pin.12621

[116] Foukas PG, de Leval L. Recent advances in intestinal lymphomas. Histopathology. 2015;**66**(1):112-136. DOI: 10.1111/his.12596

[117] Yamamoto S, Nakase H, Yamashita K, et al. Gastrointestinal follicular lymphoma: Review of the literature. Journal of Gastroenterology.

2010;**45**(4):370-388. DOI: 10.1007/s00535-009-0182-z

[118] Swerdlow SH, Jaffe ES, Brousset P, et al. Cytotoxic T-cell and NK-cell lymphomas: Current questions and controversies. The American Journal of Surgical Pathology. 2014;**38**(10):e60-e71. DOI: 10.1097/pas.0000000000000295

[119] Attygally AD, Cabeçadas J, Gaulard P, et al. Peripheral T-cell and NK-cell lymphomas and their mimics; taking a step forward—Report on the lymphoma workshop of the XVIth meeting of the European Association for Haematopathology and the Society for Hematopathology. Histopathology. 2014;**64**(2):171-199. DOI: 10.1111/his.12251

[120] Hart M, Thakral B, Yohe S, et al. EBV-positive mucocutaneous ulcer in organ transplant recipients: A localized indolent posttransplant lymphoproliferative disorder. The American Journal of Surgical Pathology. 2014;**38**(11):1522-1529. DOI: 10.1097/pas.0000000000000282

[121] Perry AM, Warnke RA, Hu Q, et al. Indolent T-cell lymphoproliferative disease of the gastrointestinal tract. Blood. 2013;**122**(22):3599-3606. DOI: 10.1182/blood-2013-07-512830

[122] Carbonnel F, d'Almagne H, Lavergne A, et al. The clinicopathological features of extensive small intestinal CD4 T cell infiltration. Gut. 1999;**45**(5):662-667. DOI: 10.1136/gut.45.5.662

[123] Ruskoné-Fourmestraux A, Dragosics B, Morgner A, et al. Paris staging system for primary gastrointestinal lymphomas. Gut. 2003;**52**:912-916. DOI: 10.1136/gut.52.6.912

[124] Al-Akwaa AM, Siddiqui N, Al-Mofleh IA. Primary gastric lymphoma. World Journal of Gastroenterology. 2004;**10**:5-11. DOI: 10.3748/wjg.v10.i1.5

[125] George MK, Ramachandran V, Ramanan SG, Sagar TG. Primary esophageal T-cell non-Hodgkin's lymphoma. Indian Journal of Gastroenterology. 2005;**24**(3):119-120

[126] Gaskin CM, Low VH, Ho LM. Isolated primary non-hodgkin's lymphoma of the esophagus. American Journal of Roentgenology. 2001;**176**:551-552. DOI: 10.2214/ajr.176.2.1760551

[127] Taal BG, Burgers JM. Primary non-Hodgkin's lymphoma of the stomach: Endoscopic diagnosis and the role of surgery. Scandinavian Journal of Gastroenterology. Supplement. 1991;**188**:33-37. DOI: 10.3109/00365529109111227

[128] Zinzani PL, Broccoli A. Marginal zone B-cell lymphomas. In: Press OW, Lichtman MA, Leonard JP, editors. Williams Hematology Malignant Lymphoid Diseases. McGraw Hill; 2017. pp. 1-14

[129] Myung SJ, Joo KR, Yang SK, et al. Clinicopathologic features of ileocolonic malignant lymphoma: Analysis according to colonoscopic classification. Gastrointestinal Endoscopy. 2003;**57**:343-347. DOI: 10.1067/mge.2003.135

[130] Byun JH, Ha HK, Kim AY, et al. CT findings in peripheral T-cell lymphoma involving the gastrointestinal tract. Radiology. 2003;**227**:59-67. DOI: 10.1111/j.1440-1827.2010.02538.x

[131] Gonzalez QH, Heslin MJ, Dávila-Cervantes A, et al. Primary colonic lymphoma. The American Surgeon. 2008;**74**:214-216. DOI: 10.1177/000313480807400306

[132] Chung HH, Kim YH, Kim JH, et al. Imaging findings of mantle cell lymphoma involving gastrointestinal tract. Yonsei Medical Journal. 2003;**44**:49-57. DOI: 10.3349/ymj.2003.44.1.49

[133] Tomizawa Y, Seki M, Mori M. Unusual presentation of localized gastric mucosa-associated lymphoid tissue

lymphoma mimicking poorly differentiated gastric adenocarcinoma. Case Reports in Gastroenterology. 2012;**6**(1):47-51. DOI: 10.1159/000336322

[134] Pennazio M. Small-intestinal pathology on capsule endoscopy: Spectrum of vascular lesions. Endoscopy. 2005;**37**(9):864-869. DOI: 10.1055/s-2005-870212

[135] Lee HJ, Han JK, Kim TK, et al. Primary colorectal lymphoma: Spectrum of imaging findings with pathologic correlation. European Radiology. 2002;**12**:2242-2249. DOI: 10.1007/s00330-002-1307-4

[136] Gollub MJ. Imaging of gastrointestinal lymphoma. Radiologic Clinics of North America. 2008;**46**(2): 287-312. DOI: 10.1016/j.rcl.2008.03.002

[137] Iwamuro M, Kondo E, Takata K, et al. Diagnosis of follicular lymphoma of the gastrointestinal tract: A better initial diagnostic workup. World Journal of Gastroenterology. 2016;**22**(4):1674-1683. DOI: 10.3748/wjg.v22.i4.1674

[138] Chouhan J, Batra S, Gupta S, Guha S. Gastrointestinal follicular lymphoma: Using primary site as a predictor of survival. Cancer Medicine. 2016;**5**(10):2669-2677. DOI: 10.1002/cam4.763

[139] Wirth A, Ritchie D. The management of gastrointestinal follicular lymphoma: Some observations on a rare disease. Leukemia & Lymphoma. 2013;**54**:9-10. DOI: 10.3109/10428194.2012.713952

[140] Ahuja S, Bharati V, Gupta A, et al. Reed Sternberg-Like Cells in an Aggressive Lymphoma: Report of a Rare Case and Review of Literature. EMJ Hematology US. 2020;**1**(1):65-69

[141] Ghimire P, Wu GY, Zhu L. Primary esophageal lymphoma in immunocompetent patients: Two case reports and literature review. World Journal of Radiology. 2010;**2**:334-338. DOI: 10.4329/wjr.v2.i8.334

[142] Ghai S, Pattison J, Ghai S, O'Malley ME, Khalili K, Stephens M. Primary gastrointestinal lymphoma: Spectrum of imaging findings with pathologic correlation. Radiographics. 2007;**27**(5):1371-1388. DOI: 10.1148/rg.275065151

[143] Lupescu IG, Grasu M, Goldis G, et al. Computer tomographic evaluation of digestive tract non-Hodgkin lymphomas. Journal of Gastrointestinal and Liver Diseases. 2007;**16**:315-319

[144] Chou CK, Chen LT, Sheu RS, et al. MRI manifestations of gastrointestinal lymphoma. Abdominal Imaging. 1994;**19**:495-500. DOI: 10.1007/BF00198248

[145] Boot H. Diagnosis and staging in gastrointestinal lymphoma. Best Practice & Research. Clinical Gastroenterology. 2010;**24**:3-12. DOI: 10.1016/j.bpg.2009.12.003

[146] Radan L, Fischer D, Bar-Shalom R, et al. FDG avidity and PET/CT patterns in primary gastric lymphoma. European Journal of Nuclear Medicine and Molecular Imaging. 2008;**35**:1424-1430. DOI: 10.1007/s00259-008-0771-8

[147] Paes FM, Kalkanis DG, Sideras PA, Serafini AN. FDG PET/CT of extranodal involvement in non-Hodgkin lymphoma and Hodgkin disease. Radiographics. 2010;**30**:269-291. DOI: 10.1148/rg.301095088

[148] Ahmad A, Govil Y, Frank BB. Gastric mucosa-associated lymphoid tissue lymphoma. The American Journal of Gastroenterology. 2003;**98**(5):975-986. DOI: 10.1111/j.1572-0241.2003.07424.x

[149] Stolte M, Bayerdörffer E, Morgner A, et al. Helicobacter and gastric MALT

lymphoma. Gut. 2002;**50**(Suppl. 3): iii19-iii24. DOI: 10.1136/gut.50.suppl_3.iii19

[150] Stathis A, Chini C, Bertoni F, et al. Long-term outcome following Helicobacter pylori eradication in a retrospective study of 105 patients with localized gastric marginal zone B-cell lymphoma of MALT type. Annals of Oncology. 2009;**20**:1086-1093. DOI: 10.1093/annonc/mdn760

[151] Raderer M, Valencak J, Österreicher C, et al. Chemotherapy for the treatment of patients with primary high grade gastric B-cell lymphoma of modified Ann Arbor Stages IE and IIE. Cancer. 2000;**88**:1979-1985. DOI: 10.1002/(sici)1097-0142(20000501)88:9<1979::aid-cncr1>3.0.co;2-l

[152] Zhang S, Wang L, Yu D, et al. Localized primary gastrointestinal diffuse large B cell lymphoma received a surgical approach: An analysis of prognostic factors and comparison of staging systems in 101 patients from a single institution. World Journal of Surgical Oncology. 2015;**13**(1):246. DOI: 10.1186/s12957-015-0668-5

[153] Ferreri AJ, Govi S, Raderer M, et al. Helicobacter pylori eradication as exclusive treatment for limited-stage gastric diffuse large B-cell lymphoma: Results of a multicenter phase 2 trial. Blood. 2012;**120**(18):3858-3860. DOI: 10.1182/blood-2012-06-438424

[154] Nagashima R, Takeda H, Maeda K, et al. Regression of duodenal mucosa-associated lymphoid tissue lymphoma after eradication of Helicobacter pylory. Gastroenterology. 1996;**111**(6):1674-1678. DOI: 10.1016/s0016-5085(96)70032-x

[155] Dunleavy K. Approach to the diagnosis and treatment of adult Burkitt's lymphoma. Journal of Oncology Practice/ American Society of Clinical Oncology. 2018;**14**(11):665-672. DOI: 10.1200/JOP.18.00148

[156] Dozzo M, Carobolante F, Donisi PM, et al. Burkitt lymphoma in adolescents and young adults: Management challenges. Adolescent Health, Medicine and Therapeutics. 2017;**8**:11-29. DOI: 10.2147/AHMT.S94170

[157] Dasappa L, Babu MCS, Sirsath NT, et al. Primary gastrointestinal mantle cell lymphoma: A retrospective study. Journal of Gastrointestinal Cancer. 2014;**45**(4):481-486. DOI: 10.1007/s12029-014-9655-2

[158] Ganapathi KA, Pittaluga S, Odejidi OO, et al. Early lymphoid lesions: Conceptual, diagnostic, and clinical challenges. Haematologica. 2014;**99**(9):1421-1432. DOI: 10.3324/haematol.2014.107938

[159] Tari A, Asaoku H, Takata K, et al. The role of "watch and wait" in intestinal follicular lymphoma in Rituximab era. Scandinavian Journal of Gastroenterology. 2016;**51**(3):321-328. DOI: 10.3109/00365521.2015.1087589

[160] Küçük C, Wei L, You H. Indolent T-cell lymphoproliferative disease of the GI tract: Insights for better diagnosis, prognosis, and appropriate therapy. Frontiers in Oncology. 2020;**10**:1276. DOI: 10.3389/fonc.2020.01276

[161] Choi WWL, Weisenburger DD, Greiner TC, et al. A new immunostain algorithm classifies diffuse large B-cell lymphoma into molecular subtypes with high accuracy. Clinical Cancer Research. 2009;**15**(17):5494-5502. DOI: 10.1158/1078-0432.CCR-09-0113

[162] Nijeboer P, de Baaij LR, Visser O, et al. Treatment response in enteropathy associated T-cell lymphoma; survival in a large multicenter cohort. American Journal of Hematology. 2015;**90**(6):493-498. DOI: 10.1002/ajh.23992

Chapter 4

Splenic B-Cell Lymphoma/Leukemia, Unclassifiable

Parastou Tizro, Rami Abdulbaki, Anita Aggarwal, Aaron Auerbach and Victor E. Nava

Abstract

Splenic B-cell lymphoma/leukemia, which is unclassifiable, includes low-grade B-cell lymphoproliferative disorders that do not fit into any other splenic lymphoid neoplasm based on current WHO classification. Presently, two provisional entities, splenic diffuse red pulp small B-cell lymphoma (SDRPL) and hairy-cell leukemia variant (HCL-v), are the most recognizable members of this group. SDRPL is an uncommon malignancy representing less than 1% of all non-Hodgkin lymphomas. Frequent clinical manifestations include splenomegaly and lymphocytosis. SDRPL is currently considered a diagnosis of exclusion and requires clinical and paraclinical correlation, including blood smear, bone marrow and spleen morphology, and the correct immunophenotype (typically positive for CD20, DBA.44, and IgG; and negative for CD5, CD10, CD23, CD43, annexin A1, CD11c, CD25, CD103, and CD123), and cytogenetic findings. Cyclin D3 is expressed in the majority of SDRPL in contrast to other types of small B-cell lymphomas. HCL-v is a less common disease accounting for 0.4% of all chronic lymphoproliferative disorders. It resembles classical HCL and SDRPL by diffusely infiltrating the splenic red pulp but is considered biologically unrelated. Splenomegaly and atypical lymphocytosis without monocytopenia are common. Distinguishing features of HCL-v include morphology, immunophenotype (the absence of CD25, CD200, CD123, annexin A1, and TRAP), genotype (wild-type *BRAF*), and prognosis.

Keywords: spleen, lymphoma, splenic B-cell lymphoma/leukemia unclassifiable, splenic diffuse red pulp small B-cell lymphoma, hairy cell leukemia-variant

1. Introduction

Splenic B-cell lymphoma/leukemia, unclassifiable, is a rare category of spleen neoplasm with unknown etiology that lacks established, precise diagnostic criteria and remains a diagnosis of exclusion. This category includes the two relatively rare entities of splenic diffuse red pulp small B-cell lymphoma (SDRPL) and hairy cell leukemia variant (HCL-v), which are provisionally recognized in the current World Health Organization (WHO) classification. Other splenic small B-cell lymphomas that do not fit into the current diagnostic scheme can also be part of this category [1].

2. Splenic diffuse red pulp small B-cell lymphoma

SDRPL is an indolent but incurable non-Hodgkin lymphoma (NHL) composed of small mature B-lymphocytes that involve the red pulp of the spleen, as well as bone marrow and peripheral blood. Therefore, it is usually diagnosed at stage IV [1]. The cell of origin is believed to be an unidentified B-cell precursor. SDRPL was first classified as a provisional entity in the 2008 WHO classification of lymphoid neoplasms [2] and was later grouped under splenic B-cell lymphoma/leukemia, unclassifiable in the 2016 revision [1]. In the older literature, this entity may overlap with splenic marginal zone lymphoma (SMZL)-diffuse variant, SMZL with diffuse red pulp involvement, and splenic red pulp lymphoma with numerous basophilic villous lymphocytes, which are terms largely abandoned.

2.1 Epidemiology

The true incidence of SDRPL is unknown, as it is a new part of the spleen lymphoma classification. In general, it has been reported to represent 1–2% of all lymphoid malignancies [3] and may account for up to 10% of the B-cell lymphomas diagnosed in splenectomy specimens [4, 5]. In a single-center case series of 37 patients, SDRPL reportedly represented 0.5% of all chronic lymphoid malignancies diagnosed by peripheral blood examination [6]. SDRPL has a slight male predominance with a male/female ratio of 1.5–2.5:1. The patients are usually older than 40 years of age with a median age of 65–77 years [6, 7].

2.2 Clinical presentation

Patients with SDRPL usually present with mild lymphocytosis and abdominal pain due to massive splenomegaly. Leukopenia and thrombocytopenia due to hypersplenism and bone marrow infiltration are frequent [1]. Almost all cases are diagnosed at clinical stage IV with involvement of peripheral blood and bone marrow, as mentioned above. Splenic hilar lymphadenopathy is frequently reported. However, peripheral lymph node involvement is very uncommon. B symptoms are reported only in one-third of cases. In a retrospective study of 17 cases with SDRPL, liver involvement was reported in 18% of cases while erythematous and pruritic skin papules were seen in 10% of patients [7]. Concurrent chronic hepatitis B infection has also been described in two cases of SDRPL [8].

Imaging studies often show diffuse splenic enlargement without discrete splenic lesions, and increased FDG-avidity may be seen on PET/CT [4]. Rarely, normal splenic size/appearance and FDG uptake are present [3].

2.3 Diagnosis

Diagnosis of SDRPL rests mainly on the exclusion of other lymphomas by correlating histopathology of spleen and bone marrow/peripheral blood, if available, with ancillary studies assessing immunophenotypic and genetic characteristics, which are not always constant in the literature. Although unequivocal diagnostic criteria for SDRPL are still being developed, generally, the combination of morphology and immunohistochemistry in the correct clinical setting allows definitive categorization. Bone marrow examination showing a purely intrasinusoidal pattern in combination with villous lymphocytosis in peripheral blood smears, together with appropriate immunophenotypic/molecular findings excluding other low-grade B-cell lymphomas, may be sufficient for diagnosis. However, splenic biopsy or splenectomy identifying a diffuse infiltration of the red pulp by neoplastic B cells with a characteristic immunophenotype may also be necessary for unequivocal classification [7]. Genetic studies are increasingly being performed and may facilitate the subclassification of difficult cases or those with limited tissue.

2.3.1 Laboratory findings

The most common laboratory finding in SDRPL is low-grade lymphocytosis (median lymphocyte count of (5.4×10^9/L), which can be a useful diagnostic hint to differentiate it from HCL-v that classically shows higher lymphocytosis. Although not present uniformly among all studies, thrombocytopenia (median platelet count <100×10^9/L) and leukopenia have been frequently reported in SDRPL. However, anemia is a rare finding [7]. Other laboratory results are usually unremarkable except for hepatitis B virus tests [8].

2.3.2 Morphologic findings

Splenectomy specimens show diffusely enlarged spleen with a homogenous red-brown cut surface (described as "beefy") and occasional wedge-shaped subscapular infarcts. Spleen nodularity has not been reported in SDRPL cases, and its presence should warn against this diagnosis. However residual lymphoid nodules composed of T-cells may be found [7].

Splenic histology reveals a purely diffuse pattern of infiltration of the red pulp cords and sinusoids by monomorphous small to medium-size mature B cells with regular ovoid nuclei, clumped chromatin, and pale cytoplasm, which spares the white pulp [9]. Focal plasmacytic differentiation can be present as in other low-grade B-cell lymphomas. Reactive T-cell lymphoid nodules or residual B-cell lymphoid follicles are occasionally present in early disease [9]. Sinusoidal disruption results in erythrocyte collections surrounded by tumor cells, which form the characteristic blood lakes seen in some cases. These so-called true blood lakes tend to be smaller (**Figure 1**) than those seen in HCL. In contrast, pseudo-blood lakes formed by sinusoidal dilation, which can also be present in other splenic lymphomas, are lined by littoral cells (CD8-positive/CD34-negative) and vascular endothelial cells (CD8-negative/CD34-positive) [7, 10]. The absence of white pulp involvement by follicular or nodular proliferation is a supportive finding to allow correct categorization [10].

The peripheral blood smear shows villous lymphocytes (**Figure 2**) in variable degrees, which may be indistinguishable from those present in other small B-cell lymphomas. However, complete circumferential distribution or longer villi should not be seen, in contrast with HCL and HCL-v.

Bone marrow trephine core biopsy typically reveals a predominantly intrasinusoidal infiltration, but occasionally interstitial and nodular aggregates may also be present. This sinusoidal pattern is considered more specific for the diagnosis but is not pathognomonic, and can also be seen in SMZL and HCL-v [10]. Neoplastic lymphoid follicles have not been reported in bone marrow specimens with SDRPL unlike in other low-grade B-cell neoplasms, such as SMZL and follicular lymphoma.

Skin involvement may be seen in advanced cases showing an unspecific patchy peri adnexal/perivascular pattern of infiltration [7].

2.3.3 Immunophenotypic findings

Based on immunophenotyping, SDRPL belongs to the group of CD5/CD10 double negative B-cell lymphomas, but phenotypic variability has been reported [11]. The

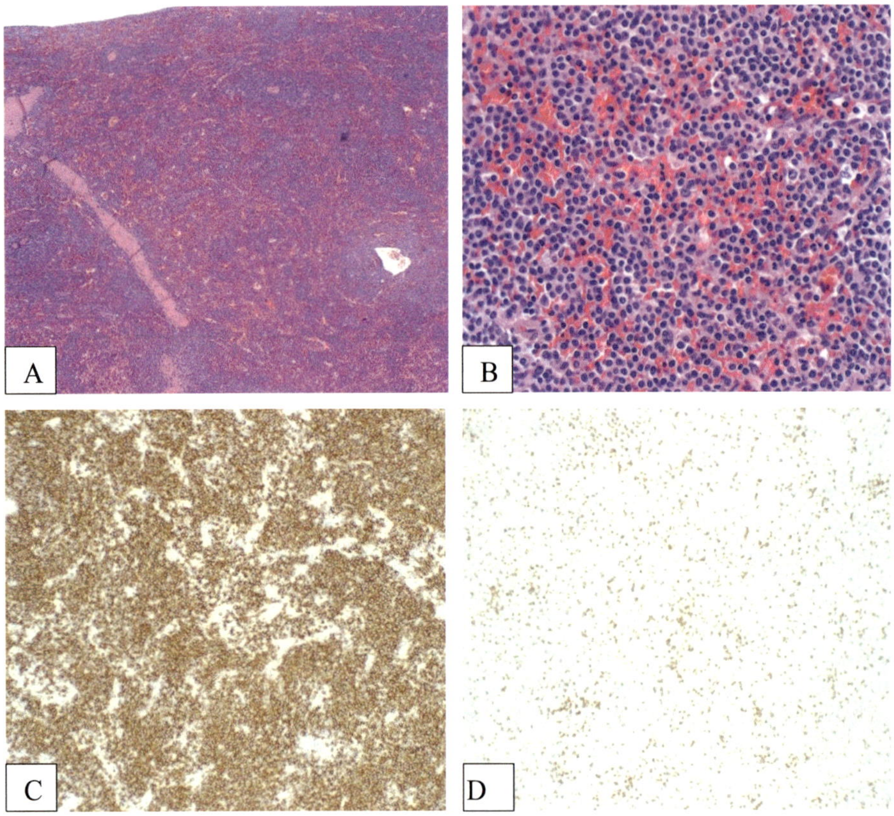

Figure 1.
(A) SDRPL in the red pulp of the spleen showing blood lakes (H&E, 40X). (B) Higher magnification of infiltrating monomorphic small B-lymphocytes with regular nuclei, clumped chromatin, and pale cytoplasm (H&E,400X). The lymphoma cells are strongly positive for CD20 (C) and negative for CD5 (D) by immunohistochemistry (200X).

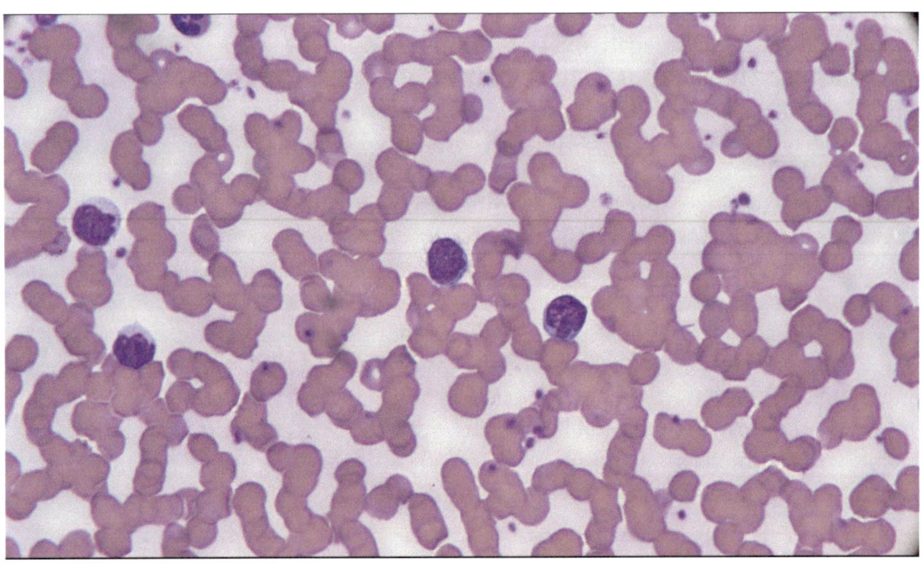

Figure 2.
Peripheral blood smear shows villous lymphocytes in SDRPL (Wright-Giemsa, 1000X).

classic immunophenotype of the neoplastic cells usually includes positivity for CD19, CD20, IgG, and BCL2; and negativity for CD5, CD23, CD43, cyclin D1, CD10, BCL6, MUM1, CD11c, CD25, CD103, CD123, and annexin A1. DBA.44 is positive in 20–90% of cases [7, 9, 10, 12]. IgD, IgM, CD103, CD11c, CD5, CD123, and CD43 positivity has been described infrequently, although expression of IgD is more commonly associated with marginal zone B-cell lymphoma. A recent study showed cyclin D3 expression in 24 out of 33 (72%) patients with SDRPL [13]. However, this marker is not readily available in most laboratories, limiting its clinical utility. Cases with plasmacytic differentiation commonly show positivity for CD38 and/or CD138, as expected.

Flow cytometry demonstrates restricted B lymphocytes based on the expression of surface light chain immunoglobulins (kappa or lambda), which could be biclonal (IgM and IgG or IgM and IgD) or monoclonal (IgG or IgM alone) based on heavy chain type. In addition, CD103 expression can be detected in up to a third of cases [14].

2.3.4 Genetic findings

Immunoglobulin heavy chain (*IGHV*) somatic hypermutation analysis shows alterations in up to 70% of the cases with selective usage of VH3 and VH4 gene families [6, 15], as is commonly also seen in HCL. VH1 usage is uncommon, in contrast with SMZL. Complex cytogenetic alterations including t(9,14) (p13;q32), involving *PAX5* and *IGH* genes have been reported. Chromosome 7q deletion, trisomy 18, and partial trisomy 3q have been rarely published. *TP53* alterations are seen only in 5–15% of cases [8, 12, 13].

A recent whole-exome sequencing (WES) study identified mutations in the *CCND3* PEST domain in a high proportion of SDRPL cases, whereas no mutations in *NOTCH2* or *BRAF* V600E were reported [12, 13]. A distinct mutational landscape has been observed in 42 SDRPL samples as compared with eight and 46 samples from HCL and SMZL patients, respectively [15]. WES identified recurrent *BCOR* (*BCL6* corepressor) mutations or losses in 10 of 42 SDRPL cases (24%). In contrast, *BCOR* alterations were rare in SMZL (one of 46) and absent in HCL (0 of eight). *CCND3* mutations were also detected in 21% of SDRPL and 13% of SMZL cases. *BRAF* V600E mutation was present in all HCL samples (eight of eight) but only in one of 42 SDRPL and one of 46 SMZL specimens. In contrast, mutations in the NOTCH (*NOTCH2*, *NOTCH1,* and *SPEN*) and NF-κB pathways (*KLF2*, *TNFAIP3,* and *MYD88*) were rare (0–2%) in SDRPL as opposed to SMZL. These molecular findings could aid in the differential diagnosis of primary splenic lymphomas with ambiguous morphology.

2.4 Treatment

Since SDRPL is a very rare disease there is a paucity of clinical studies evaluating different management strategies. Therefore, treatment modalities for SDRPL are evolving and usually rely on the experience with other primary splenic lymphomas, such as SMZL. The most utilized therapeutic approaches for SDRPL include splenectomy, rituximab monotherapy, or expectant management. Although splenectomy can achieve durable remission, it is by definition non-curative since residual disease remains in the bone marrow and peripheral blood compartments [7, 12].

2.5 Prognosis

Patients with SDRPL as a rule have a chronic clinical course with a median survival compared to those of individuals with SMZL (8–10 years), but significantly superior to those with HCL-v. Although standard treatment is still unavailable, splenectomy is an excellent alternative to producing durable remission in most cases. However, around 25% of patients follow a more progressive course, which may be related to genetic alterations in *NOTCH1*, *MAP2K1*, and *TP53* [12].

Transformation to a large B-cell lymphoma with aggressive behavior has been described rarely [7, 8, 16], and unusual transformation to B-cell prolymphocytic leukemia (B-PLL) is also possible [17, 18].

Future genetic profiling is necessary to discover alterations with prognostic significance in SDRPL, and consequently, molecular testing may be particularly indicated in young patients [9].

3. Hairy cell leukemia variant

HCL-v is a provisional diagnostic entity in the WHO classification since 2001 and was later included in the broader category of splenic B-cell lymphoma/leukemia, unclassifiable [1]. HCL-v was formally first described by Cawley et al. [19] as an indolent lymphoproliferative disorder with some resemblance to HCL, but biologically divergent based on the postulated cell of origin (activated late-stage B cell for HCL-v vs. mature B cell of unknown type for HCL). This divergence is reflected in its variant histomorphologic, immunophenotypic, genotypic, and clinical features. Accordingly, HCL-v does not respond well to HCL therapeutic regimens and tends to behave more aggressively [20].

As in HCL, the spleen, bone marrow, and peripheral blood are usually involved in HCL-v, which commonly present with splenomegaly due to red pulp infiltration. However, absolute lymphocytosis without monocytopenia is the norm, as opposed to the cytopenias, especially monocytopenia, observed in HCL.

3.1 Epidemiology

HCL-v has an annual incidence of approximately 0.03 cases per 100,000 population [1]. It accounts for 10–20% of lymphoproliferative disorders initially diagnosed as HCL and 0.4% of all chronic lymphoproliferative disorders, accounting for 60–75 new HCL-v cases reported annually in the United States alone [20]. The patients are usually middle-aged to elderly with a slight (1.6:1) male predominance [21]. Although a geographical predilection has not been reported so far, the disease may be more prevalent in Asian populations [21, 22].

3.2 Clinical presentation

The typical initial manifestations, including abdominal discomfort, anemia, bleeding, or infection, are usually related to splenomegaly and/or the presence of cytopenias. In earlier stages of the disease, cytopenias are mainly related to hypersplenism rather than some form of bone marrow failure. A small proportion of cases are identified incidentally by routine hematology (cell blood counts and/or peripheral blood smear reviews) [21], since leukocytosis (on average 30×10^9/L) with an absolute lymphocytosis and atypical lymphocytes may be detected before the onset of symptoms. However, the absolute number and proportion of monocytes are not decreased in contrast with the usual type of HCL [22]. While thrombocytopenia can be seen in almost half of the patients, anemia is reported in 25% of them [23]. A single institute case series study of 52 patients showed splenomegaly in most (85%) and hepatomegaly in less than a third of the patients. However, lymphadenopathy was rare [22]. Autoimmune hemolytic anemia and extra-splenic involvement (including skin, brain, and terminal ileum) have been reported rarely [23].

3.3 Morphologic findings

The HCL-v cells display morphologic heterogeneity in the peripheral blood. In most cases, identification of villous lymphocytes is possible, however, the cytoplasmic projections tend to be more polarized, less frequent (**Figure 3**), and more robust than the typical hair-like long circumferential "pseudopods" of classical HCL. In fact, these projections may be missing completely and when present may be indistinguishable from those seen in SDRPL, SMZL, and HCL. Nuclear features may also be inconsistent and include prominent central prolymphocytoid nucleolus, convolution (instead of round to oval nuclei), and condensed or blastic chromatin, which justifies the published terminology of "hybrid form of HCL" for this entity [1, 24]. Large cells with convoluted nuclei are prominent when HCL-v transforms to high-grade B-cell lymphoma, which is uncommon [25]. In contrast with HCL, insignificant bone marrow fibrosis is detected on reticulin stains, which allows successful aspiration. The lymphomatous burden is usually minimal, vague, and interstitial (**Figure 4**). However, sometimes an intrasinusoidal growth pattern is present in common with SMZL and SDRPL [26, 27]. Similar to SDRPL and HCL, the splenic infiltrate by neoplastic B cells diffusely expand the red pulp and spares the white pulp, which appears atretic [26].

3.4 Immunophenotypic findings

A cardinal difference between HCL-v and classic HCL is the absence of expression of CD25, CD200, CD123, and annexin A1 [28–30]. Immunohistochemical stains (**Figure 5**), show positivity for CD103, DBA.44 (CD72), and CD11c in most cases, which overlaps with HCL. However, the

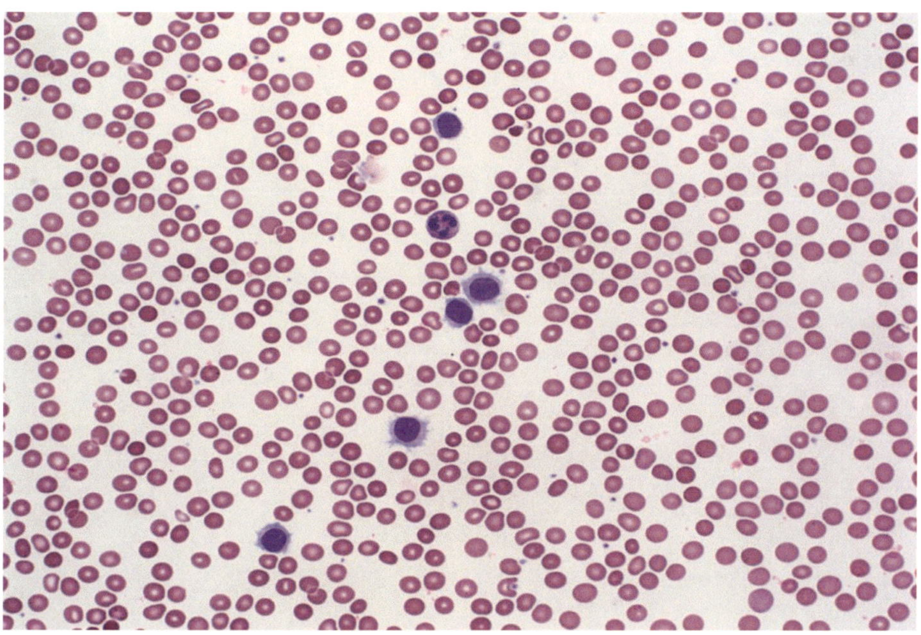

Figure 3.
Peripheral blood smear shows villous lymphocytes in HCL-v (Wright-Giemsa, 400X).

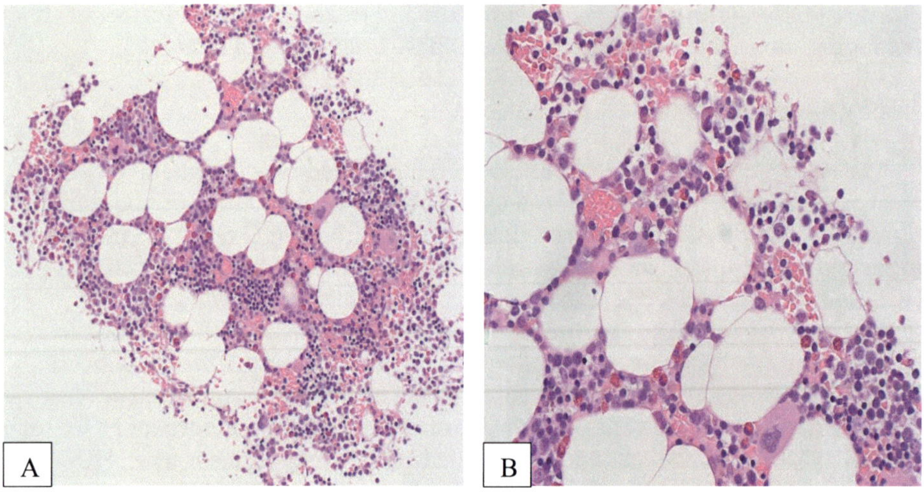

Figure 4.
(A) Bone marrow biopsy of HCL-v shows subtle interstitial lymphomatous involvement (H&E, 200X). (B) Higher magnification of the bone marrow demonstrating involvement by atypical lymphocytes with convoluted nuclei (H&E, 400X).

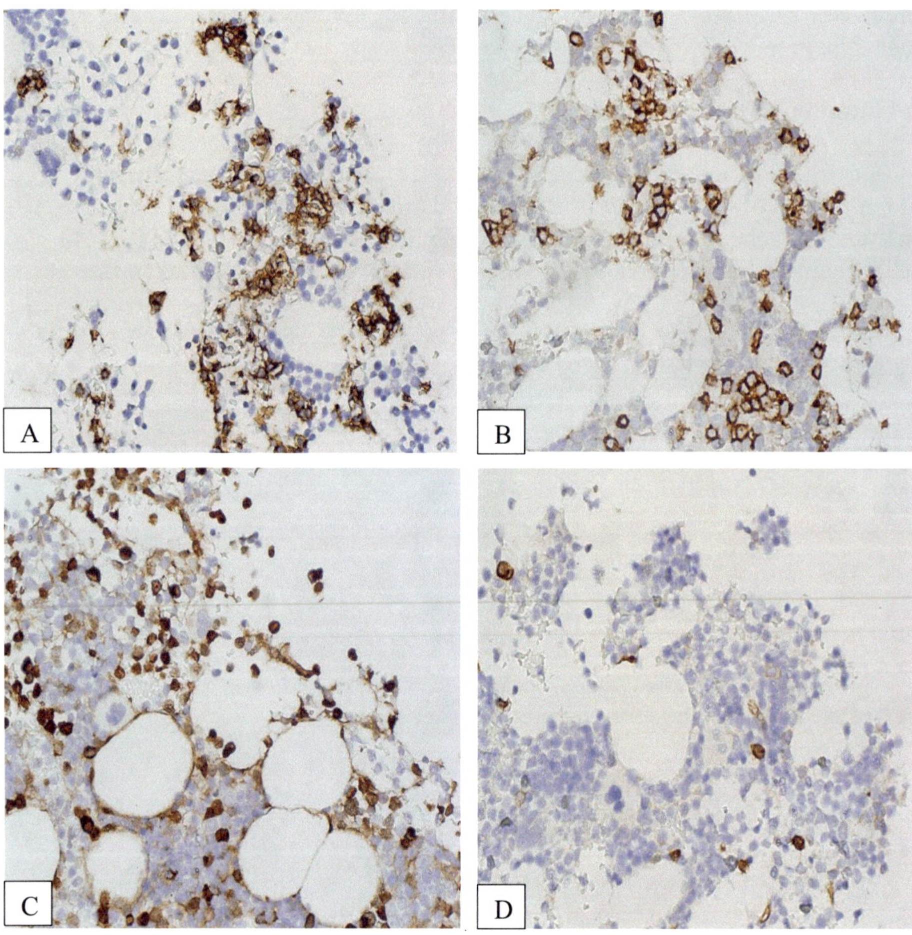

Figure 5.
Immunohistochemistry of bone marrow biopsy from HCL-v showing neoplastic cells positive for CD20 (A) and DBA44 (B). Annexin a is negative on the atypical lymphocytes and highlights myeloid cells (C). CD123 is also negative on neoplastic cells (D) (400X).

expression of CD11c and CD103 can separate HCL-v from SMZL and SDRPL. As with any mature B-cell neoplasm, the immunophenotypic profile of HCL-v also demonstrates positivity for pan-B-cell markers (CD19, CD20, and CD22) and is usually strongly positive for surface immunoglobulins expression, most commonly IgG and lambda light chain. In addition, the majority of cases express FMC7 and HLA-DR, one-third expresses CD24 and CD79a, and only a minority express CD10 and CD138. Lastly, CD5 and CD23 have been reported negative in almost every case [19, 21, 28].

3.5 Genetic findings

Although HCL-v shares classic pathologic features with other splenic lymphomas, the signaling pathways involved are different at the molecular level. For instance, alterations in TP53 are more frequent in HCL-v when compared with classical HCL. Likewise, *IGHV* somatic hypermutation is more common in HCL-v (33%) than in HCL (15%), and preferentially affects the VH4–34 gene segment (40% in HCL-v and 10% in HCL). Of interest, 44% of *TP53*-mutated HCL-v cases had unmutated *IGHV* [23]. Furthermore, a British DNA copy number analysis study demonstrated more abnormalities in HCL-v predominantly representing gains of chromosome 5 and losses of chromosomes 7p and 17p. [31]. However, emerging data from a Chinese cohort suggests a more complex picture with a higher ratio of large chromosomic alteration and a lower copy number variation in HCL versus HCL-v [32]. Regarding the prototypical *BRAF* V600E mutation present in HCL, multiple studies demonstrate its absence in HCL-v [33–35]. In contrast, *MAP2K1* alterations have been documented in the majority of HCL-v, and only in rare classical HCL with *IGHV*4–34 usage and wild-type *BRAF*, which suggests a common pathogenic MAPK activation in a subset of cases [36].

Additional studies are necessary to clarify the genomic landscape of HCL-v, including further analysis of the reported mutations in U2AF1, *ARID1A,* and *TTN* [37], and to identify meaningful biological features possibly leading to novel therapy. To that effect, it may also be beneficial to further investigate the role of cytokines (Fibroblast growth factor and transforming growth factor beta) and adhesion molecules preferentially expressed in HCL but not in HCL-v, which promote bone marrow fibrosis in the former [38].

3.6 Treatment

The treatment of HCL-v is challenging due to the rarity of the disease, which has hampered the development of definitive guidelines. Although expectant management (active observation) is an option, most patients will eventually require therapy, ranging from splenectomy to chemoimmunotherapy [23]. Indications for treatment include the development of progressive splenomegaly, rapid increase in lymphocyte count, or symptoms related to cytopenias [22]. Splenectomy alone can lead to long-lasting partial remission in about two-thirds of patients [28] and maybe the best option because it not only removes the bulk of the disease but also corrects hypersplenism alleviating cytopenias. Moreover, splenectomy followed by Rituximab may be an additional treatment option [39]. HCL-v is resistant to agents effective against HCL, such as cladribine and pentostatin [24]. However, adding rituximab to cladribine as a combination therapy has shown promising results, achieving a complete response in nine of 10 patients, of whom only two showed minimal residual disease (MRD) [40]. Anti-CD22 recombinant immunotoxin, an agent used in refractory HCL, has also been utilized successfully [22, 41].

Alemtuzumab, a monoclonal antibody effective for chronic lymphocytic leukemia with mutated *TP53*, achieved morphologic remission after 8 weeks of treatment in one patient with HCL-v. However, flow cytometry detected MRD with 1.5% malignant cells [42]. The B-cell receptor inhibitor, Ibrutinib, failed to induce complete remission in 28 patients (1 treatment-naive HCL-v, 10 relapsed HCL-v, and 17 relapsed HCL) and showed a better overall response rate in subjects with HCL [43].

3.7 Prognosis

HCL-v is a treatable but still incurable chronic disease. The median survival is 9 years, and 42% of patients die of unrelated causes. Transformation to large-cell lymphoma is seen in 6% of patients [21]. A study of 35 cases of HCL-v showed a significantly shorter five-year survival in HCL-v compared with SMZL (57% vs. 84%). In contrast, classical HCL has a good response to purine analogs with a five-year and 10-year survival reaching 90%. Poor prognostic indicators in HCL-v include *TP53* mutation, older age, and severe anemia. For example, the five-year survival was 11% in patients with *TP53* mutation compared with 73% in patients without it [23].

4. Differential diagnosis

SDRPL and HCL-v must be differentiated from each other and other low-grade B-cell lymphomas/leukemias in the spleen, in particular SMZL, HCL, and lymphoplasmacytic lymphoma (LPL). This task can be a challenge even for experienced hematopathologists since these entities may present clinical and pathologic overlap. Splenomegaly may be the principal clinical finding, and the neoplastic B cells in these four malignancies are generally double negative for CD5 and CD10. In addition, HCL-v displaying prominent nucleoli could be confused with B-PLL. However, clinicopathological correlation, including immunohistochemistry, should allow a categorical differentiation from B-PLL. Salient differential features are highlighted below focusing on distinctions among SMZL, HCL, and LPL (**Table 1**). Finally, a brief differential between HCL-v and B-PLL are presented.

4.1 Splenic marginal zone lymphoma

The key differentiating trait of classic SMZL from other diseases is nodular involvement of the white pulp frequently showing a microscopic targetoid appearance composed of a darker central zone with small lymphocytes surrounded by a peripheral zone of larger paler marginal zone cells. This pattern is better appreciated on Ki-67 immunohistochemistry. Blood lakes are absent, unlike in SDRPL, HCL, and HCL-v, which all grossly show a characteristic "beefy" red cut splenic surface (correlated with red pulp infiltration and atrophic white pulp). The bone marrow involvement may also be nodular, but interstitial and intrasinusoidal patterns are also common. Notably, well-formed reactive follicles can be seen, which are typically absent in the other entities.

Immunohistochemistry may be of limited value to diagnose CD5/CD10-negative lymphomas due to variable expression of possible differentiating markers. Ideally, both CD25 and CD103 are positive in SMZL and HCL, while CD25 and CD103 are absent in HCL-v and LPL, respectively. In contrast, SDRPL should be double negative for CD25 and CD103. However, this routine clinicopathologic information may

DOI: http://dx.doi.org/10.5772/intechopen.101418

	Peripheral Blood	Spleen	Bone marrow	Immunophenotype	Chromosomal Aberrations	Altered Genes
SDRLP	Polar broad base small villous projections, condensed chromatin	Red pulp, blood lakes (possible)	Intrasinusoidal, interstitial ±, nodular ± (no follicles)	CD25-, CD103±, CD123-, DBA44±, Annexin A1-, Cyclin D3+, IgG+	Uncommon: Trisomy 3q, Trisomy 18, del 7q	*CCND3*, *IGHV3–4*, *BCOR*, *MAP2K1*
HCL-v	Circumferential shorter villous projections, prominent nucleoli (subset)	Red pulp, white pulp effacement, blood lakes (uncommon)	Interstitial, Intrasinusoidal, no increased fibrosis	CD25-, CD103+, CD123-, DBA44+, Annexin A1-, TRAP±	del 17p, del 7q, Gain of 5	*MAP2K1*, *IGHV4–34*, *U2AF1*, *ARID1A*, *TP53*
HCL	Circumferential long (hairy) projections, oval nucleus, inconspicuous nucleolus	Red pulp, blood lakes (common)	Interstitial, diffuse, prominent fibrosis (dry tap)	CD25+, CD103+, CD123+, DBA44+, Annexin A1+, CD200+, CyclinD1±	Chromosomes 5 and 7 abnormalities	*BRAF* V600E
SMZL	Polar shorter villi (or similar to SDRPL), condensed chromatin.	White pulp with marginal zone expansion	Nodular±, intrasinusoidal ±, interstitial± (residual follicles)	CD25±, CD103±, CD123-, DBA44±, Annexin A1-, IgD+	Gain of 3q, del 7q	*NOTCH2*, *IGHV1–2*, *KLF2*

Table 1.
Differential diagnosis for splenic B-cell leukemia/lymphoma-unclassifiable.

be equivocal, and therefore, esoteric testing including cytogenetic and molecular analysis may be necessary. Cytogenetic abnormalities including deletion 7q, trisomy 3q, trisomy 12q, and *IGH* mutation are more common in SMZL than in the other diseases considered [36]. In addition, *NOTCH2*, the most commonly mutated gene in SMZL, has been detected in 20–25% of cases and is classified as a recurrent alteration in this disease [37]. Furthermore, *IGHV* mutation with a predilection for VH1–2 usage, present in SMZL, is so far absent in SDRPL, which may be of diagnostic value [7].

4.2 Hairy cell leukemia

Although HCL shares with SDRPL and HCL-v a diffuse pattern of red pulp involvement accompanied by atrophy of the white pulp, its clinicopathologic/molecular features are usually very distinctive. HCL frequently presents with significant pancytopenia and monocytopenia without lymphocytosis. In the contrast, HCL-v and SDRPL are often associated with lymphocytosis without monocytopenia. Bone marrow morphology may show focal or diffuse involvement with characteristic cytology demonstrating round/oval nuclei and somewhat abundant well-demarcated cytoplasm (conferring a "fried-egg" appearance). However, a sinusoidal pattern, which is possible in the other diseases, would make the diagnosis of HCL improbable. Furthermore, significantly increased reticulin fibrosis delineating every neoplastic cell is characteristic and almost always presents in HCL [1]. Immunophenotypically, triple-positivity for CD25, CD103, and CD123 (or quadruple-positivity considering CD11c), is very helpful for solidifying the diagnosis of HCL. In addition, expression of tartrate-resistant acid phosphate and annexin A1 may also be seen, which tend to be negative in the other entities in the differential diagnosis. Of interest, DBA.44 is a nonspecific marker that can also be expressed in SDRPL, HCL-v, and SMZL, limiting its diagnostic power. Finally, the vast majority of HCL cases harbor the *BRAF* V600E mutation, which can allow a definitive diagnosis in difficult cases [36]. Notably, BRAF can be detected by immunohistochemistry and can be present in 2% of SMZL [44, 45].

4.3 Lymphoplasmacytic lymphoma

LPL is a bone marrow disease typically recognized by the combination of an IgM gammopathy (with possible hyperviscosity/Waldenstrom macroglobulinemia) and the characteristic *MYD88* L265P mutation, which is present in more than 90% of cases [1, 22]. However, approximately 15–30% of cases can show progressive nodal and/or extranodal involvement resembling other low-grade splenic lymphomas involving red pulp (SDRLP, HCL, and HCL-v). Some of the distinguishing characteristics have been described in the preceding sections, including the nodular white pulp splenic involvement also seen in SMZL. In addition, double negativity for CD103 and CD123 should allow the exclusion of HCL and HCL-v. Therefore, the remaining diagnostic dilemma may be between rare *MYD88*-unmutated/IgM-negative LPL (exceedingly rare) and SDRPL, which is frequently positive for DBA.44, IgG (up to 66% of cases) and cyclin D3 by immunohistochemistry. In addition, molecular analysis may be contributory in equivocal situations, revealing *CCDN3* and *BCOR* mutations in SDRPL versus del6q in LPL [22, 46].

4.4 B-cell prolymphocytic leukemia

B-PLL is an extremely rare disease that may present de novo, mimicking HCL-v. B-PLL shows B cells with prominent nucleoli and without villous projections.

DOI: http://dx.doi.org/10.5772/intechopen.101418

However, B-PLL usually follows a more aggressive course with massive splenomegaly and accelerated lymphocytosis above 100×10^9/L. CD103 expression in HCL-v should resolve this quandary. However, due to variable immunophenotypes and genetic profiles, differentiation of B-PLL from HCL-v may be difficult, especially when a splenectomy specimen is unavailable (since B-PLL may show white pulp or red pulp involvement, while HCL-v is restricted to the red pulp) [1, 22, 28]. Specific molecular markers have not been identified yet to resolve this differential diagnosis. *TP53* alterations have been detected in both entities [1, 28], but *MYC* alterations have been described only in a subset to B-PLL [45].

5. Conclusion

In summary, a review of splenic B-cell lymphoma/leukemia, unclassifiable has been presented, focusing on the differential diagnosis of SDRPL and HCL-v, the two most recognizable members of this group.

Conflict of interest

The authors reported no potential conflicts of interest.

Author details

Parastou Tizro[1]*, Rami Abdulbaki[2], Anita Aggarwal[3], Aaron Auerbach[4] and Victor E. Nava[3]

1 City of Hope Comprehensive Cancer Center, Los Angeles CA, USA

2 George Washington University Hospital, Washington, DC, USA

3 Veterans Affairs Medical Center, Washington DC, USA

4 The Joint Pathology Center, Silver Spring, MD, USA

*Address all correspondence to: ptizro@coh.org

References

[1] Swerdlow SH, Campo E, Harris NL, Jaffe ES, Pileri SA, Stein H, et al. WHO Classification of Tumours of Haematopoietic and Lymphoid Tissues. Revised 4th ed. Lyon: IARC; 2017

[2] Swerdlow SH, Campo E, Harris NL, Jaffe ES, Pileri SA, Stein H, et al. editors. WHO Classification of Tumours of Haematopoietic and Lymphoid Tissues. 4th ed. Lyon: IARC; 2008

[3] Saboo SS, Krajewski KM, O'Regan KN, Giardino A, Brown JR, Ramaiya N, et al. Spleen in haematological malignancies: Spectrum of imaging findings. The British Journal of Radiology. 2012;**1009**:81-92. DOI: 10.1259/bjr/31542964

[4] Shimizu-Kohno K, Kimura Y, Kiyasu J, Miyoshi H, Yoshida M, Ichikawa R, et al. Malignant lymphoma of the spleen in Japan: A clinicopathological analysis of 115 cases. Pathology International. 2012;**62**(9):577-582. DOI: 10.1111/j.1440-1827.2012.02844.x

[5] Li M, Zhang L, Wu N, Huang W, Lv N. Imaging findings of primary splenic lymphoma: A review of 17 cases in which diagnosis was made at splenectomy. PLoS One. 2013;**8**(11): e80264. DOI: 10.1371/journal.pone.0080264

[6] Traverse-Glehen A, Baseggio L, Bauchu EC, Morel D, Gazzo S, Ffrench M, et al. Splenic red pulp lymphoma with numerous basophilic villous lymphocytes: A distinct clinicopathologic and molecular entity? Blood. 2008;**111**:2253-2260

[7] Kanellis G, Mollejo M, Montes-Moreno S, Rodriguez-Pinilla SM, Cigudosa JC, Algara P, et al. Splenic diffuse red pulp small B-cell lymphoma: Revision of a series of cases reveals characteristic clinico-pathological features. Haematologica. 2010;**95**(7):1122-1129. DOI: 10.3324/haematol.2009.013714

[8] Kerbauy MN, Fernandes CM, Bezerra ED, Lage LA, Siqueira SA, Pereira J. Splenic diffuse red-pulp small B-cell lymphoma associated with hepatitis B virus: A report of two cases. São Paulo Medical Journal. 2016;**134**(4):359-365. DOI: 10.1590/1516-3180.2016.0035130416

[9] Medeiros LJ, Miranda RN. Splenic Diffuse Red Pulp Small B-Cell Lymphoma. Diagnostic Pathology: Lymph Nodes and Extranodal Lymphomas. Second ed. Philadelphia, USA: Elsevier; 2018. pp. 574-581

[10] Ponzoni M, Kanellis G, Pouliou E, Baliakas P, Scarfò L, Ferreri AJ, et al. Bone marrow histopathology in the diagnostic evaluation of splenic marginal-zone and splenic diffuse red pulp small B-cell lymphoma: A reliable substitute for spleen histopathology? The American Journal of Surgical Pathology. 2012;**36**(11):1609-1618. DOI: 10.1097/PAS.0b013e318271243d

[11] Traverse-Glehen A, Baseggio L, Salles G, Coiffier B, Felman P, Berger F. Splenic diffuse red pulp small-B cell lymphoma: Toward the emergence of a new lymphoma entity. Discovery Medicine. 2012;**13**(71):253-265

[12] Martinez D, Navarro A, Martinez-Trillos A, Molina-Urra R, Gonzalez-Farre B, Salaverria I, et al. NOTCH1, TP53, and MAP2K1 mutations in splenic diffuse red pulp small b-cell lymphoma are associated with progressive disease. The American Journal of Surgical Pathology. 2016;**40**(2):192-201. DOI: 10.1097/PAS.0000000000000523

[13] Curiel-Olmo S, Mondéjar R, Almaraz C, Mollejo M, Cereceda L,

Marès R, et al. Splenic diffuse red pulp small B-cell lymphoma displays increased expression of cyclin D3 and recurrent CCND3 mutations. Blood. 2017;**129**:1042-1045. DOI: 10.1182/blood-2016-11-751024

[14] Baseggio L, Traverse-Glehen A, Callet-Bauchu E, Morel D, Magaud JP, Berger F, et al. Relevance of a scoring system including CD11c expression in the identification of splenic diffuse red pulp small B-cell lymphoma (SRPL). Hematological Oncology. 2011;**29**(1): 47-51. DOI: 10.1002/hon.957

[15] Jallades L, Baseggio L, Sujobert P, Huet S, Chabane K, Callet-Bauchu E, et al. Exome sequencing identifies recurrent BCOR alterations and the absence of KLF2, TNFAIP3 and MYD88 mutations in splenic diffuse red pulp small B-cell lymphoma. Haematologica. 2017;**102**:1758

[16] Wang R-C et al. Villous lymphocytes in splenic large B-cell lymphoma with diffuse red pulp infiltration. International Journal of Hematology. 2019;**109**(2):133-134

[17] Hoehn D, Miranda RN, Kanagal-Shamanna R, Lin P, Medeiros LJ. Splenic B-cell lymphomas with more than 55% prolymphocytes in blood: Evidence for prolymphocytoid transformation. Human Pathology. 2012;**43**(11):1828-1838. DOI: 10.1016/j.humpath.2012.01.003

[18] Cheng WY, Zhu YM, Cheng S, Chen YS, Shen Y. Development of B-cell prolymphocytic leukemia in a patient with splenic diffuse red pulp small B-cell lymphoma. Leukemia & Lymphoma. 2018;**59**(8):1990-1993. DOI: 10.1080/10428194.2017.1405397

[19] Cawley JC, Burns GF, Hayhoe FG. A chronic lymphoproliferative disorder with distinctive features: A distinct variant of hairy-cell leukaemia. Leukemia Research. 1980;**4**(6):547-545

[20] Wang X, Spielberger R, Huang Q. Hairy cell leukemia variant, a new entity of the WHO 2008. Journal of Clinical Oncology. 2011;**29**(36):e864-e866

[21] Matutes E, Wotherspoon A, Catovsky D. The variant form of hairy cell leukaemia. Best Practice & Research. Clinical Haematology. 2003;**16**(1):41-56. DOI: 10.1016/s1521-6926(02)00086-5

[22] Matutes E. Diagnostic and therapeutic challenges in hairy cell leukemia-variant: Where are we in 2021? Expert Review of Hematology. 2021;**14**(4):355-363. DOI: 10.1080/17474086.2021.1908121

[23] Hockley SL, Else M, Morilla A, Wotherspoon A, Dearden C, Catovsky D, et al. The prognostic impact of clinical and molecular features in hairy cell leukaemia variant and splenic marginal zone lymphoma. British Journal of Haematology. 2012;**158**(3):347-354. DOI: 10.1111/j.1365-2141.2012.09163.x

[24] Robak T. Current treatment options in hairy cell leukemia and hairy cell leukemia variant. Cancer Treatment Reviews. 2006;**32**(5):365-376. DOI: 10.1016/j.ctrv.2006.04.010

[25] Zanelli M, Ragazzi M, Valli R, Piattoni S, Alvarez De Celis MI, Farnetti E, et al. Transformation of IGHV4-34+ hairy cell leukaemia-variant with U2AF1 mutation into a clonally-related high grade B-cell lymphoma responding to immunochemotherapy. British Journal of Haematology. 2016;**173**(3):491-495. DOI: 10.1111/bjh.13627

[26] Kanellis G, Garcia-Alonso L, Camacho FI, Garcia JF, Mollejo M, Montes-Moreno S, et al. Hairy cell leukemia, blastic type: Description of spleen morphology and immunophenotype of a distinctive case. Leukemia & Lymphoma. 2011;**52**(8): 1589-1592. DOI: 10.3109/10428194.2011.575488

[27] Cessna MH, Hartung L, Tripp S, Perkins SL, Bahler DW. Hairy cell leukemia variant: Fact or fiction. American Journal of Clinical Pathology. 2005;**123**(1):132-138. DOI: 10.1309/8qytyq1clqmhq9cl

[28] Matutes E, Wotherspoon A, Brito-Babapulle V, Catovsky D. The natural history and clinico-pathological features of the variant form of hairy cell leukemia. Leukemia. 2001;**15**(1):184-186. DOI: 10.1038/sj.leu.2401999

[29] Alapat D, Coviello-Malle J, Owens R, Qu P, Barlogie B, Shaughnessy JD, et al. Diagnostic usefulness and prognostic impact of CD200 expression in lymphoid malignancies and plasma cell myeloma. American Journal of Clinical Pathology. 2012;**137**(1):93-100. DOI: 10.1309/AJCP59UORCYZEVQO

[30] Matutes E. Immunophenotyping and differential diagnosis of hairy cell leukemia. Hematology/Oncology Clinics of North America. 2006;**20**(5):1051-1063. DOI: 10.1016/j.hoc.2006.06.012

[31] Hockley SL, Morgan GJ, Leone PE, Walker BA, Morilla A, Else M, et al. High-resolution genomic profiling in hairy cell leukemia-variant compared with typical hairy cell leukemia. Leukemia. 2011;**25**(7):1189-1192

[32] Zhang R, Wu Y, Wang X, Lu X, Li Y, Li S, et al. Difference of genomic copy numbers alterations between hairy cell leukemia-variant and classical hairy cell leukemia: A pilot retrospective study in Chinese. International Journal of Medical Sciences. 2020;**17**(3):325-331. DOI: 10.7150/ijms.39307

[33] Laurini JA, Aoun P, Iqbal J, Chan W, Greiner TC. Investigation of the BRAF V600E mutation by pyrosequencing in lymphoproliferative disorders. American Journal of Clinical Pathology. 2012;**138**:877-883

[34] Tiacci E, Schiavoni G, Forconi F, Santi A, Trentin L, Ambrosetti A, et al. Simple genetic diagnosis of hairy cell leukemia by sensitive detection of the BRAF-V600E mutation. Blood. 2012;**119**(1):192-195. DOI: 10.1182/blood-2011-08-371179

[35] Tiacci E, Trifonov V, Schiavoni G, Holmes A, Kern W, Martelli MP, et al. BRAF mutations in hairy-cell leukemia. The New England Journal of Medicine. 2011;**364**(24):2305-2315. DOI: 10.1056/NEJMoa1014209

[36] Waterfall JJ, Arons E, Walker RL, Pineda M, Roth L, Killian JK, et al. High prevalence of MAP2K1 mutations in variant and IGHV4-34-expressing hairy-cell leukemias. Nature Genetics. 2014;**46**(1):8-10. DOI: 10.1038/ng.2828

[37] Dufresne SD, Felgar RE, Sargent RL, Surti U, Gollin SM, McPhail ED, et al. Defining the borders of splenic marginal zone lymphoma: A multiparameter study. Human Pathology. 2010;**41**(4):540-551. DOI: 10.1016/j.humpath.2009.09.007

[38] Shehata M, Schwarzmeier JD, Hilgarth M, Hubmann R, Duechler M, Gisslinger H. TGF-beta1 induces bone marrow reticulin fibrosis in hairy cell leukemia. The Journal of Clinical Investigation. 2004;**113**(5):676-685. DOI: 10.1172/JCI19540

[39] Yoshida T, Mihara K, Sugihara S, Arihiro K, Mino T, Sasaki N, et al. Splenectomy followed by administration of rituximab is useful to treat a patient with hairy cell leukemia-variant. Annals of Hematology. 2013;**92**(5):711-713. DOI: 10.1007/s00277-012-1612-1

[40] Kreitman RJ, Wilson W, Calvo KR, Arons E, Roth L, Sapolsky J, et al. Cladribine with immediate rituximab for the treatment of patients with variant hairy cell leukemia. Clinical Cancer Research. 2013;**19**(24):6873-6881. DOI: 10.1158/1078-0432.CCR-13-1752

[41] Kreitman RJ, Wilson WH, Bergeron K, Raggio M, Stetler-Stevenson M, FitzGerald DJ, et al. Efficacy of the anti-CD22 recombinant immunotoxin BL22 in chemotherapy-resistant hairy-cell leukemia. The New England Journal of Medicine. 2001;**345**(4):241-247. DOI: 10.1056/NEJM200107263450402

[42] Telek B, Batár P, Udvardy M. Atipusos vonásokat mutató hajas sejtes leukémiavariáns sikeres alemtuzumab-(Campath 1H) kezelése [Successful alemtuzumab treatment of a patient with atypical hairy cell leukaemia variant]. Orvosi Hetilap. 2007;**148**(38): 1805-1807. DOI: 10.1556/OH.2007.28169

[43] Troussard X, Grever MR. The revised guidelines for the diagnosis and management of hairy cell leukaemia and the hairy cell leukaemia variant. Br J Haematology. 2021;**193**(1):11-14. DOI: 10.1111/bjh.17201

[44] Turakhia S, Lanigan C, Hamadeh F, Swerdlow SH, Tubbs RR, Cook JR. Immunohistochemistry for BRAF V600E in the Differential Diagnosis of Hairy Cell Leukemia vs Other Splenic B-Cell Lymphomas. Am J Clin Pathol. 2015 Jul;**144**(1):87-93. DOI: 10.1309/AJCP5WVXJ2KTLODO. PMID: 26071465

[45] Flatley E, Chen AI, Zhao X, Jaffe ES, Dunlap JB, Pittaluga S, et al. Aberrations of MYC are a common event in B-cell prolymphocytic leukemia. American Journal of Clinical Pathology. 2014;**142**(3):347-354. DOI: 10.1309/AJCPUBHM8U7ZFLOB

[46] Cook JR, Aguilera NI, Reshmi S, Huang X, Yu Z, Gollin SM, et al. Deletion 6q is not a characteristic marker of nodal lymphoplasmacytic lymphoma. Cancer Genetics and Cytogenetics. 2005;**162**(1):85-88

Chapter 5

Testicular Lymphoma: Primary and Secondary Involvement

Alberto Artiles Medina, Javier Lorca Álvaro, Inés Laso García, César Mínguez Ojeda, Marina Mata Alcaraz, Marta Santiago González, Mariam Bajawi Carretero, Juan José Gordillo Perdomo, Victoria Gómez Dos Santos and Francisco Javier Burgos Revilla

Abstract

This chapter explores the testicular involvement of lymphoma. Testicular lymphoma may either represent secondary involvement by systemic disease or primary malignancy. Regarding primary testicular lymphoma (PTL), it is a rare form of extranodal lymphoma and the most frequent malignant testicular neoplasm in men over the age of 60 years. The diffuse large B-cell lymphoma (DLBCL) accounts for the majority of cases. The morphologic manifestation of PTL on imaging may be in the form of a localized mass or a diffuse enlargement of the testis. On ultrasonography, PTL usually appears as a hypoechoic area with hypervascularity. MRI and positron emission tomography with computed tomography (PET/CT) are useful diagnostic tools. The latter is crucial in staging and follow-up of these patients. The treatment of PTL is based on orchiectomy, chemotherapy, and radiotherapy. The prognosis is poor and PTL exhibits a propensity to relapse in the central nervous system (CNS) and in the opposite testis. Secondary involvement of the testis by non-Hodgkin lymphoma (NHL) is more frequent than PTL. Patients may develop the relapsed or refractory disease in the testis in the context of disseminated lymphomas due to the existence of the blood-testis barrier. This chapter discusses the treatment of secondary involvement by lymphoma.

Keywords: testicular lymphoma, non-Hodgkin lymphoma, testis, sanctuary sites, primary testicular lymphoma

1. Introduction

Approximately 30% of all non-Hodgkin lymphomas (NHL) arise from extranodal sites. The management of primary extranodal presentation often implies site-specific diagnostic and therapeutic strategies [1].

Testicular lymphoma often represents secondary involvement, although primary testicular lymphoma (PTL) may occur. Secondary testicular involvement is frequent in advanced NHL cases and is observed in up to 20% of patients in autopsy findings [2]. Furthermore, the testis is considered a "sanctuary" site for chemotherapy and is commonly the site of residual cancer after adequate treatment with chemotherapy [3].

IntechOpen

PTL is the most common malignant testicular neoplasm in men over sixty years. It is an aggressive and rare form of extranodal lymphoma and represents 1–2% of NHL and 1–9% of all testicular tumors [4].

2. Primary testicular lymphoma

2.1 Histological subtypes

There are several histological subtypes of PTL, such as follicular lymphoma, Burkitt's lymphoma, and diffuse large B-cell lymphoma (DLBCL). Primary DLBCL is the most common subtype of lymphoma (80%) in the adult testis, whereas most of testicular lymphomas in children consist of secondary involvement by lymphoblastic lymphoma, DLBCL, or Burkitt's lymphoma [5].

Infrequent histological subtypes in testis include mantle cell lymphoma, the extranodal natural killer–cell lymphoma, peripheral T-cell lymphoma, extranodal marginal zone lymphoma, and activin receptor-like kinase-1–negative anaplastic large cell lymphoma. **Table 1** summarizes PTL subtypes and their frequency.

Patients with HIV (human immunodeficiency virus) infection often exhibit more aggressive variants of PTL [6]. Follicular lymphoma (FL) of the testis is very uncommon and has been reported mainly in childhood.

2.2 Epidemiology

Regarding the incidence of extranodal NHLs, it is similar to other lymphomas: in countries with high NHL incidence, there is an increased incidence of extranodal disease. An important geographic variation of the distribution across the diverse anatomic sites of onset as well as the overall frequency of the extranodal presentation has been reported.

Extranodal lymphomas can derive from practically each and every organ. The published data from large series have shown bone, skin, brain, and gastrointestinal (GI) tract to be the most frequent sites of extranodal involvement. Ann Arbor staging system classifies the Waldeyer's ring and tonsils as lymphatic locations, so their designation as extranodal sites remains a controversy. However, when they are included in the extranodal lymphoma series, the neck and head are the second most frequent locations. Furthermore, the incidence of primary extranodal presentation is variable across the different B-cell histologic subtypes, including less than 10% of follicular lymphomas (FL), up to 50% of DLBCL, and the majority of Burkitt's

Subtype	Frequency (according to SEER data) [7]
Diffuse large B-cell lymphoma (DLBCL)	78.1%
DLBCL, immunoblastic variant	3.7%
Burkitt's lymphoma	1.3%
Diffuse non-Hodgkin's mixed small and large cell lymphoma	1.2%
Small lymphocytic lymphoma	0.8%
Lymphoplasmacytic lymphoma	0.6%
Mantle cell lymphoma	0.4%
Others/not specified	8.8%

Table 1.
Histological subtypes of PTL.

lymphomas (BL). The histologic subtypes can be site-specific for some localizations such as central nervous system (CNS) or testis, where the majority of cases are DLBCL. Contrarily, in the GI tract, a wide spectrum of lymphoma types can be found, including mantle cell lymphoma (MCL), marginal zone lymphoma of mucosa-associated lymphoid tissue (MALT) BL, FL, and DLBCL [1].

The annual incidence of PTL is 0.09–0.26/100,000 per year and the median age at diagnosis of PTL is 67 years old [7]. Moreover, PTL is both the most common testicular malignancy in men age > 60 years and the most frequent bilateral testicular neoplasm [6].

2.3 Risk factors and genetics

Despite the fact that there are limited data about risk factors for PTL, HIV infection is a well-known risk factor for aggressive NHL, with lymphomas in HIV-positive patients more frequently developing in extranodal sites, such as the testis.

HIV-infected patients with PTL are younger (36 years is the median age). In these patients, Burkitt-like, plasmablastic and immunoblastic histological types are more habitual [6].

With regard to genetic risk factors for lymphoma, plasmacytoid differentiation, that is shown in some cases of PTL, with somatic hypermutation of immunoglobulin heavy-chain genes (IgH) and the presence of a high rate of T-cell infiltrate, suggest that antigen-driven stimulation could be implicated, as well as in extranodal marginal zone lymphoma of mucosa-associated lymphoid tissue (eMZL of MALT).

Other characteristics usually observed in PTL that raise the possibility of an antigen-driven mechanism in their pathogenesis are a higher frequency of the loss of HLA-DR and DQ expression, along with homozygous deletions of the corresponding genes, and the frequency of HLA-DRB1–15 and HLA-DRB1–12 [8].

2.4 Clinical features

Testicular lymphoma can be the initial presentation of clinically occult disease or a primary extranodal disease. It must be considered in the differential diagnosis of a testicular mass, especially in patients over 60 years old [9].

The classic presentation consists of a painless, swollen, and hard testis or a testicular mass, without preference for either side. An associated hydrocele is found in about 40% and synchronous bilateral involvement occurs in approximately 6% of cases. Systemic B symptoms are usually present only in an advanced stage. Moreover, patients can present abdominal pain or ascites. In addition to the contralateral testis, the disease typically spreads to other extranodal sites such as the skin and subcutaneous tissue, the lungs, the bone, and mainly the CNS [1].

2.5 Diagnosis and stages

In clinical practice, ultrasonography and magnetic resonance imaging (MRI) are the most commonly used imaging modalities, which allow simultaneous evaluation of both testicles, paratesticular space, and spermatic cord.

Staging workup is the same as used for other forms of aggressive NHL. It consists of bone marrow biopsy and FDG PET/CT, with the addition of specific CNS staging with a lumbar puncture for cerebrospinal fluid analysis and cranial MRI. CNS is the most frequent metastatic location with a reported incidence of 45%. Furthermore, 64% of CNS relapses involve the brain parenchyma [10].

Stage I: Involvement of a single extralymphatic organ or site or of a single lymph node region.
Stage II: Localized involvement of an extralymphatic organ or site or involvement of two or more lymph node regions on the same side of the diaphragm.
Stage III: Involvement of lymph node regions or structures on both sides of the diaphragm.
Stage IV: Diffuse or disseminated involvement of one or more extralymphatic organs, or either: • Involvement of the liver, bone marrow, pleura or cerebrospinal fluid. • Isolated extralymphatic organ involvement without adjacent regional lymph node involvement, but with the disease in distant sites.
Additional sub staging variables include: • **A:** Asymptomatic • **B:** Presence of B symptoms (including fever, night sweats, and weight loss of ≥10% of body weight over 6 months.) • **E**: Involvement of a single, extranodal site, contiguous or proximal to a known nodal site (stages I to III only; additional extranodal involvement is stage IV). • **S**: Splenic involvement. • **X:** Bulky nodal disease: nodal mass > 1/3 of intrathoracic diameter or 10 cm in dimension.

Table 2.
Ann-Arbor staging system used in PTL.

The Ann Arbor staging system is the most widely utilized for lymphoma staging, for both HL and NHL. It is named after the town of Ann Arbor in the US state of Michigan where the Committee on Hodgkin's Disease Staging Classification met in 1971 to agree on it. It updated and replaced the earlier Rye staging system (**Table 2**) [11].

The disease is limited to the testis (stage IE) in the majority of patients and nearly 20% of patients have stage II disease. Disseminated disease is rare. A stage IV testicular lymphoma is virtually indistinguishable from a nodal one with testicular involvement [1].

2.5.1 Ultrasound scan

Scrotal ultrasound is useful to confirm the diagnosis of a solid intratesticular tumor, but it does not provide sufficiently reliable information to precisely determine the T stage: whether the tunica albuginea, tunica vaginalis, epididymis, or spermatic cord are affected [12].

Generally, ultrasonography demonstrates focal or diffuse areas of hypoechogenicity with hypervascularity in an enlarged testis. MRI allows detailed evaluation of both testes, paratesticular spaces, and spermatic cord [6].

In the series of Bertolotto et al., these authors described a group of 43 patients with pathologically proven testicular lymphoma investigated with grayscale and Doppler ultrasound scan. Doppler ultrasound findings confirmed that testicular lymphomas present as hypoechoic lesions of the testis, either focal or diffuse, predominantly with a hypervascular appearance. In 72% of cases, normal testicular vessels traversing the lesion can be found. This sonographic feature is only indicative of the infiltrative nature of the pathologic process, but it is not specific for lymphoma, because it has been reported in other infiltrative neoplasms, such as plasmacytoma and leukemia infiltration. On the other hand, non-neoplastic disorders and other inflammatory diseases, such as chronic granulomatous orchitis, may present as hypervascularity of the entire testis or a striated pattern, decreased echogenicity, diffuse enlargement, or multifocal hypoechoic hypervascular lesions,

DOI: http://dx.doi.org/10.5772/intechopen.101505

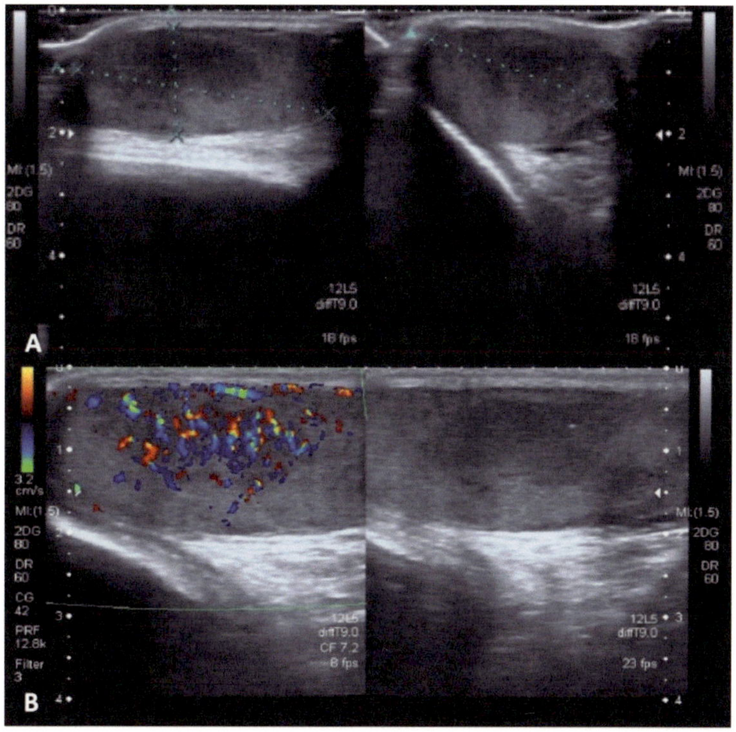

Figure 1.
Testicular ultrasound scan of a patient with suspected testicular lymphoma showing an enlarged right testicle (11 cc) with heterogeneous echogenicity, with poorly defined hypoechoic areas (A). The Doppler study (B) shows increased vascularity of the testicular parenchyma.

identical to the grayscale and Doppler sonographic characteristics of lymphoma. An accurate interpretation of these findings could be difficult if clinical features of inflammation are absent. In these cases, biopsy should be considered, and often orchidectomy is performed to establish the final diagnosis (**Figure 1**) [13].

2.5.2 Magnetic resonance imaging

MRI of the testes seems to be more accurate than ultrasound for detecting involvement of the tunica albuginea, the epididymis and the spermatic cord (**Figures 2** and **3**) [12].

2.5.3 PET/CT

PET/CT and bone marrow biopsy, along with the specific CNS staging (lumbar puncture for cerebrospinal fluid analysis by cytology and flow cytometry and brain MRI) are used at the initial staging of patients with PTL [6].

Nowadays, PET with glucose analog 18F-fluorodeoxyglucose (18F-FDG) is the most commonly used imaging modality for evaluating tumor metabolism. PTL usually shows increased 18F-FDG uptake. Despite the growing use in clinical practice of FDG PET/CT, its role in PTL has neither been clearly defined (**Figures 4** and **5**) [10].

2.5.4 Bone marrow biopsy and lumbar puncture

Because of the high tendency of PTL to disseminate to particular extranodal sites, some specific diagnostic procedures are required for complete staging. The

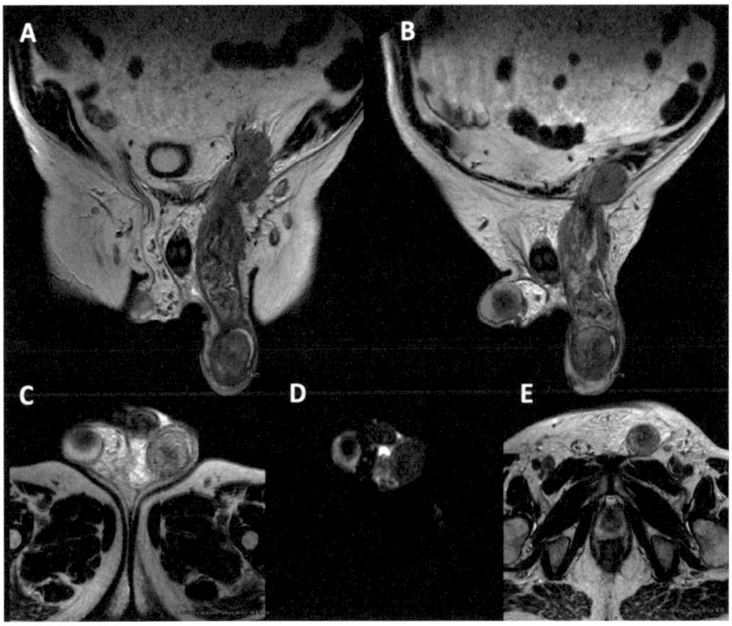

Figure 2.
Coronal and axial MRI in a patient with diffuse large cell lymphoma B (activated phenotype). The images show thickening of the left spermatic cord from its intra-abdominal segment to the interior of the scrotum, with involvement of the epididymis and testis (A and B). The right testis shows a low signal, hyper-uptake lesion, 3 cm in size (C-E).

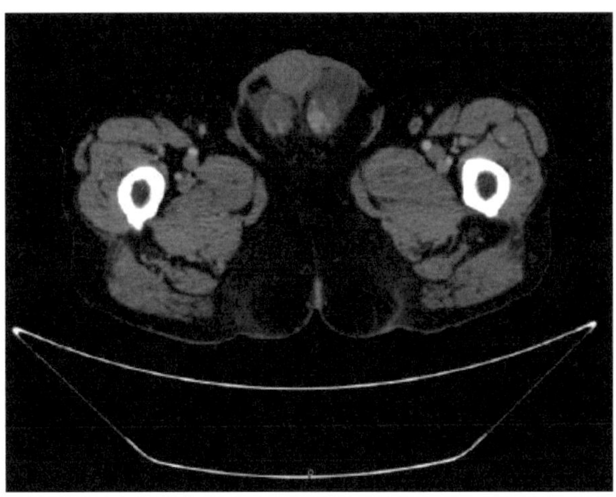

Figure 3.
An axial MRI image shows a testicular nodule in a patient with generalized lymphadenopathy.

presence of pulmonary mass, pleural effusion, skin, or Waldayer's ring lesions needs histological confirmation.

An accurate examination of the skin is recommended due to the association of PTL with cutaneous "leg-type DLBCL" and testicular DLBCL. Additionally, skin is a frequent site of extranodal relapse of PTL, especially in HIV-positive patients.

Lumbar puncture with cytological and flow cytometric analysis on CSF is mandatory to exclude CNS involvement. Benevolo et al. conducted a study comparing the diagnostic and prognostic value of conventional cytological (CC) examination and flow cytometry (FCM) of a base-line sample of cerebrospinal fluid in 174

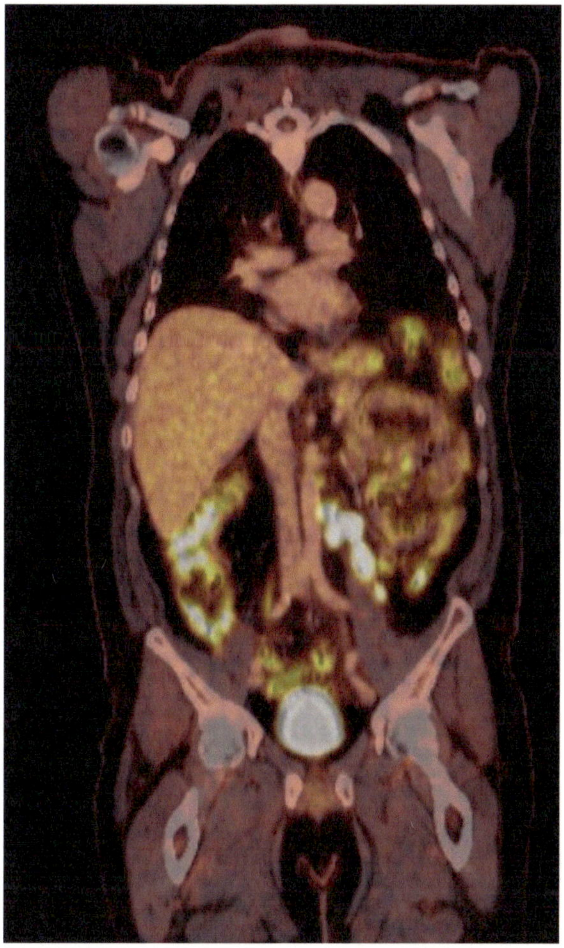

Figure 4.
PET/CT in a patient diagnosed with a PTL (diffuse large B-cell lymphoma). Numerous hypermetabolic left paraaortic lymphadenopathy (16 mm and SUVmax: 18), located in the anterior aspect of the psoas.

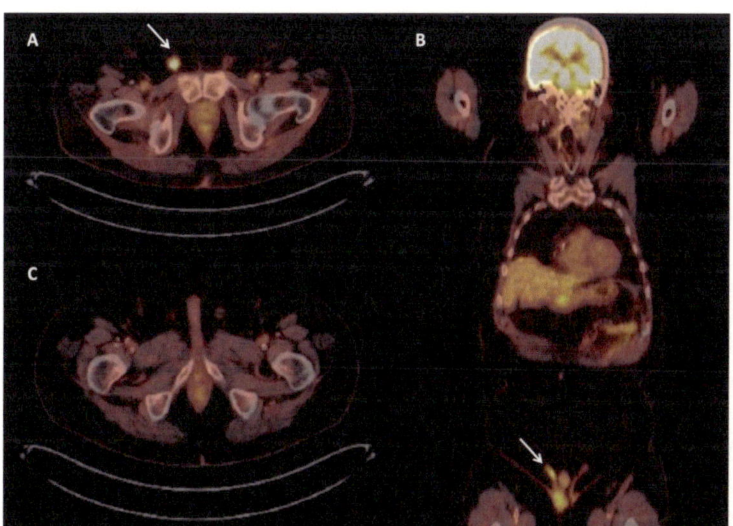

Figure 5.
Burkitt's lymphoma relapse in the testicle. Radiotracer uptake is observed in the right inguinal canal (arrow, A and B). The last image (C) corresponds to the control PET/CT after right orchiectomy.

patients with aggressive NHL. The results showed a significantly higher risk of CNS progression in patients with FCM-positive and CC-negative patients, compared to patients who are both FCM- and CC-negative. Therefore, FCM is a highly sensitive test to rule out CNS involvement, and it should be recommended in all NHL patients at high risk of CNS relapse, including testicular lymphoma. Moreover, HIV serology should be checked in all cases, because testicular lymphoma is more frequent in HIV-positive patients [8].

2.6 Differential diagnosis

Bacterial epididymal-orchitis, primary testicular tumors, testicular infarction, and genitourinary tuberculosis must be considered in the differential diagnosis of PTL. Several germ cell tumors, such as classic seminoma, spermatocytic seminoma, and embryonal carcinoma, should be included in the differential diagnosis of primary testicular DLBCL. Granulomatous and viral orchitis can also mimic lymphoma. Unlike the majority of lymphoma cells, seminoma cells have a distinctive histologic pattern, including rounded but focally flattened central nuclei, glycogen-rich cytoplasms, and distinct cell membranes. The cells of spermatocytes seminoma are polymorphous and they can be divided into three types. Embryonal carcinoma has a classic epithelioid appearance that usually forms papillary, tubular, or glandular structures. Lymphomas usually consist of smaller cells with a higher nucleo-cytoplasmic ratio. Furthermore, these neoplasms exhibit diffuse intertubular infiltration with recognizable tubular remnants. This characteristic intertubular growth pattern of lymphoma is initially suggestive of the diagnosis in numerous cases. Contrary to seminoma and embryonal carcinoma, lymphomas lack precursor intratubular germ cell neoplasia. Viral and granulomatous orchitis have heterogeneous and benign-appearing inflammatory cellular infiltrates, in contrast to the more homogeneous and malignant-appearing infiltrate of lymphoma [5].

2.7 The role of testicular biopsy

The diagnosis of primary testicular lymphoma is often confirmed through orchiectomy or testis biopsy [14]. Over the past decades, there has been a trend towards primary orchidectomy [15].

Coad et al. found needle biopsy to be a safe and simple method of examining the testes of patients with acute leukemia and non-Hodgkin's lymphoma. The procedure is quickly carried out under a short general anesthetic on an outpatient basis. Only one out of 102 cases provided insufficient material for histological examination. Using needle biopsy, a good correlation between clinical assessment and histological appearance was found. Out of 70 clinically normal testes, in 6 (8.5%) cases testicular infiltration was detected [16].

2.8 Pathology

According to prior work, lymphoma can infiltrate the epididymis and spermatic cord. The macroscopic observations showed that the cut surface of the tumor is usually solid, and testicular masses measures around 5.5 cm (range: 2.5–9 cm). Regarding macroscopic tumor appearance, they were gray or gray-red in color, tender, and spongy, and had clear boundaries [17].

The large majority of PTLs (80–98%) are DLBCLs, although patients with HIV infection commonly present with more aggressive variants. B-cell markers, such as CD19, CD20, CD79a, and PAX5 are typically expressed by DLBCL-type PTL. Bcl-2 protein is expressed in 70% of cases, but Bcl-6 is rarely positive.

The median MIB1 proliferative index is 40%, and in the non-HIV population, Epstein–Barr virus is usually negative (**Figure 6**) [6].

2.9 Treatment

The treatment of primary testicular lymphoma is based on orchiectomy, chemotherapy, and occasionally radiotherapy, but there is not a standardized regimen. It is an extremely aggressive neoplasm with poor progression-free survival and overall survival [14]. A study from the International Extranodal Lymphoma Study Group (IELSG) has reported that R-CHOP chemoimmunotherapy with intrathecal methotrexate prophylaxis and radiotherapy to the contralateral testis could reduce CNS relapse (6%) [18].

Orchiectomy is usually required for the pathological diagnosis and its removal avoids the potential chemotherapy "sanctuary" site as a consequence of the blood-testis barrier.

In the largest series of patients with testicular lymphoma, the IELSG observed a 10- and 5-year incidence of CNS relapse of 35% and 20%, respectively. Therefore, CSF cytology should be included in the staging. Nevertheless, the pattern of CNS involvement is characterized by parenchymal involvement and late relapses. This contrasts with primary nodal DLBCL, in which the CNS relapse rate is lower (approximately 5%) and relapses are common of early-onset and leptomeningeal presentation.

Testicular lymphomas are very aggressive malignancies, with a poor outcome. Indeed, in spite of initial chemoradiation (CR), patients with stage I-II disease

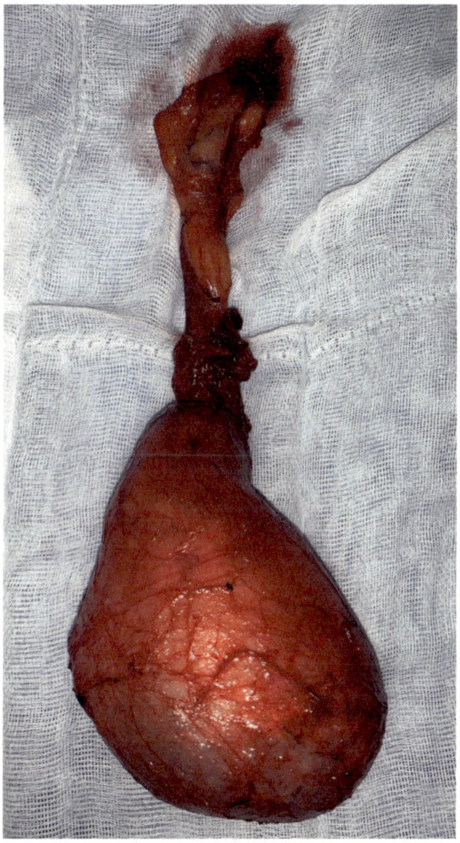

Figure 6.
Macroscopic findings in a surgical specimen (orchiectomy) of PTL.

frequently relapse. The large retrospective IELSG series, that enrolled 373 patients, reported a 10- and 5-year OS rate of 27% and 48%, respectively. The OS and PFS survival curves showed no clear evidence of plateau, suggesting no cure for these patients, including those with stage I-II disease. The majority of patients did not receive CNS prophylactic chemotherapy, but in patients who received anthracycline-based chemotherapy plus intrathecal prophylaxis and scrotal irradiation, a reduction of the risk of progression by administering CNS prophylaxis was observed (5-year PFS, 72%). IELSG-10 phase II trial showed that combined treatment with six cycles of R-CHOP-21, intrathecal MTX, and contralateral testis irradiation was associated with better outcomes in stage I-IIE disease (5-year PFS and OS rates were 74% and 85%, respectively). Moreover, radiation therapy reduced the risk of contralateral testis relapse.

According to the guidelines for the treatment of advanced stage nodal DLBCL, patients with disseminated PTL should be treated with the addition of prophylactic scrotal radiotherapy and intrathecal chemotherapy. Routine CNS prophylaxis is recommended in testis lymphoma of any stage because of the high rate of CNS relapse (**Figure 7**) [1].

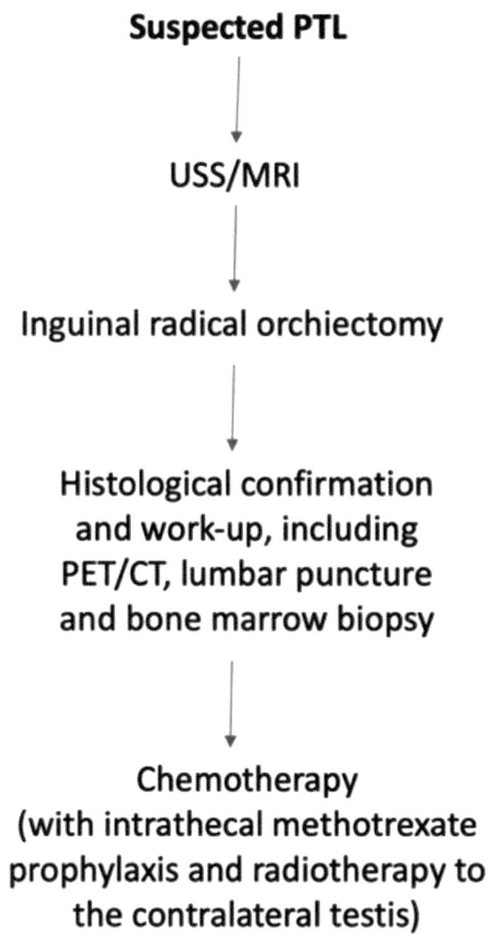

Figure 7.
Diagnostic algorithm and treatment of the PTL. USS, Ultrasound scan; MRI, Magnetic resonance imaging.

2.10 Prognosis

Historically, PTL has been associated with poor prognosis with an overall 5-year survival rate ranging from 17 to 48%, mainly primary testicular DLBCL, which is a very aggressive neoplasm with a clear tendency to spread to the skin and the CNS at presentation and relapse [5].

Testicular lymphoma has been reported to have a poor prognosis compared to other extranodal lymphomas and NHL and may need a more prolonged course of chemotherapy. Pathologic grading and stage are the main predictive factors for outcome. Early-stage and younger age, which are part of the International Prognostic Index (IPI), have been shown to be independent prognostic factors affecting the overall and disease-free survival (**Table 3**) [19].

3. Secondary involvement of the testis

3.1 Testicular involvement at diagnosis or relapse

Three types of presentation of testicular lymphoma have been documented:

- Primary extranodal: very rare, most cases are primary testicular DLBCLs.
- Extranodal relapse after chemotherapy: usually in aggressive lymphomas, such as Burkitt. The testicle is a "sanctuary organ" thanks to the blood-gonad barrier, which inhibits the accumulation of chemotherapeutic agents. This phenomenon has been described most frequently in children with acute lymphoblastic leukemia; however, it has also been documented in patients with lymphomas.
- The primary manifestation of unknown systemic disease [20].

>1 extranodal site
Adverse prognostic factors for PFS in studies of PTL
Age > 70 years
Advanced stage
ECOG performance status >1
B symptoms
Hypoalbuminemia
Involvement of extranodal sites other than testis
Involvement of the left testis
Raised serum LDH
Raised serum β2-microglobulin
Tumor diameter > 10 cm

Table 3.
Prognostic factors for PFS identified in PTL [6]. ECOG, eastern cooperative oncology group; LDH, lactate dehydrogenase.

Overall, secondary involvement of the testis by NHL is more common than primary extranodal disease [19].

3.2 Testicles as "sanctuary sites" for chemotherapy

The testis is an immunologically privileged site. The blood-testis barrier interferes with the delivery of chemotherapeutic agents, making the testicle a potential site for relapse or residual disease.

Testicular relapse of leukemia and lymphoma is a well-recognized phenomenon: testicular relapse of lymphoma is more frequent in the adult population, whereas leukemia relapse is most commonly seen in the pediatric population. With the advent of F-18 fluoro-2-deoxyglucose (FDG) positron emission tomography (PET) in the evaluation of lymphoma, it is possible to detect PTL or testicular relapse on the FDG-PET examination. Testicular relapse of NHL detected on FDG-PET has been reported previously. Prior studies have examined normal standardized uptake value maximum (SUVmax) values in the testicle, with normal values ranging from 2.81 (30–39 years) to 2.18 (80–89 years), depending upon age. Elevated activity in one testicle or lateralizing activity should be deemed suspicious, and etiologies can include primary testicular tumor, primary or secondary testicular lymphoma, and metastatic disease with other etiologies less likely.

Autopsy findings have demonstrated testicular involvement is identified in 64.3% of male patients with acute leukemia, in 22.4% of male patients with chronic leukemia, and in 18.6% of patients with lymphosarcoma (NHL) [21].

3.3 Management of residual testicular disease

Lymphoma and leukemia are the predominant secondary tumors of the testis. Acute lymphoblastic leukemia (ALL) is a frequent cause of prepuberal testicular mass. Indeed, microscopic involvement of the testis has been found in autopsy in 66% of patients with ALL.

The management of testicular lymphoma and leukemia relapses is similar. The finding of a palpable mass on physical examination in a patient with recently diagnosed lymphoma or leukemia should prompt a scrotal ultrasound scan. This commonly demonstrates a homogeneous hypoechoic mass.

Currently, literature discourages testicular biopsy in patients before initiating chemotherapy as no survival benefit has been reported. However, a patient with new or persistent enlarged testis undergoing chemotherapy, especially in leukemia, could imply a relapse while on therapy. This scenario should prompt a biopsy to guide therapeutic decisions. In this case, additional chemotherapy is typically needed to eradicate the residual disease in "sanctuary" sites and possible systemic disease, as well as radiation to the affected testis.

In 25% of cases, testicular lymphoma is a manifestation of widespread systemic involvement, another 25% present with Ann Arbor stage II disease and the remaining 50% have disease confined to the testis (Ann Arbor I) [22].

If residual tumor within the gonad after chemotherapy persists, delayed orchiectomy should be considered, because the blood-testis barrier limits anticancer drug penetration [3].

For example, in the management of testicular relapse of BL, radical orchiectomy is indicated in cases in which the testicle has been completely replaced by a tumor, or is persistent after chemotherapy. Additionally, this procedure can be beneficial in tissue diagnosis and staging (**Figure 8**) [23].

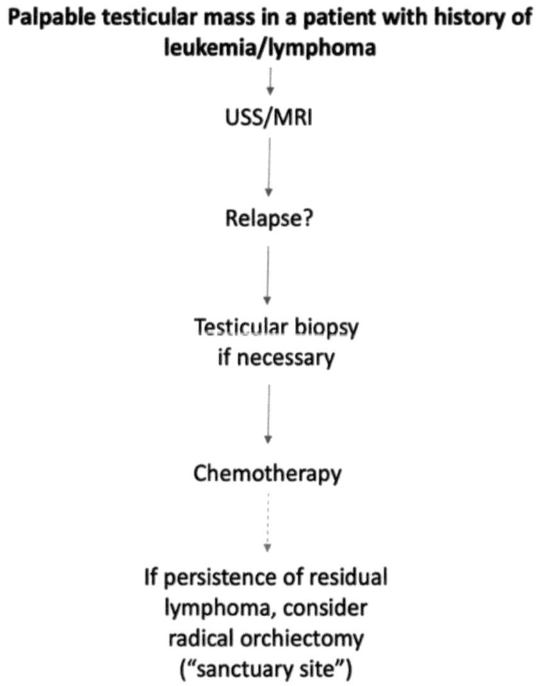

Figure 8.
Management of suspected testicular relapse in systemic lymphoma.

4. Conclusions

Testicular lymphoma is the most common testicular tumor in patients over the age of 60 years. The clinical and radiologic features of PTL should be known because it is the most common secondary testicular cancer. A painless, swollen, and hard testis or a testicular mass are the most common presenting signs and symptoms of PTL. The imaging studies used to diagnose and evaluate the stage of PTL are ultrasonography, MRI, and PET/CT. After diagnosis of PTL, lumbar puncture for cerebrospinal fluid analysis and brain MRI provide information regarding CNS staging.

PTL may mimic germ cell tumors and other diseases, such as orchiepididymitis or testicular tuberculosis. The treatment includes radical orchiectomy, chemotherapy, and occasionally radiotherapy, although there is not a well-established regimen. PTL is an extremely aggressive neoplasm with poor progression-free survival and overall survival. According to the results from the study by IELSG, the recommended therapeutic strategy of primary testicular DLBCL should include R-CHOP chemoimmunotherapy with intrathecal methotrexate prophylaxis and radiotherapy to the contralateral testis in order to reduce the risk of CNS and testicular relapses.

Regarding secondary involvement of the testis, testicular relapse of leukemia and lymphoma usually occur due to the existence of a blood-testis barrier. If residual tumor within the testis after an adequate course of chemotherapy persists, delayed orchiectomy should be considered.

Conflict of interest

The authors declare no conflict of interest.

Author details

Alberto Artiles Medina[1*], Javier Lorca Álvaro[1], Inés Laso García[1], César Mínguez Ojeda[1], Marina Mata Alcaraz[1], Marta Santiago González[1], Mariam Bajawi Carretero[2], Juan José Gordillo Perdomo[3], Victoria Gómez Dos Santos[1] and Francisco Javier Burgos Revilla[1]

1 Urology Department, Ramón y Cajal University Hospital, Alcalá University, IRYCIS, Madrid, Spain

2 General and Digestive Surgery Department, Ramón y Cajal University Hospital, Alcalá University, Madrid, Spain

3 Clinical Analysis Department, Dr. Negrín University Hospital, Las Palmas de Gran Canaria, Spain

*Address all correspondence to: alberc.artiles@gmail.com

References

[1] Vannata B, Zucca E. Primary extranodal B-cell lymphoma: Current concepts and treatment strategies. Chinese Clinical Oncology. 2015;**4**(1): 10-10

[2] Bhatia K, Vaid AK, Gupta S, Doval DC, Talwar V. Primary testicular non-Hodgkin's lymphoma: A review article. São Paulo Medical Journal. 2007;**125**(5):286-288

[3] Dave DS, Leppert JT, Rajfer J. Is the Testis a Chemo-privileged site? Is there a blood-testis barrier? Revista de Urología. 2007;**9**(1):28

[4] Artiles Medina A, Lorca Álvaro J, Carretero Barrio I, García-Cosío M, Burgos Revilla FJ. Primary testicular lymphoma. Medicina Clínica Práctica. 2021;**4**:3

[5] Kim H-S. Primary testicular diffuse large B-cell lymphoma: A case report focusing on touch imprint cytology and a non-germinal center B-cell-like phenotype. Experimental and Therapeutic Medicine. 2013;**6**(1):33-36

[6] Cheah CY, Wirth A, Seymour JF. Primary testicular lymphoma. Blood. 2014;**123**(4):486-493

[7] Xu H, Yao F. Primary testicular lymphoma: A SEER analysis of 1,169 cases. Oncology Letters. 2019;**17**(3): 3113-3124

[8] Castellino A, Vitolo U. DLBCL in unusual locations. The management and treatment of primary testicular lymphoma. 19th Congress of the European Hematology Association. Hematology Education: the education program for the annual congress of the European Hematology Association. 2014;**8**:123-132

[9] Chen WJ, Kuo JY, Lin CC, Chung HJ, Huang WJS, Wu HHH, et al. Primary testicular lymphoma—A single center experience and review of literature. Urological Science. 2016;**27**(2):96-100

[10] Okuyucu K, İnce S, Alagöz E, Ataş E, Arslan N. Utility of FDG PET/ CT in the management of primary testicular Lymphoma. Molecular Imaging and Radionuclide Therapy. 2018;**27**(2):61

[11] Ann Arbor staging system | Radiology Reference Radiopaedia.org. Available from: https://radiopaedia.org/articles/ann-arbor-staging-system

[12] Brunereau L, Bruyère F, Linassier C, Baulieu JL. The role of imaging in staging and monitoring testicular cancer. Diagnostic and Interventional Imaging. 2012;**93**(4):310-318

[13] Bertolotto M, Derchi LE, Secil M, Dogra V, Sidhu PS, Clements R, et al. Grayscale and color Doppler features of testicular Lymphoma. Journal of Ultrasound in Medicine. 2015;**34**(6):1139

[14] Chen B, Cao DH, Lai L, Guo JB, Chen ZY, Huang Y, et al. Adult primary testicular lymphoma: clinical features and survival in a series of patients treated at a high-volume institution in China. BMC Cancer. 2020;**20**(1):220

[15] Shaida N, Berman LH. Percutaneous testicular biopsy for indeterminate testicular lesions. The British Journal of Radiology. 2012;**85**(SPEC. ISSUE 1):S54

[16] Coad N, Oakhill A, Cameron A, Gornall P, Mann J. Needle biopsy of the testes in boys with leukaemia and non-Hodgkin's lymphoma. European Paediatric Haematology and Oncology; 2009;**2**(1):183-188

[17] Wang Q, Zheng D, Chai D, Wu S, Wang X, Chen S, et al. Primary testicular diffuse large B-cell lymphoma: Case series. Medicine (Baltimore). 2020;**99**(12):e19463

[18] Kim J, Yoon DH, Park I, Kim S, Park JS, Lee SW, et al. Treatment of primary testicular diffuse large B cell lymphoma without prophylactic intrathecal chemotherapy: A single center experience. Blood Research. 2014;**49**(3):170-176

[19] Lantz AG, Power N, Hutton B, Gupta R. Malignant lymphoma of the testis: A study of 12 cases. Canadian Urological Association Journal. 2009;**3**(5):393

[20] Singh C, Sierra D. Testicular Lymphoma: Case series. Findings in ultrasound mode B, color and spectral Doppler. Rev. Colomb. Radiol. 2020;**31**(3):5403-7

[21] Scotti SD, Laudadio J. Testicular relapse of non-Hodgkin Lymphoma noted on FDG-PET. Journal of Radiology Case Reports. 2009;**3**(8):18

[22] Coran AG, Caldamone A, Adzick NS, Krummel TM, Laberge J-M, Shamberger R. Pediatric Surgery. Seventh ed. Philadelphia: Elsevier Saunders; 2012. Vol. 1. p. 553

[23] Kwon YS, Munshi F, Patel NR, Serei V, Patel N, Drachtman RA, et al. An isolated testicular relapse of Burkitt's Lymphoma. Glob Pediatr Health; 2019;**6**

Chapter 6

Hydroa Vacciniforme-Like Cutaneous T-Cell Lymphoma

Carmen Ximena Gallegos Riofrio and Juan Daniel Garzon Gallegos

Abstract

Hydroa vacciniforme (HV)-like cutaneous T-cell lymphoma (HVLL) is a controversial skin pathology because some cases appear as hydroa vacciniforme, whereas others progress to cutaneous T-cell lymphoma with or without angiocentricity. It is usually associated with infections of Epstein Barr viruses and NK-cell lymphomas and typically affects the pediatric population. Symptoms include facial edema, papules, vesicles, and blisters in the facial region, arms, legs, and areas exposed to sunlight that leave varioliform scars. There may be infiltration of the lips, eyelids, and nose, usually accompanied by comorbid infections and hypersensitivity to insect bites. Frequency is rare, but HVLL more commonly affects patients from South America and Asia. Its clinical management can be difficult and accompanied by a high index of malignancy, thus early diagnosis is essential for effective and timely management.

Keywords: hydroa vacciniforme, T-cell cutaneous lymphoma, angiocentric lymphoma, nasal-type NK lymphoma, varioliform scars

1. Introduction

Hydroa vacciniforme-like lymphoma (HVLL) has an uncommon presentation that appears in young patients, especially those of Asiatic or indigenous race. It mimics the clinical profile of hydroa vacciniforme (HV) belonging to a special subtype of T-cell cutaneous lymphoma characterized by extreme photosensitivity with appearance of vesicles in the facial region that leave varioliform scars.

Several authors have studied this pathology in depth and despite presenting a great diagnostic difficulty due to nonspecific clinical findings and histopathology, it has been concluded with the help of immunohistochemistry that HVLL corresponds to a true T-cell lymphoma with its own characteristics that is very difficult to recognize and requires effective treatment to avoid fatal results since it can demonstrate high lethality.

2. Discussion

In 1995, Ruiz Maldonado et al. described an entity called "edematous scarring vasculitic panniculitis" in pediatric patients. It resembled hydroa vacciniforme (HV) clinically, but the researchers considered it more of a malignant evolution [1].

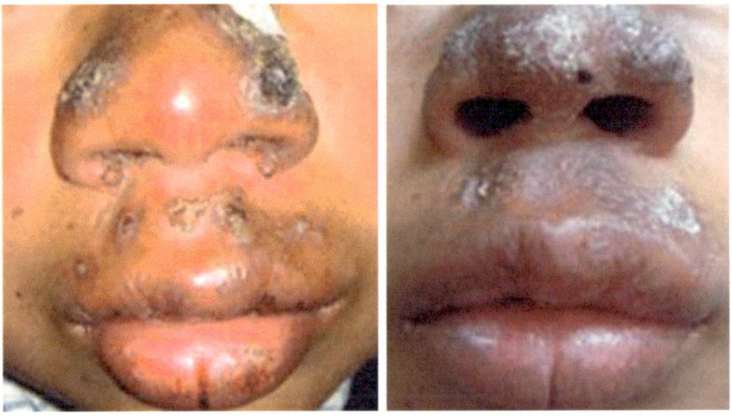

Figure 1.
Edematous and infiltrating ulcerocostrous lesions on the lip and nasal pyramid.

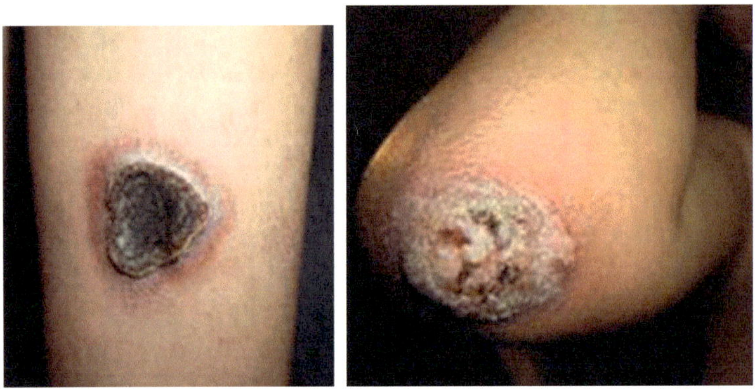

Figure 2.
Ulcerative plate covered with necrotic crust and erythematous halo on the forearm and ulcerative keratotic plate on the elbow.

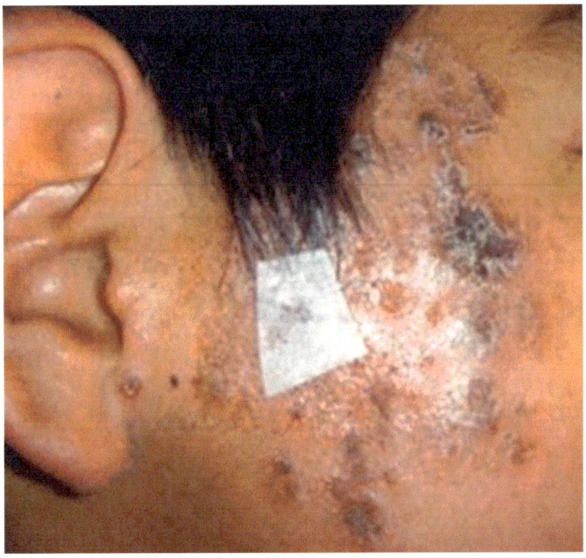

Figure 3.
Eroded and crusty lesions on cheeks.

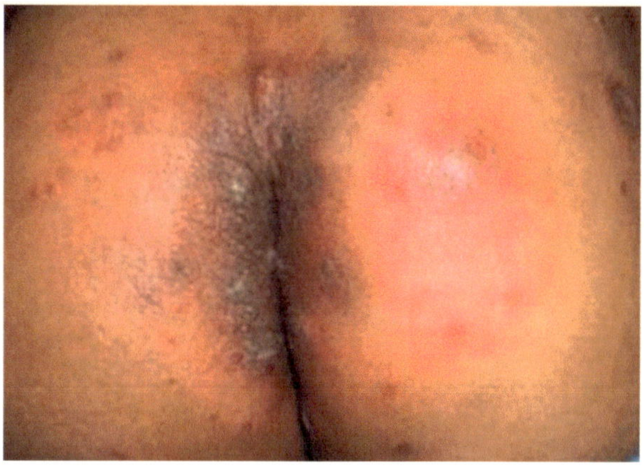

Figure 4.
Ulcerated and suppurative nodules on the buttocks.

Those who suffer from this dermatosis manifest facial edema and recurrent outbreaks of papules, infiltrate and erythematous nodules, vesicles, blisters, ulcers, skin necrosis, and scabs that leave varioliform scars (**Figures 1–4**). These injuries occur on the face, back of the hands, arms, and legs, in areas both exposed and not exposed to sunlight. These injuries are accompanied by fever, asthenia, weight loss, hepatosplenomegaly, lymphadenopathy, and increased lactate dehydrogenase (LDH) level. High fever has been associated with hypersensitivity to insect bites [2–4]. At present, HVLL is considered within the spectrum of lymphoproliferative disorders (LPDs) of Epstein-Barr virus (EBV)–positive T cells in childhood [5]. Accumulating evidence indicates that these skin disorders could be of the T-cell/natural killer (NK)-type [2, 6, 7], are difficult to diagnose, and have a high rate of malignancy and resistance to chemotherapeutic agents (**Table 1**) [5, 8–12]. HVLL is a rare EBV+ NK variant/T-cell lymphoma, most seen in Central and South America. The illness shows a predilection for young adults and children. Often the disease runs a long course leading to an aggressive phase (concurrent infections and diseases). Histologically, an atypical small-to-medium-sized lymphocyte infiltrate with nuclei-dense chromatin and/or central necrosis is observed, especially of T cells throughout the skin. Exocytosis, necrotic epidermis (**Figures 5–7**), and lobular or septal panniculitis and vasculitis, usually with angiocentricity, are also present. On occasion, numerous reactive cells such as eosinophils, plasma cells, and histiocytes. It may be associated with pseudoepitheliomatous hyperplasia [13].

Although differential diagnosis may be difficult, cutaneous NK-cell lymphoma, mycosis fungoides (MF), subcutaneous panniculitis-like T-cell lymphoma, precursor T-cell lymphoblastic lymphoma, peripheral T-cell lymphoma, and cutaneous anaplastic lymphoma of large cells should be considered. HVLL can be confused with leishmaniasis, syphilis, tuberculosis, paracoccidioidomycosis, and other deep mycoses such as rhinosporidiosis or mucormycosis. It is important to differentiate it from hepatocutaneous porphyrias, erythropoietic protoporphyria, light polymorphic eruption, actinic prurigo, and lupus erythematosus (**Table 2**) [14].

The 2016 revision of the World Health Organization classification of lymphoid neoplasms is used to diagnose lymphomas (**Table 1**) [3, 15]. In lymphomas derived from T and NK cells, major modifications in classification continues to be a challenge. Anaplastic large cell lymphoma (ALCL) negative can already be reliably differentiated from other CD30-positive T lymphomas; genetic studies allow viewing of prognostic heterogeneity and category lymphoma—the TP63 mutation being notable for its bad outcome and rearrangement of 6p25 for its best forecast. Primary

Classic presentations	Mycosis fungoides Sézary syndrome
Lymphoproliferative disorders	Childhood EBV1 T-cell systemic lymphoma Hydroa vacciniforme (HV) lymphoproliferative disorder
Rare and aggressive forms	Adult T-cell leukemia/lymphoma Nasal-type extranodal T/NK cell lymphoma
Lymphomas associated with gastrointestinal pathology	T-cell lymphoma-associated enteropathy Monomorphic intestinal epitheliotropic T-cell lymphoma Indolent T-cell lymphoproliferative disorders of the gastrointestinal tract Hepatosplenic T-cell lymphoma
Panniculitis	Subcutaneous T-cell lymphoma resembling panniculitis
Others	Primary cutaneous CD301 T-cell lymphoproliferative disorders Lymphomatoid papulosis Primary cutaneous anaplastic large cell lymphoma Primary cutaneous gd T-cell lymphoma Cutaneous epidermal primal cytoplasmic T lymphoma CD81 Primary cutaneous CD81 T-cell lymphoma Primary cutaneous lymphoproliferative disorder of CD41 T lymphocytes Peripheral T-cell lymphoma NOS Angioimmunoblastic T-cell lymphoma Follicular T-cell lymphoma Peripheral T-cell lymphoma with TFH phenotype Anaplastic large cell lymphoma, ALK1 Anaplastic large cell lymphoma, ALK2

Table 1.
Classification of mature, histiocytic, and dendritic lymphoid neoplasms (WHO, 2016 revision).

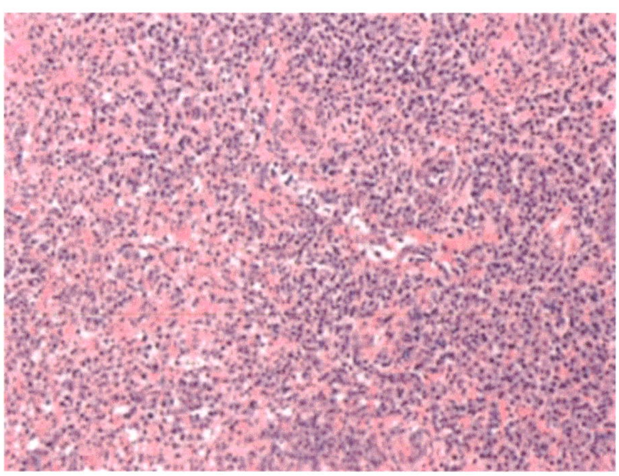

Figure 5.
Atypical lymphoid infiltrate.

cutaneous lymphomas correspond to a heterogeneous group of lymphocytic neoplasms with characteristic clinical, histological, immunophenotypic, and specific genetics [16]. Cutaneous T-cell lymphoma is recognized as a neoplastic process with clonal malignant T cells leading to regional and sometimes visceral lymph node metastasis [17, 18].

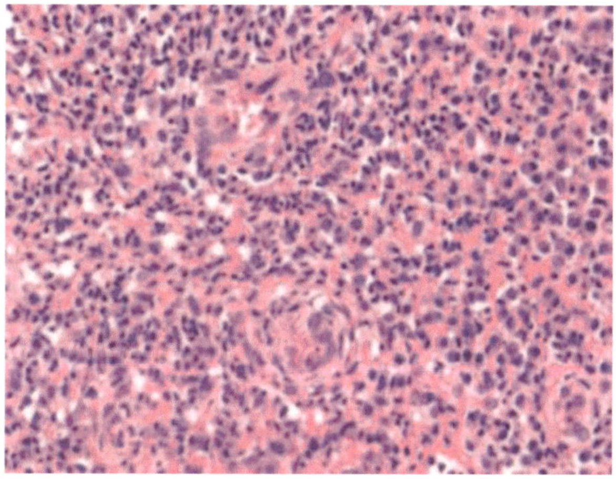

Figure 6.
Abundant infiltration of malignant atypical lymphocytes.

A often originate from CD4+ T cells, such as mycosis fungoides (MF), generally indolent in the behavior, [18, 19] and Sézary syndrome (SS), an aggressive variant; comprise about 53% of all cutaneous lymphomas. MF almost always affects older people, with a median age at diagnosis of 55–60 years old and a male-to-female ratio of 2:1. However, it can also be seen in populations of younger people, including children. Most patients (70%) are white, with Blacks, Hispanics, and Asians representing 14%, 9%, and 7% of MF cases in the United States, respectively [3].

Sometimes rarer forms of cutaneous lymphomas, such as HVLL, can disfigure anatomical structures and cause secondary infections if there are ulcers. The lesions have a complex immune environment; recent clinical data suggest that the presence of CD8+ T cells may be correlated with a better prognosis, whereas detection of macrophages is associated with a poor prognosis [20, 21].

Given advances in tumor biology, changes have been made to many of the lymphoma classification categories [3]. In the *International Classification of Diseases, 10th Revision* (ICD-10), codes C81–C96 categorize malignant neoplasms of lymphoid, hematopoietic and related tissue [22]. Nasal-type extranodal NK/T lymphomas are a rare aggressive form of primary cutaneous lymphoma that show strong expression of CD56 and cytotoxic proteins such as perforin, granzyme B, or TIA-1. The TCR/CD3 complex is not expressed on the surface. The episodic episomal presence of EBV is typically found. Angiocentric and angiodestructive growth is observed, resulting in necrosis and ulceration. Mitoses are common. In a Peruvian series of 16 patients, 10 died in an average of 11.6 months. There are few current reports on cutaneous EBV+ NK/lymphoid T-cell proliferations that are phenotypically different or clinically unusual, both in classic NK-/T-cell lymphoma as in the nasal type and in HVLL, suggesting that the spectrum of these conditions could be broader [13, 23].

Most cases have a CD81 T-cell lymphocyte phenotype; a small proportion of cases have an NK-cell phenotype. Only rare cases of CD41 T cells have been described. Lymphoid cells are positive for cytotoxic markers such as granzyme B and T-cell intracellular antigen 1 (TIA-1); CD30 expression is found in some reported cases [2, 24].

Since the incorporation of HVLL into the WHO's classification of lymphomas, some controversies have arisen that have yet to be clarified. It is not known whether HVLL represents a true lymphoma or a preneoplastic disorder with risk of

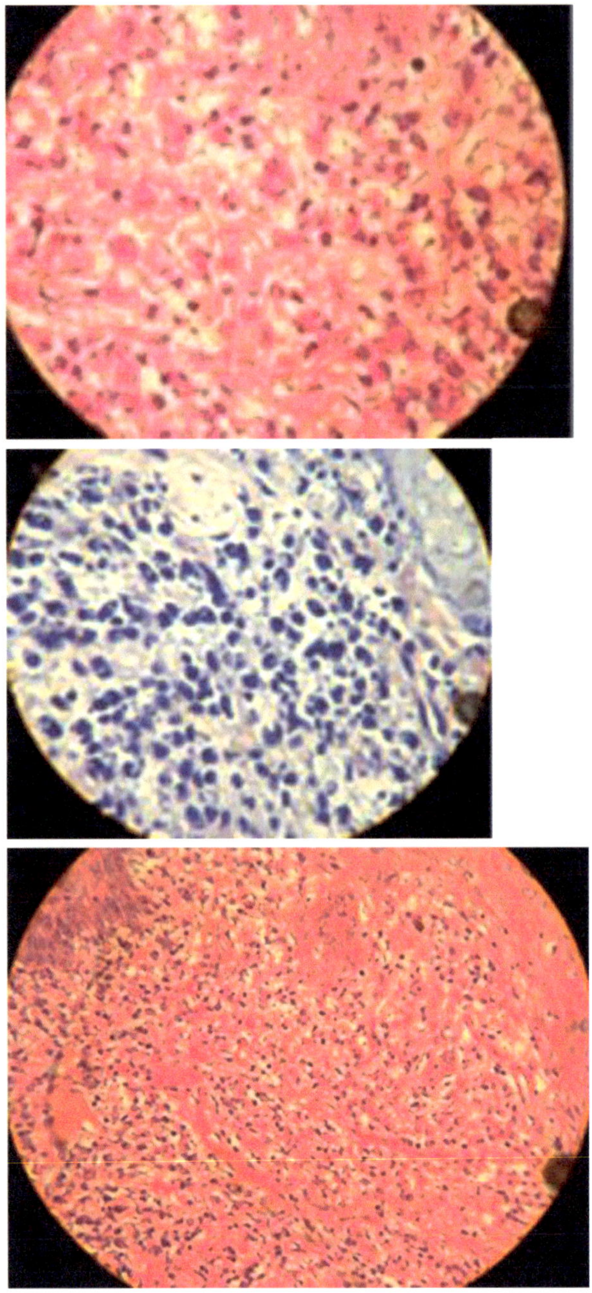

Figure 7.
Histopathological images with abundant lymphoplasmacytic infiltration.

developing into systemic lymphoma. It is also uncertain whether HVLL is a de novo disease or develops with long-term HV disease [2, 24].

Studies in Asian populations showed that “classic” HV is also associated with EBV, thus it was proposed to include HV as part of the spectrum of chronic, active EBV infection. However, it is not clear whether what has been called "classic" HV in Asian populations corresponds to the same disease described in Western populations and Mexico where the disease is self-limited and no progression to HVLL has been observed. This discrepancy has contributed to

Age of onset		Evolution	Cells involved
Lymphoid pathologies			
Cutaneous NK cell lymphoma	Adult	Aggressive	CD2+, CD3+/−, CD56+, CD8+/−
Mycosis fungoides	Adult	Torpid	CD2+, CD3+, CD4+, CD8−
Cutaneous T-lymphoma resembling subcutaneous panniculitis	Adult	Aggressive	CD3+, CD4−, CD8+TIA1+
Precursor T-cell lymphoblastic lymphoma	Adult	Aggressive	CD3+/−, CD7+, CD4+/−, CD8+/−, TdT+
Peripheral T-cell lymphoma	Childhood	Aggressive	CD2+, CD3+, CD4+, CD8−
Cutaneous anaplastic large cell lymphoma	Adult	Torpid	CD3+, CD4+, CD30+, EMA−, ALK1−, TIA1+/−
Cutaneous hydroa vacciniform T-cell lymphoma	Childhood	Aggressive	CD2+, CD3+, CD56−, CD8+, TIA1+, CD30+/−
Nonlymphoid pathologies			
Infectious pathologies	Syphilis Tuberculosis Paracoccidioidomycosis Leishmaniasis Rhinosporidiosis Mucormycosis		
Cutaneous porphyrias	Erythropoietic protoporphyria Congenital erythropoietic porphyria Porphyria cutanea tarda Hepatoerythrocytic porphyria Hereditary coproportion Porphyria variegata		
Autoimmune pathologies	Lupus erythematosus		

Table 2.
Differential diagnoses of HVLL.

uncertainty in differential diagnosis between classic HV and HVLL. It has been proposed that the most useful criterion for separating these two entities is the monoclonality of TCR.2 genes. Accumulating evidence indicates that these two cutaneous disorders could represent different manifestations within the spectrum of those encompassed under the setting of chronic, active infection by type-T EBV/NK [14, 15].

A study of severity in 20 Mexican children revealed that HV-type LPD of EBV1, regardless of the presence or absence of systemic symptoms of skin lesions, is a monoclonal T- and/or NK-cell disorder with a broad clinical spectrum, prolonged clinical course, and long-term risk of progressing to a systemic lymphoma. Later work showed that these lesions often have monoclonal rearrangements of TCR genes; thus the term "*hydroa vacciniforme-like lymphoma*" was proposed [2]. The relatively long clinical course before patients sought medical attention (range: 1–5 years) underlines the nature of this chronic disorder.

Apparently, monoclonality and clonal persistence are not predictive of aggressive disease or a progressive clinical course. Kimura et al. [4] reported four cases of "classic" HV, defined as patients with a characteristic dermatosis without systemic symptoms or cellular atypia, which were reclassified as having HVLL based on the monoclonality of the TCR-g genes. This suggests that EBV1 HV often is monoclonal, regardless of the presence or absence of systemic symptoms. Furthermore, no difference in the number of EBER1 infiltrators among these disorders has been found.

The Alpha and Beta or Gamma Cell Controversy and delta2 could be related to racial differences or reflect EBV-infected cells in peripheral blood and the skin. All HVLL cases revealed a phenotype of NK cells [4], indicating that one third of all HVLLs are from NK phenotype cells, which is more than has been observed before.

Morphologically, these lesions can mimic subcutaneous panniculitis-like T-cell lymphoma (SPTCL), primary cutaneous gamma and delta T-cell lymphoma, or skin involvement by extranodal NK/T lymphoma of nasal-type cells. Without clinical information, diagnosing the latter is almost impossible because the morphology and phenotype of the cells that infiltrate EBV1 are indistinguishable. Patients with the NK-cell phenotype rarely present with systemic symptoms despite alarming histology. Consequently, these patients show a relatively indolent clinical course compared to those with a T-cell phenotype [2, 3]. For any other autors, patients with an NK-cell phenotype appear have an increased risk of developing systemic lymphoma [13]. The severity of the clinical picture has been proposed to predict progression to systemic disease.

Some of those diagnosed with severe HV developed NK-/T-cell lymphoma 2–14 years after onset of the disease. It should be noted that all cases were associated with NK-cell lymphocytosis, HMB, and/or hemophagocytosis. "Subcutaneous lymphomas" without further specification raise the possibility that these injuries represent more manifestations of the disease and not a progression of the same. Although HVLL is characterized by a proliferation of monoclonal T cells or NK cells, treatment remains uncertain. Chemotherapy and/or radiation therapy are of little or no benefit. Their effects are usually transitory and do not induce sustained remission [13]. In addition, patients seem to have a worse prognosis and shorter survival due to sepsis and liver failure, with only slight improvement of skin lesions. In contrast, immunomodulatory therapies (prednisolone, cyclosporine, interferon A, chloroquine, and thalidomide) can sometimes improve symptoms temporarily.

3. Conclusions

HVLL is considered an EBV1 cutaneous T-cell lymphoma. This is based only on the demonstration of a proliferation of monoclonal T cells. However, its clinical evolution and relatively good response to immunomodulatory therapy challenge the concept of a lymphoma full malignant startup.

Criteria such as the presence of systemic symptoms, T-cell clonality, number of EBV1cells, and/or infiltrate density do not help predict who will progress to systemic disease. To avoid aggressive treatment and the stigma of a lymphoma diagnosis, the term HV-like EBV1 lymphoma, which encompasses the different manifestations and clinical signs of HV-like skin lesions with EBV, both from T cells and NK cells, is preferable for clinical use. The challenge remains to identify morphological or clinical markers to predict which patients are or are not at risk of progressing to a systemic lymphoma [25].

We believe the best term for this pathology is hydroa vacciniforme like type cutaneous T- cell lymphoma (LCCTHVL). LCCTHVL is a rare disease that is more prevalent in low-income pediatric populations. It is difficult to diagnose, and its clinical evaluation is vitally important for timely treatment due to its malignant potential and lethal prognosis. LCCTHVL is a diagnostic challenge, especially if it is not an entity well known to specialists; hence the importance of emphasizing its existence in Latin American countries and Asia where it is more prevalent, especially among young adults and children [1, 2, 5, 8, 10–12, 14], and in tropical locations where it could easily be mistaken for a infectious disease such as leishmaniasis, tuberculosis, syphilis, paracoccidioidomycosis, or some other deep mycosis.

Although this malignant lymphoproliferative entity is highly aggressive and difficult to diagnose, it has been studied and described by multiple authors. Early diagnosis is essential for planning effective treatment (e.g., chemotherapy) to improve patient survival. However, it is important to note that comorbidities and the high degree of malignancy of this cutaneous variant of lymphoma can lead to a fatal outcome.

Conflict of interest

"The authors declare no conflict of interest."

Author details

Carmen Ximena Gallegos Riofrio* and Juan Daniel Garzon Gallegos
Hospital Metropolitano, Quito, Ecuador

*Address all correspondence to: cxgr2004@yahoo.es

References

[1] Ruiz-Maldonado R, Parrilla FM, Orozco-Covarrubias ML, Ridaura C, Tamayo-Sánchez L, Duran-McKinster C. Edematous, scarring vasculitic panniculitis: A new multisystemic disease with malignant potential. Journal of the American Academy of Dermatology. 1995;**32**(1): 37-44

[2] Quintanilla-Martinez L, Ridaura C, Nagl F, Sáez-de-Ocariz M, Durán-McKinster C, Ruiz-Maldonado R, et al. Hydroa vacciniforme-like lymphoma: A chronic EBV+ lymphoproliferative disorder with risk to develop a systemic lymphoma. Blood. 2013;**122**(18): 3101-3110

[3] Jawed SI, Myskowski PL, Horwitz S, Moskowitz A, Querfeld C. Primary cutaneous T-cell lymphoma (mycosis fungoides and Sézary syndrome): Part I. Diagnosis: Clinical and histopathologic features and new molecular and biologic markers. Journal of the American Academy of Dermatology. 2014;**70**(2): 205.e1-16; quiz 221-222

[4] Kimura H, Hoshino Y, Kanegane H, Tsuge I, Okamura T, Kawa K, et al. Clinical and virologic characteristics of chronic active Epstein-Barr virus infection. Blood. 2001;**98**(2):280-286

[5] Durán-McKinster C, Ruiz-Maldonado R. Hidroa vacciniformelike o enfermedad de Ruiz Maldonado. Dermatologia Revista Mexicana. 2013;**57**(6):464-467

[6] Kanazawa T, Hiramatsu Y, Iwata S, Siddiquey M, Sato Y, Suzuki M, et al. Anti-CCR4 monoclonal antibody mogamulizumab for the treatment of EBV-associated T- and NK-cell lymphoproliferative diseases. Clinical Cancer Research. 2014;**20**(19): 5075-5084

[7] Florencia-Fernández M, Bettina-Cervini A, Chantada G, Pierini AM. Linfoma cutáneo de células T hidroa vacciniforme-like. Archivos Argentinos de Dermatología. 2013;**63**(6):219-225

[8] Ramos RC, Cortez F, Quijano E, Carayhua D, Jiménez H, Rivera A. Linfoma tipo hidroa: Presentación de un caso. Rev Soc Peruana de Dermatología. 2011;**21**(3):126-129

[9] Lim MS, de Leval L, Quintanilla-Martinez L. Commentary on the 2008 WHO classification of mature T- and NK-cell neoplasms. Journal of Hematopathology. 2009;**2**(2):65-73

[10] Beltrán BE, Maza I, Moisés-Alfaro CB, Vasquez L, Quiñones P, Morales D, et al. Thalidomide for the treatment of hydroa vacciniforme-like lymphoma: Report of four pediatric cases from Peru. American Journal of Hematology. 2014;**89**(12):1160-1161

[11] Maldonado-García CA, Beirana-Palencia A. Hidroa vacciniforme, revisión del tema. Revista del Centro Dermatológico Pascua. 2006;**15**(3):198-202

[12] Wang RC, Chang ST, Hsieh YC, Huang WT, Hsu JD, Tseng CE, et al. Spectrum of Epstein-Barr virus-associated T-cell lymphoproliferative disorder in adolescents and young adults in Taiwan. International Journal of Clinical and Experimental Pathology. 2014;**7**(5):2430-2437

[13] Kempf W, Kazakov DV, Kerl K. Cutaneous lymphomas: An update. Part 1: T-cell and natural killer/t-cell lymphomas and related conditions. The American Journal of Dermatopathology. 2014;**36**(2):105-123

[14] Di Martino-Ortiz B, Barboza G, Moreno T, Valiente C, Buongermini A, Boggino H. Linfoma cutáneo tipo hidroa

vacciniforme. Desorden linfoproliferativo asociado a infección por virus del Epstein-Barr en la infancia. Piel. 2015;**30**(7):420-423

[15] Sorigue M, Sancho JM. The 2016 revision of the WHO classifi cation of lymphoid neoplasms: The clinician's view. Medicina Clínica (Barcelona). 2018;**150**(2):64-66

[16] Kempf W, Mitteldorf C. Pathologic diagnosis of cutaneous lymphomas. Dermatologic Clinics. 2015;**33**(4): 655-681

[17] Sawada A, Inoue M, Koyama-Sato M, Kondo O, Yamada K, Shimizu M, et al. Umbilical cord blood as an alternative source of reduced-intensity hematopoietic stem cell transplantation for chronic Epstein-Barr virus-associated T or natural killer cell lymphoproliferative diseases. Biology of Blood and Marrow Transplantation. 2014;**20**(2):214-221

[18] Hwang ST, Janik JE, Jaffe ES, Wilson WH. Mycosis fungoides and Sézary syndrome. Lancet. 2008; **371**(9616):945-957

[19] Dummer R, Urosevic M, Kempf W, Kazakov D, Burg G. Imiquimod induces complete clearance of a PUVA-resistant plaque in mycosis fungoides. Dermatology. 2003;**207**(1):116-118

[20] Kim EJ, Hess S, Richardson SK, Newton S, Showe LC, Benoit BM, et al. Immunopathogenesis and therapy of cutaneous T cell lymphoma. The Journal of Clinical Investigation. 2005;**115**(4): 798-812

[21] Sugaya M, Miyagaki T, Ohmatsu H, Suga H, Kai H, Kamata M, et al. Association of the numbers of CD163(+) cells in lesional skin and serum levels of soluble CD163 with disease progression of cutaneous T cell lymphoma. Journal of Dermatological Science. 2012;**68**(1):45-51

[22] Fritz A, Percy C, Jack A, Shanmugaratnam K, Sobin L, Parkin DM, et al. International Classifi cation of Diseases for Oncology. 3rd ed. Malta: WHO; 2013. Available from: http://apps.who.int/iris/bitstream/10665/96612/1/9789241548496_eng.pdf?ua=1

[23] Barrionuevo C, Anderson VM, Zevallos-Giampietri E, Zaharia M, Misad O, Bravo F, et al. Hydroa-like cutaneous T-cell lymphoma:a clinicopathologic and molecular genetic study of 16 pediatric cases from Peru. Applied Immunohistochemistry & Molecular Morphology. 2002;**10**(1):7-14

[24] Swerdlow SH, Campo E, Pileri SA, Harris NL, Stein H, Siebert R, et al. The 2016 revision of the World Health Organization classification of lymphoid neoplasms. Blood. 2016;**127**(20): 2375-2390

[25] Fauci AS, Haynes BF, Katz P, Wolff SM. Wegener's granulomatosis: Prospective clinical and therapeutic experience with 85 patients for 21 years. Annals of Internal Medicine. 1983; **98**(1):76-85

Chapter 7

Clinical and Laboratory Data Which Are Not Typical of De Novo Diffuse Large B-Cell Lymphoma

Aminat Magomedova, Anna Misyurina, Sergey Kravchenko, Fatima Babaeva and Andrey Vorobiev

Abstract

Diffuse large B-cell lymphoma (DLBCL) is a heterogeneous group of diseases of the lymphatic system, which is represented by de novo and secondary tumors resulting from the transformation of indolent lymphomas. In the absence of a long history of the disease at the stage of histological transformation (HT), it is difficult to distinguish between de novo and secondary diffuse large B-cell lymphoma. According to the data of a randomized study, we obtained clinical and laboratory data that are not typical for de novo diffuse large B-cell lymphoma. These include exclusive, predominant retroperitoneal localization, compression of the ureters/kidneys with or without the development of acute renal failure (ARF), unilateral lymphostasis of the leg due to compression of the inguinal, iliac lymph nodes by the conglomerate, intratumor in the central nervous system (CNS) at the onset/relapse/progression of the disease, discordant bone marrow involvement, blood involvement, paraprotein secretion.

Keywords: DLBCL, ARF, retroperitoneal localization, asymmetric lymphostasis of the leg, CNS intratumor, paraprotein, discordant involvement of bone marrow, blood involvement, relapses

1. Introduction

Diffuse large B-cell lymphoma (DLBCL) was isolated from the general group of lymphatic tumors by histological and immunotypic features—diffuse proliferation of large B-cells, which either can form a structure of diffuse growth or be diffusely scattered among nontumor cells of a specific organ [1, 2].

In the past, lymphomas were classified solely for histological features. The advent of immunophenotyping of tumor cells changed the situation, but it turned out that some lymphoproliferative diseases (LPD), including DLBCL, do not have an unambiguous specific immunophenotype. All markers (pan B-cell, CD10, Bcl-2, Bcl-6, CD5, MUM1, CD30, CD23, ALK, and CD138) occurring in DLBCL also found in other LPD [3–5]. Subsequently, cytogenetic disorders made it possible to distinguish a number of diseases of the lymphatic system into separate nosological forms. These include *c-MYC gene* rearrangement and 11q aberration, characteristic of Burkitt's lymphoma; rearrangement of gene *BCL-2*, characteristic of follicular lymphoma (FL); the *CYCLIN D1* gene, characteristic of mantle cell lymphoma; t(2;5) (p23;p35); characteristic of anaplastic T-cell lymphoma, etc. The combination of rearrangement of the *c-MYC* gene with rearrangement of the *BCL2* and/or *BCL6 genes* in the recent past made it possible to isolate a separate form of high-grade B-cell lymphoma from DLBCL [6–11]. However, de novo DLBCL, unspecified, stands apart from all B-cell lymphomas, due to the absence of immunophenotype characteristic only of it, cytogenetic and molecular markers. Therefore, the diagnosis was made after excluding all other large B-cell lymphomas.

Although the "boundaries" of DLBCL are defined in the World Health Organization (WHO) classification, it is currently overdiagnosed. Moreover, the latter affects the tactics of choosing an induction course and therapy at the end of treatment.

The absence of clear clinical, morphological, immunophenotypic, cytogenetic, and molecular differential diagnostic signs puts the clinician in a difficult position, who needs to determine the polychemotherapy program, avoiding the appointment of the so-called R-CHOP to all patients, and in turn, without exposing patients unjustified risk, the appointment of high-dose therapy. Moreover, in cases of DLBCL because of the transformation of indolent lymphomas, patients remain without maintenance therapy with rituximab for 2 years, which is currently mandatory.

All of the above dictate the need to highlight the decisive differential diagnostic clinical and laboratory data of the disease; therefore, clinicians have to take into account all the details that are of key importance for differential diagnosis.

1.1 Medical history

Many mature cell LPDs transformed in DLBCL with varying frequency, in some cases. A carefully collected history helps to find out whether it is a de novo tumor or the result of the transformation of indolent lymphomas. Although the history of the disease is a purely subjective sign, and not all patients pay attention to some minor changes in the state of health or the results of the study, doctors must scrupulously find out all the details of the history. This is the time from the first manifestations of the disease to the diagnosis, independent reduction in the size of the tumor before starting treatment, multiple biopsies, and ambiguous data of histological, immunohistochemically studies; study medical documentation, correctly interpret the results of previous studies. Despite the absence of clear criteria regarding the duration of the history, it is known that de novo DLBCL does not proceed for years and has an aggressive course if this is not a local process. In the terminal stage, the histological picture of any indolent lymphomas may look like DLBCL, which leads to an error diagnosis by pathologists. Therefore, a carefully collected anamnesis, in some cases, helps to establish an accurate diagnosis, to identify cases of indolent lymphomas.

1.2 Clinical manifestations

In patients with DLBCL, there is no clinical picture typical only for it; it all depends on the localization of the tumor, the extent of the lesion, the presence of B-symptoms, etc. Therefore, the diagnosis is based on histological and immunohistochemically studies. However, at the same time, at present, some clinical manifestations give us a clue about de novo or the transformation of DLBCL. The experience of previous years allowed us to assume that an intratumor in the central nervous system (CNS) at the time of diagnosis, progression, or recurrence does not occur with de novo DLBCL. In addition, the predominant retroperitoneal localization, asymmetric lymphostasis of the legs, compression of the ureters, kidneys by tumor and impaired urinary outflow, hydronephrosis, and acute renal failure (ARF) are not typical of de novo DLBCL. It turned out that intratumor in the central nervous system does not occur in patients with de novo DLBCL, and neuroleukemia is rare.

The most common extranodal form of de novo DLBCL is gastric DLBCL. Therefore, it was noticed that the pyloric stenosis, which persists after achieving complete remission (CR), due to the formation of fibrosis and requires bougienage or surgery, is not typical of de novo DLBCL of the stomach. Many of our assumptions were subsequently confirmed by the data of repeated biopsies and histological, immunohistochemical studies performed in progression and relapse within the framework of the DLBCL-2015 protocol. Further monitoring of patients is required to confirm some of the assumptions.

1.3 Bone marrow trephine biopsy data

Most often, 25–35%, FL transformed from indolent lymphomas in DLBCL [8]; therefore, cases with the presence of rearrangement of the *BCL2* gene are now referred to as FL. Previously, it was thought that rearrangements of the *BCL2* gene could also occur in de novo DLBCL. The assumption that such cases are a transformation of FL was made by us in 2004 and confirmed later [12]. Then, we noticed that the frequency of achieving complete remission (CR) is lower and the prognosis is worse in patients in whom the morphological picture of tumor foci and bone marrow biopsy at the same time differed from each other, that is, there was a discordant involvement of bone marrow. Therefore, we analyzed the morphological differences of tumor formations and the mitotic activity of tumor cells in different lesions. The proliferative activity of lymphoid cells of the lymph node, of the stomach, tonsil, spleen, and other foci and bone marrow was different—high in lymph node and other lesions and low in the bone marrow. The tumor in the bone marrow had signs of indolent LPD—morphologically, the cells corresponded to the structure of a normal lymphocyte, without polymorphism and atypism, and had low mitotic activity. In lymph nodes or other lesions, tumor cells had all signs of aggressiveness and high-proliferative activity. In such cases, we also noticed the retroperitoneal localization of the tumor and the complications caused by it, due to the compression of the urinary tract by the tumor, most likely due to fibrosis. Therefore, pathologists should take into account the severity of fibrosis during histological, immunohistochemically examination.

Currently, special attention paid to the transformation of lymphoma from cells of the marginal zone (LMZ) (splenic, nodal forms, and LMZ mucosa-associated lymphoid tissue (MALT-lymphoma), because it is one of the indolent lymphomas, with a similar histological picture with de novo DLBCL does not have a specific immunophenotype, cytogenetic, and molecular markers. In some cases, it is impossible to distinguish lymphoma transformation of the marginal zone from de novo DLBCL without information about the previous history. The frequency of transformation of lymphoma from cells of the marginal zone to DLBCL ranges from 8 to 10% [2, 13, 14]. According to a large retrospective study, which included 340 patients with LMZ, with a mean follow-up of 4.8 years, the mean overall survival and progression-free survival for the entire population was 14.5 and 5 years, respectively. Histological transformation (HT) observed in 13 (3.8%) cases—5% with splenic form, 4% with MALT—lymphoma, and 3% with nodal LMZ. The risk of HT was 5% at 5 and 10 years after diagnosis and 10% at 12 years. With an average follow-up of 12 months after HT, four (31%) of 13 patients died, all because of disease progression. The two-year overall survival rate after transformation was 57% [15, 16]. In 1/3 of patients with LMZ, there is an involvement of bone marrow both discordant and concordant.

It noted that the prognosis of patients with the transformation of indolent lymphomas in DLBCL is similar to the prognosis of patients with blast crisis of chronic myeloid leukemia. Therefore, young patients with HT in DLBCL may now need to undergo intensive courses of induction chemotherapy with or without subsequent transplantation in order to increase relapse-free survival.

Thus, cases with the presence of focal, focal-interstitial, and diffuse mature cell involvement of bone marrow with the histological picture of DLBCL in lymph nodes or other tumor foci are considered as an outcome of indolent lymphomas.

1.4 Laboratory data

New generation sequencing made it possible to detect tumor messenger ribonucleic acid (mRNA) in the blood, because of which DLBCL is classified into three subgroups, differing from each other in pathogenesis [17]. However, leukocytosis with the presence of tumor cells in the blood is very rare in patients with DLBCL. Even with a concordant involvement of bone marrow, in no case did we confirm the presence of tumor cells according to the data of immunophenotyping of blood by flow cytometry, as well as B-cell clonally by polymerase chain reaction (PCR). On the contrary, in patients with indolent lymphomas, such as FL and LMZ, blood involvement is more common [4, 5, 8]. Therefore, this is taken into account in the differential diagnosis of de novo DLBCL from the transformation from indolent lymphomas.

1.5 Secretion of paraprotein

The next laboratory sign of the transformation of indolent lymphomas into DLBCL is the **secretion of paraprotein**, which occurs in 1/3 of patients with LMZ, in a smaller percentage of cases of FL [4, 5, 8]

In the latest WHO classification and many publications, it is noted that the secretion of paraprotein, including an increase in the concentration of light chains, as well as lesions of intramuscular tissue, including discordant ones, are signs of a poor prognosis in patients with de novo DLBCL [2].

It has now been proven that the secretion of paraprotein is a sign of a poor prognosis in patients with DLBCL with the presence of paraprotein [18, 19].

The fact that patients with de novo DLBCL cured can be, and secondary DLBCL – is not, despite the success achieved in the treatment of LPD. The secretion of paraprotein indicates the secondary nature of DLBCL. Indolent lymphomas transformed into DLBCL relapses after anytherapy. Allogenic hematopoietic cell transplantation is the only therapeutic option for complete recovery.

1.6 Relapses after adequate induction therapy

Some forms of DLBCL were isolated from the general group by the response to therapy; therefore, in all cases of relapses, as well as the progression of DLBCL with adequate induction therapy, morphologists should pay attention to this fact when establishing the form of the disease. Since de novo DLBCL is a curable disease, treatment outcomes, namely the incidence of PR, progression, and relapse, are independent predictors of prognosis.

Relapses in patients with DLBCL with discordant involvement of bone marrow, with the secretion of paraprotein, blood involvement, as well as all the clinical manifestations described above, should suggest that these cases are the result of the transformation of indolent lymphomas and, subsequently, should receive supportive therapy.

The results of our pilot prospective study on the treatment of DLBCL patients with the modified mNHL-BFM-90 program demonstrated that all relapse cases, including late ones (two cases after 13 years) turned out to be other forms, that is, there was an overdiagnosis of de novo DLBCL.

Since 2002, we have been using a modified mNHL-BFM-90 program as an induction program for the treatment of patients with de novo DLBCL with signs of poor prognosis, which has demonstrated high efficiency, including those from the high-risk group [20]. From that moment, all our observations allowed us to identify clinical and laboratory data that are not characteristic of de novo DLBCL. These include all of the above data—a long history of the disease an independent decrease in the size of the tumor from the moment the first symptoms appear and the diagnosis is made to the start of therapy; multiple and uninformative biopsies; secretion of paraprotein; intratumor in the central nervous system initially, in relapse, in progression. Moreover, the exclusive or predominant retroperitoneal localization of the tumor with data of tumor compression of the urinary tract, as a result of which ARF, asymmetric lymphostasis of the limbs of the lower leg due to compression of the conglomerate of the inguinal and iliac lymph nodes, discordant involvement of bone marrow, blood, and relapses after adequate therapy do not occur in patients de novo DLBCL. Our pilot, prospective, and randomized studies allowed us to assume that all of the listed signs indicate the transformation of mature cell lymphomas into DLBCL, these cases are not de novo DLBCL and in such cases, patients should receive maintenance therapy with Rituximab. This is very important, especially for elderly patients.

Thus, de novo DLBCL is currently the diagnosis of exclusion among large B-cell lymphomas.

The aim of our work is to determine additional clinical and laboratory signs of differential diagnosis of de novo and transformation of indolent lymphomas into DLBCL within the framework of the DLBCL-2015 protocol.

2. Materials and methods

We are conducting a prospective multicenter randomized study on the treatment of primary patients with DLBCL with ≥2 signs of poor prognosis—the DLBCL protocol—2015 (ClinicalTrials.gov. R-DA-EPOCH-21 versus R-mNHL-BFM-90 and auto-SCT in Poor Prognosis DLBCL NCT02842931). From January 2015 to April 30, 2021, 140 patients were randomized from 13 hematology clinics in Russia. The analysis included 130 patients. Treatment was completed in 127 patients. The diagnosis of DLBCL was established according to the WHO criteria of 2008 and 2017 [2, 3].

At the diagnostic stage, all patients underwent examination according to the LPD protocol—all routine tests, positron emission tomography combined with computed tomography (PET-CT), CT scan of the brain. In the absence of time according to the severity of the patient's condition or the possibility of performing it—CT or magnetic resonance imaging (MRI) of the neck (if indicated), chest, abdominal cavity, retroperitoneal space, and small pelvis, trepan biopsy of the ilium, as well as diagnostic lumbar puncture. A Fluorescence in situ Hybridization (FISH) cytogenetic study was performed in 70 patients to determine rearrangement involving the *c-MYC, BCL2,* and *BCL6* gene loci to exclude high-grade B-cell lymphoma; in 11 patients, next generation sequencity was performed in order to determine the mutation of the *TP53* gene (4-9 exons). Analyzed separately, both the intent to treat group (**Table 1**) and the de novo DLBCL patient group (**Table 2**). This work analyzes the above described clinical and laboratory signs of differential diagnosis of de novo and a secondary result of the transformation of indolent lymphomas of DLBCL.

Characteristics of patients included by intent to treat are presented in **Table 1**. The characteristics of patients with primary DLBCL are presented in **Table 2**. The groups are compared with each other in all parameters.

Variable	**R-DA-EPOCH ± autoSCT n = 62 (48%)**	**R-mNHL-BFM-90 ± autoSCT n = 68 (52%)**	**Total n = 130 (100%)**
Age, median of years (range):			
<40	15 (24.2%)	20 (29.4%)	35 (26.9%)
40–60	39 (62.9%)	45 (66.2%)	84 (64.2%)
>=60	8 (12.9%)	3 (4.4%)	11 (8.5%)
Gender:			
M	30 (48.4%)	41 (60.3%)	71 (54.6%)
F	32 (51.6%)	27 (39.7%)	59 (45.4%)
Nodal	53 (85.5%)	58 (85.3%)	111 (85.4%)
Extranodal	9 (14.5%)	10 (14.7%)	19 (14.6%)
Stage:			
II (bulky diseases)	2 (3.2%)	5 (7.3%)	7 (5.4%)
III	12 (19.4%)	18 (26.5%)	30 (23.1%)
IV	48 (77.4%)	45 (66.2%)	93 (71.5%)
Exclusive/predominant retroperitoneal localization with compression of the ureters /kidneys/ hydronephrosis/ARF	3 (4.8%) 2 (3.2%)	2 (2.9%) 1 (1.5%)	5 (3.8%) 3 (2.3%)
Retroperitoneal localization in stage III–IV: Compression of the ureters/kidneys/ hydronephrosis/acute renal failure	22 (46.8%) 0	25 (53.2%) 0	47 (36%) 0
Asymmetric lymphostasis of the leg	1 (1.6%)	1 (1.5%)	2 (1.5%)
Involvement bone morrow:			
Histological (n = 120):	7 (5.8%)	5 (4.2%)	12 (10%)
Discordant	2 (1.7%)	1 (0.83%)	3 (25%)
Concordant	5 (4.2%)	4 (3.3%)	9 (75%)
Immunophenotyping (n = 11) Blood involvement	2 (18.2%)	0	2 (18.2%)
Mutation gene *TP53* (n = 11)	1 (9%)	2 (18.2%)	3 (27.3%)
Neuroleukemia	1 (1.6%)	0	1 (0.76%)
Intratumor	0	0	0
Paraprotein (n = 103): n = 50, R-DA-EPOCH n = 53, R-m-NHL-BFM-90	7 (14%)	5 (9.43%)	12 (11.65%)
Aa IPI:			
1	0	1 (1.5%)	1 (0.8%)
2	21 (33.9%)	19 (27.9%)	40 (30.8%)
3	41 (66.2%)	48 (70.6%)	89 (68.4)
PR	36 (58.06%)	63 (92.65%)	99 (76.15%)
Relapse	5 (14%)	6 (9.5%)	11 (11.1%)

Variable	R-DA-EPOCH ± autoSCT n = 62 (48%)	R-mNHL-BFM-90 ± autoSCT n = 68 (52%)	Total n = 130 (100%)
Progression	6 (9.7%)	0	6 (8.4%)
Death	3 (4.84%)	1 (1.47%)	4 (3.08%)
The therapy continues	3 (4.84%)	1 (1.47%)	4 (4.6%)
The diagnosis is in relapse, progression:			
DLBCL	4 (6.5%)	1 (1.47%)	5 (3.8%)
FL grade 1–2	1 (1.6%)	0	1 (0.76%)
FL grade 3 (A/B)	3 (4.8%)	1 (1.47%)	4 (3.1%)
NLPHL	1 (1.6%)	1 (1.47%)	2 (1.53%)
PMBL	0	1 (1.47%)	1 (0.76%)
AITL	1 (1.6%)	0	1 (0.76%)
NMZL	2 (3.2%)	0	2 (1.53%)
HGBL: with *c-MYC* and *BCL2*	1 (1.6%)	0	1 (0.76%)
NOS	1 (1.6%)	0	1 (0.76%)

FL-follicular lymphoma, NLPHL-nodular lymphocyte-predominant Hodgkin lymphoma, PMBL-primary mediastinal (thymic) large B-cell lymphoma, AITL-angioimmunoblastic T-cell lymphoma, NMZL-nodal marginal zone lymphoma.

Table 1.
Characteristics of patients in the intention-to-treat included in the DLBCL-2015 trial.

Variable	R-DA-EPOCH ± autoSCT n = 55 (47%)	R-mNHL-BFM-90 ± autoSCT C n = 62 (53%)	Total n = 117 (100%)
Age, median of years (range):			
<40	14 (25%)	18 (29%)	32 (27%)
40–60	35 (64%)	41 (66%)	76 (65%)
>=60	6 (11%)	3 (5%)	9 (8%)
Gender:			
M	22 (47%)	39 (63%)	65 (56%)
F	29 (53%)	23 (37%)	52 (44%)
Nodal	46 (84%)	52 (84%)	98 (84%)
Extranodal	9 (16%)	10 (16%)	19 (16%)
Stage:			
II (bulky diseases)	2 (4%)	5 (8%)	7 (6%)
III	11 (20%)	16 (26%)	27 (23%)
IV	42 (76%)	41 (66%)	83 (71%)
Exclusive/predominant retroperitoneal localization with compression of the ureters/kidneys/hydronephrosis/ARF	0	0	0
Retroperitoneal localization in stage III–IV:	22 (46.8%)	25 (53.2%)	47 (36%)
Compression of the ureters/kidneys/ hydronephrosis/acute renal failure	1 (4.5%)	0	1 (2.12%)
Asymmetric lymphostasis of the leg	0	0	0
Involvement bone marrow:			
Histological (n = 120):	5 (5.6%)	4 (3.7%)	9 (10%)
Discordant	0	0	0
Concordant	5 (5.6%)	4 (3.7%)	9 (10%)
Mutation gene *TP53* (n = 8)	1 (9%)	2 (18.2%)	3 (27.3%)
Neuroleukemia	1 (1.81%)	0	1 (0.85)
Intratumor	0	0	0

Variable	R-DA-EPOCH ± autoSCT n = 55 (47%)	R-mNHL-BFM-90 ± autoSCT C n = 62 (53%)	Total n = 117 (100%)
Paraprotein (n = 97): R-DA-EPOCH (n = 48) R-m-NHL-BFM-90 (n = 49)	2 (4.2%)	5 (10.2%)	7 (7.2%)
Aa IPI:			
1	0	1 (2%)	1 (1%)
2	19 (35%)	18 (29%)	37 (32%)
3	36 (65%)	43 (69%)	79 (67%)
CR	36 (65.45%)	59 (95.16%)	95 (81.20%)
Relapse	3 (5.45%)	2 (3.23%)	5 (4.27%)
Progression	5 (14%)	6 (9.5%)	11 (11.1%)
Death	3 (5.45%)	2 (3.23%)	5 (4.27%)
The therapy continues	3 (4.84%)	1 (1.47%)	4 (4.6%)

Table 2.
Characteristics of patients with de novo DLBCL.

3. Results

This section will discuss the clinical and laboratory signs that have differential diagnostic value, obtained in the course of a prospective study.

3.1 An intent to treat the group

As indicated in **Table 1**, generalized lesion of peripheral, intrathoracic, intra-abdominal lymph nodes with or without extranodal foci and with massive retroperitoneal conglomerate >7 cm, bulky diseases (stage III–IV), was observed in 47 (37%) patients and not in one case, ARF was not observed due to compression of the urinary tract by tumor bulky. However, five patients had preferential/exclusive retroperitoneal localization, and three of them had data of renal/ureteral compression—ARF and hydronephrosis. In two of these three cases, it combined with the presence of Mk paraprotein secretion, as well as with discordant lesion of the bone marrow. All this allows us to assume the transformation of indolent lymphomas into DLBCL. In two of 47 patients, asymmetric lymphostasis of the lower extremity was noted, due to squeezing of the iliac and/or inguinal lymph nodes by the conglomerate. Neuroleukemia was diagnosed in one patient, no one initially had intratumor, and one patient had a relapse, and this patient was diagnosed with primary mediastinal large B-cell lymphoma (PMBL). Peripheral blood immunophenotyping was performed in 11 patients with leukocytosis, and in two of them, a monoclonal population of lymphoid cells with a tumor-like immunophenotype was found. The *TP53* gene mutation was detected in three out of 11 patients studied. Paraproteinemia/paraproteinuria was found in 12 (11.65%) patients. Complete remission was achieved in 99 (76.15%)—in 36 (58.06) on R-DA-EPOCH therapy, in 63 (92.65%) on R-mNHL-BFM-90; progression was observed in six (9.65%), and all patients received R-DA-EPOCH therapy, relapse developed in 11 (11.1%) patients. At the time of progression and relapse, the patients underwent repeated tumor biopsy, histological and immunohistochemically studies. Of the 16 cases, 11 turned out to be different diagnoses (**Table 1**)—five patients diagnosed with de novo DLBCL, three of these five patients found to have a *TP53* mutation and two patients were on R-DA-EPOCH therapy. Involvement of bone marrow was observed in 12

(9.23%) patients—in three patients, the lesion was discordant and in all patients in relapse, the diagnosis was changed in favor of FL in 2 cases and indolent lymphoma, unspecified in 1 case.

3.2 De novo DLBCL

Table 2 presents the data of the group of primary DLBCL. As seen in none of the cases was there an exclusive/predominant retroperitoneal localization, as well as out of 47 cases lesions of peripheral, intrathoracic, intra-abdominal lymph nodes with or without extranodal foci and with a massive retroperitoneal conglomerate >7 cm, bulky diseases, III–IV stage, no one had data of compression by the tumor conglomerate of the kidneys/ureters, ARF. In addition, in this group, no one had asymmetric lymph stasis of the leg, intratumor in the central nervous system; one patient had neuroleukemia at the time of diagnosis. None of the patients had mature cell lesions bone marrow; large cell lesions were observed in nine (97.7%) patients. In this group, there were no cases of blood involvement. All three patients with the *TP53* mutation were in the de novo DLBCL group. Paraproteinemia/paraproteinuria was observed in only seven (7.2%) patients, five of whom received intensive induction therapy with R-mNHL-BFM-90, the effectiveness of which exceeds 90%. Complete remission was achieved in 95 (82.20%) patients—36 (65.45%) after R-DA-EPOCH therapy, in 59 (95.16%) patients after R-mNHL-BFM-90. Progression was observed in five (4.27%) patients and all of them underwent R-DA-EPOCH therapy and belonged to a high-risk group. Relapses developed only in two patients, and both had a *TP53* mutation.

4. Discussion

Thus, the obtained data indicate that currently there is an over diagnostics of de novo DLBCL. Most often, the reason for this is either a lack of some data or an incorrect interpretation of the available research results. However, the main reason remains the lack of clear diagnostic criteria.

As a rule, a carefully collected anamnesis of the disease allows you to find out the duration of the disease, whether the tumor size decreased without any treatment or not, how long they were observed or treated by doctors of other specialties. Multiple and uninformative biopsies performed by different specialists also indicate the transformation of indolent lymphomas into DLBCL. However, there are cases when both do not allow for an accurate diagnosis.

4.1 Clinical manifestations

4.1.1 Exclusive/predominant retroperitoneal localization

Even in the REAL 1994 classification, some forms of DLBCL distinguished into separate nosological forms according to the localization of the tumor. These include primary mediastinal large B-cell lymphoma, serous cavity lymphoma, and intravascular DLBCL and CNS lymphoma [1]. Therefore, there is reason to think that exclusive/predominant retroperitoneal localization with compression of the ureters/kidneys, with or without ARF in morphological diagnosis, is a separate form of B-cell lymphomas. Compression is most likely due to the development of fibrosis in the tumor tissue, as in PMBL and Hodgkin's lymphoma (HL). In the development of fibrosis, various cytokines produced by tumor cells can participate, among other mechanisms. Back in the early 90s of the last century, it was known which important role cytokines play in the pathogenesis of lymphomas. Some of the clinical and morphological features of aggressive lymphomas are partially explained by the action of cytokines, the level of which is increased in serum or tissues of patients with lymphomas. In particular, it proved that Hodgkin's lymphoma cells express IL-1, IL-5, IL-9, TNFα, M-CSF, etc., which are responsible for the enhancement of the cellular response and fibrosis observed in HL tissues [21]. In addition, the effect of blood plasma of a patient with DLBCL on the properties of mesenchymal hematopoietic stem cells through cytokines and proteins secreted by tumor cells is proven [22]. Therefore, it assumed that tumor cells of de novo and secondary DLBCL secrete "their" cytokines, and it causes different clinical manifestations. Recently, for the first time, large changes were obtained in mesenchymal stem cells in patients with DLBCL without the involvement of bone marrow. It assumed that tumor cells that do not populate the bone marrow have a humoral, pathological effect on the stromal progenitor cells of the bone marrow. The tumor process in one way or another affects the entire body. Recently, for the first time, it has been shown that the precursors of the stromal microenvironment—multipotent mesenchymal stromal cells—change in DLBCL patients without involvement of bone marrow due to the humoral effect of the tumor and the body's response to it. A comprehensive analysis of the results showed that when remission is achieved in patients with DLBCL, the composition of plasma cytokines normalizes, but does not reach the level observed in healthy donors [23].

As it can be seen from the results of the study, in almost 40% of patients, the dimensions of the retroperitoneal conglomerate with generalized lesions are larger than 7 cm and, in only one case, was hydronephrosis. The same patient had paraproteinemia Mƙ. In this case, too, we assume the transformation of indolent lymphoma. The patient is under our supervision.

4.1.2 Asymmetric lymphostasis

Asymmetric lymphostasis of the leg was observed in two patients from the intent to treat group, and when the diagnosis was revised at the reference center, the diagnosis changed in favor of type 3 FL. The pathogenesis of lymphostasis due to compression of the inguinal and/or iliac lymph nodes by a tumor conglomerate is most likely to be the same as in retroperitoneal localization.

We have cases of gastric DLBCL with pyloric stenosis. As a rule, in such cases, they need to bougienage or surgery. I think that these cases are similar and represent the transformation of indolent lymphomas in DLBCL.

4.1.3 Intratumor and neuroleukemia

No cases of intratumor in CNS at the time of diagnosis/relapse/progression was observed in de novo DLBCL. All patients underwent a CT scan of the brain. In one case, an intratumor was detected in a relapse, and when the diagnosis was revised at the reference center, the patient was found to have PMBL [24]. Therefore, when conducting a differential diagnosis of primary DLBCL with other lymphomas, it is necessary to consider this. Neuroleukemia was diagnosed at the time of diagnosis in one patient.

The US National Multidisciplinary Cancer Network (NCCN) recommends the use of IPI-CNS to determine the likelihood of a relapse involving the CNS. This predictive model is based on data from the German non-Hodgkin lymphoma research group [25]. It assumed that the IPI-CNS would allow stratification of patients into groups with a low, medium, and high risk of recurrence with involvement of the CNS. The same German research group for the study of non-Hodgkin lymphomas published the updated results in 2016, which showed that the rate of recurrence in the central nervous system during the first 2 years in the high-risk group was 10%, in the moderate-risk group—2.9%, and low risk—0.8% [26]. Based on these data, it is recommended to prevent the development of relapse with the involvement of the central nervous system in patients with high-risk DLBCL. At the same time, the pathogenesis mechanism of the development of relapses with the involvement of the central nervous system is unknown.

The registry of DLBCL patients of the German research group for the study of non-Hodgkin's lymphomas began long before the change in the diagnostic criteria for DLBCL and before the isolation of new forms of aggressive B-cell lymphomas. In 2008 WHO classification, an unclassified B-cell lymphoma was isolated from the heterogeneous group of DLBCL, which occupies an intermediate position between DLBCL and Burkitt's lymphoma, based on the determination of the gene expression profile, characterized by an aggressive clinical course and poor prognosis [3]. In the 2017 revised WHO classification, based on the detection of molecular breakdowns—translocations involving the *c-MYC, BCL2,* and/or *BCL-6* gene loci, it was given a new name—high-grade B-cell lymphoma—double-/triple-hit lymphoma (HGBL, DHL/THL), and without these translocations—high-grade B-cell lymphoma, unspecified (HGBL, NOS) [2]. It is known from the literature that it is in these two groups that the intratumor of the central nervous system is more common. The likelihood of developing relapses with involvement of the central nervous system exceeds 10–20% in the medium and high-risk groups, respectively [27, 28]. Relapses with isolated involvement of the brain substance also occur in patients with primary mediastinal B-cell large cell and follicular lymphoma [29].

4.2 Bone marrow trephine biopsy data

Discordant involvement of the bone marrow in patients with DLBCL in 2017 WHO classification remains as a manifestation of DLBCL and indicated as a sign of a poor prognosis. Everyone understands that the signs of prognosis are considered within the framework of a specific program, and adverse signs on R-CHOP leveled out on intensive care. Since de novo DLBCL is an aggressive and curable disease, and indolent lymphomas constantly recur and cannot be cured, discordant involvement of bone marrow indicates the transformation of indolent lymphomas into DLBCL.

According to the concept of tumor progression, hemoblastoses, including lymphomas, usually go through two stages—monoclonal (indolent) and polyclonal (malignant); a tumor can sequentially go through different stages of progression, but it can also start directly from the malignant stage [16, 30].

4.3 Laboratory data

4.3.1 Paraprotein secretion

Paraprotein secretion is characteristic of indolent lymphomas. However, like discordant involvement of bone marrow in the WHO classification in 2017, indicated that patients with de novo DLBCL can occur and is a sign of a poor prognosis. Therefore, all that said regarding discordant involvement bone marrow applies to the secretion of paraprotein. Paraprotein M is usually secreted. However, there are isolated cases of secretion of paraprotein G and, it is a laboratory sign indicating the secondary nature of DLBCL. However, we must not forget that some of these cases may be a manifestation of Monoclonal gammopathy of undetermined significance (MGUS), especially in elderly patients.

According to a large retrospective study, which included 599 patients with de novo DLBCL, an immunochemical study was performed in 245 patients, of whom the secretion of paraprotein M was detected in 12.5%, and the latter turned out to be an independent sign of a poor prognosis, the reason for which the authors could not explain. In another retrospective study, which included 245 patients, the predominant paraprotein isotype was immunoglobulin G and this was explained either by the different methodology used to determine the paraprotein isotype or by racial differences. The authors of both studies indicated that the presence of paraprotein, regardless of isotype, was an independent sign of lower overall and event-free survival [19]. The authors of one of these works attributed the reason for the poor results to thc presence of the *MYD88 L265p* mutation.

In another large retrospective study involving 382 patients who underwent an immunochemical analysis of blood and urine, of which 225 (59%), patients had M paraprotein secretion and Waldenstrom's macroglobulinemia was diagnosed. Of the remaining 157 (41%) cases, 77 (49%) had Chronic lymphocytic leukemia (CLL)/ small lymphocyte lymphoma, 27 (17.2%) LMZ, 18 (11.5%) FL, 11 (7%)—lymphoma from cells of the mantle zone, in 5 (3.2%)—DLBCL as a result of transformation of mature cell lymphomas, in 7 (4.5%)—de novo DLBCL, in 4 (2.5%)—angioimmunoblastic T-cell lymphoma, in another 8 (5%) people—unspecified B-cell lymphoma [31]. Thus, the percentage of paraproteinemia, paraproteinuria in patients with DLBCL is small, but when examining patients, an immunochemical study of blood and urine is mandatory.

According to Gavrilina OA, significant differences in survival were obtained in the group with involvement of the bone marrow. Monoclonal paraprotein secretion was typical for DLBCL with involvement of the bone marrow ($p < 0.0001$) [32].

All of the above allows us to assume that cases with the secretion of paraprotein are also the transformation of indolent lymphomas in DLBCL.

4.4 Relapses

Response to therapy should be considered an independent predictor of the prognosis within any protocol. All patients with de novo DLBCL who received R-mNHL-BFM-90 at the Federal State Budgetary Institution of the National Medical Research Center of Hematology are under our supervision. Of 86 patients from the high- and intermediate-risk group included in the pilot study from 2002 to 2010 with a diagnosis of de novo nodal DLBCL, unspecified, relapses within 3 years developed in 11 people, 2 morc patients developed relapses after 13 years. Only two cases out of the 11 indicated that there was de novo DLBCL. When reviewing histological preparations in nine patients, the diagnoses were revised in favor of FL, LMZ, nodular lymphocyte-predominant Hodgkin lymphoma (NLPHL), and high-grade B-cell lymphoma. The five-year disease-free survival rate was 86%.

The histological results of relapses of patients in a randomized trial are presented above. As it can be seen from **Table 2**, relapses for primary DLBCL are not typical, including on R-CHOP therapy, even in high-risk patients if CR is achieved and there is no *TP53* gene mutation. However, there is an assumption that cases with the presence of a mutation in the *TP53* gene are also the result of the transformation of indolent lymphomas. This assumption arose from the theoretical concepts of tumor progression that the changing signs of a tumor during its growth, the emergence of resistance to previously effective antitumor drugs are explained by repeated mutations of tumor cells, the appearance of subclones, and the selection of more resistant forms among them. Therefore, given the aggressiveness of de novo DLBCL, there is no time for changes in tumor signs during its growth, as well as for the selection of the most resistant forms. In our two patients with de novo

DLBCL with relapse and the presence of a *TP53 gene* mutation, in one case, paraprotein secretion took place, indirectly indicating the transformation of indolent lymphoma. In the second case, it has an exceptional lesion of extranodal organs—at the onset of the mammary gland, in the first relapse - of the pleura involvement. The second relapse was represented by mammary gland involvement.

In the case of achieving CR, with the exception of cases with a mutation in the *TP53* gene, in patients with primary DLBCL, including extranodal, including DLBCL of the testes and mammary gland, relapses are casuistic.

It is currently difficult to distinguish de novo DLBCL from nodular LMZ, as well as MALT - lymphoma in the case of histological transformation if there is no long history of the disease.

Finally, in recent years, there are fewer and fewer cases of de novo DLBCL with Germinal center (GC) molecular type, which indicates that all cases from B-cells of the germinal center are either FL or high-grade B-cell lymphoma.

Conflict of interest

The authors declare no conflict of interest.

Dedication

The work is dedicated to the memory of my deceased Teacher, Academician Andrei Vorobyov.

Author details

Aminat Magomedova*, Anna Misyurina, Sergey Kravchenko, Fatima Babaeva and Andrey Vorobiev†
Federal State Institution "National Research Center for Hematology", Ministry of Health, Moscow, Russian Federation

*Address all correspondence to: maminat@mail.ru

† Deceased author

References

[1] Harris NL, Jaffe ES, Stein H, et al. A revised European-American classification of lymphoid neoplasm's: A proposal from the international lymphoma study group. Blood. 1994;**84**(5):1301-1392. DOI: 10.1182/84.5.1361.1361

[2] Gascoyne RD, Campo E, Jaffe ES, Chan WC, et al. Diffuse large B-cell lymphoma, NOS. In: WHO Classification of Tumours of Haematopoietic and Lymphoid Tissues. 4nd ed. Lyon: International Agency for Research on Cancer; 2017. pp. 291-3253

[3] Stein H, Warnke RA, Chan WC, Jaffe ES. Diffuse large B-cell Lymphoma. In: WHO Classification of Tumours of Haematopoietic and Lymphoid Tissues. Lyon: International Agency for Research on Cancer; 2008. pp. 233-257

[4] Campo E, Pileri SA, Jaffe ES, Nathwani BN, Stein H, Muller-Hermelink HK. Nodal marginal zone lymphoma. In: WHO Classification of Tumours of Haematopoietic and Lymphoid Tissues. Lyon: International Agency for Research on Cancer; 2017. pp. 263-266

[5] Cook JR, Isaacson PG, Chott A, Nakamura S, Muller-Hermelink HK, Harris NL, et al. Extranodal marginal zone lymphoma of mucosa-associated lymphoid tissue (MALT lymphoma). In: WHO Classification of Tumours of Haematopoietic and Lymphoid Tissues. Lyon: International Agency for Research on Cancer; 2017. pp. 259-263

[6] Leoncini L, Campo E, Stein H, Harris NL, Jaffe ES, Kluin PM. Burkitt lymphoma. In: WHO Classification of Tumours of Haematopoietic and Lymphoid Tissues. 4nd ed. Lyon: International Agency for Research on Cancer; 2017. pp. 330-334

[7] Leoncini L, Campo E, Stein H, Harris NL, Jaffe ES, Kluin PM. Burkitt-like lymphoma with 11q aberration. In: WHO Classification of Tumours of Haematopoietic and Lymphoid Tissues. 4nd ed. Lyon: International Agency for Research on Cancer; 2017. pp. 334-335

[8] Jaffe ES Harris NL Swerdlow SH. H Ott G. Nathwani BN. de Jong D. Yoshino T. Spagnolo D. Gascoyne RD. Follicular lymphoma. WHO Classification of Tumours of Haematopoietic and Lymphoid Tissues,International Agency for Research on Cancer, Lyon 2017. 266-282

[9] Swerdlow SH, Campo E, Seto M, Muller-Hermelink HK. Mantle cell lymphoma. In: WHO Classification of Tumours of Haematopoietic and Lymphoid Tissues. 4nd ed. Lyon: International Agency for Research on Cancer; 2017. pp. 285-344

[10] Falini B, Lamant-Rochaix L, Campo E, Jaffe ES, Gascoyne RD, Stein H, et al. Anaplastic large cell lymphoma, ALK-positive. In: WHO Classification of Tumours of Haematopoietic and Lymphoid Tissues. 4nd ed. Lyon: International Agency for Research on Cancer; 2017. pp. 413-418

[11] Kluin PM, Harris NL, Stein H, Leoncini L, Campo E, Jaffe ES, et al. High-grade B-cell lymphoma. In: WHO Classification of Tumours of Haematopoietic and Lymphoid Tissues. Lyon: International Agency for Research on Cancer; 2017. pp. 335-341

[12] Magomedova A, Kremenetskay A, Kravchenko S, et al. Prognostic value of focal bone marrow lesions in diffuse large B-cell lymphosarcoma. Therapeutic Archives. 2004;7:60-63

[13] Maeshima AM, Taniguchi H, Toyoda K, Yamauchi N, et al. Clinicopathological features of histological transformation from extranodal marginal zone B-cell

lymphoma of mucosa-associated lymphoid tissue to diffuse large B-cell lymphoma: An analysis of 467 patients. British Journal of Haematology. 2016;**174**:923-931. DOI: 10.1111/bjh.14153, Epub 2016 Jul 27

[14] Camacho FI, Mollejo M, Mateo MS, et al. Progression to large B-cell lymphoma in splenic marginal zone lymphoma: A description of a series of 12 cases. The American Journal of Surgical Pathology. 2001;**25**:1268-1276. DOI: 10.1097/00000478-200110000-00007

[15] Conconi A, Franceschetti S, Aprile von Hohenstaufen K, Margiotta-Casaluci G, et al. Histologic transformation in marginal zone lymphomas. Annals of Oncology. 2015;**26**:2329-2335. DOI: 10.1093/annonc/mdv368, Epub 2015 Sep 23

[16] Parry-Jones N, Matutes E, Gruszka-Westwood AM, et al. Prognostic features of splenic lymphoma with villous lymphocytes: A report on 129 patients. British Journal of Haematology. 2003;**120**:759-764. DOI: 10.1046/j.1365-2141.2003.04165.x

[17] Dubois S, Viailly P-J, Mareschal S, Bohers E, et al. Next-generation sequencing in diffuse large B-cell lymphoma highlights molecular divergence and therapeutic opportunities: A LYSA study. Clinical Cancer Research. 2016;**22**(12):2919-2928. DOI: 10.1158/1078-0432.CCR-15-2305

[18] Christina Cox M, Di Napoli A, Fabbri A, Ruco ECL. The significance of serum immunoglobulin paraprotein in diffuse large B-cell lymphoma. British Journal of Haematology. 2018;**182**(5):741-742. DOI: 10.1111/bjh.14873, Epub 2017 Aug 17

[19] Li Y, Wang L, Zhu H-Y, Liang J-H, Wu W, et al. Prognostic significance of serum immunoglobulin paraprotein in patients with diffuse large B cell lymphoma. British Journal of Haematology. 2018;**182**(1):131-134. DOI: 10.1111/bjh.14735, Epub 2017 May 11

[20] Magomedova A, Kravchenko S, Kremenetskay A, Zvonkov E, et al. Nine years of experience in the treatment of patients with diffuse large B-cell lymphosarcoma. Therapeutic Archives. 2011;7:5-10

[21] Hsu SM, Hsu PL. Autocrine and paracrine functions of cytokines in malignant lymphomas. Biomedicine & Pharmacotherapy. 1994;**48**(10):433-444. DOI: 10.1016/0753-3322(94)90004-3

[22] Petinati N, Bigildeev A, Karpenko D, Sats N, et al. Humoral effect of a B-cell tumor on the bone marrow multipotent mesenchymal stromal cells. Biochemistry. 2021;**86**(2):207-216. DOI: 10.1134/S0006297921020097

[23] Fastova A, Magomedova A, Petinati N, Sats N, et al. Multipotent mesenchymal bone marrow stromal cells in patients with diffuse large B-cell lymphoma. Cell Technologies in Biology and Medicine. 2019;**1**:33-36. DOI: 10.1007/s10517-019-04480-6, Epub 2019 Jun 10

[24] Magomedova A, Misiurina A, Mangasarova J, Gorenkova L, et al. Involvement of the central nervous system and the feasibility of preventing recurrence in the central nervous system in patients with nodal diffuse large B-cell lymphoma, NOS. Prospective study data. Therapeutic Archives. 2019;**91**(7):35-40. DOI: 10.26442/00403660.2019.07.000323

[25] Boehme V, Zeynalova S, Kloess M, Loeffler M, et al. Incidence and risk factors of central nervous system recurrence in aggressive lymphoma: a survey of 1693 patients treated in protocols of the German high-grade non-Hodgkin's lymphoma study group

(DSHNHL). Annals of Oncology. 2007;**18**(1):149-157. DOI: 10.1093/annonc/mdl327

[26] Schmitz N, Zeynalova S, Nickelsen M, Kansara R, et al. CNS international prognostic index: A risk model for CNS relapse in patients with diffuse large B-cell lymphoma treated with RCHOP. Journal of Clinical Oncology. 2016;**34**(26):3150-3156. DOI: 10.1200/JCO.2015.65.6520

[27] Savage KJ, Slack GW, Mottok A, Sehn LH, et al. Impact of dual expression of MYC and BCL2 by immunohistochemistry on the risk of CNS relapse in DLBCL. Blood. 2016;**127**(18):2182-2188. DOI: 10.1182/blood-2015-10-676700, Epub 2016 Feb 1

[28] Horn H, Ziepert M, Becher C, Barth TF, et al. MYC status in concert with BCL2 and BCL6 expression predicts outcome in diffuse large B-cell lymphoma. Blood. 2013;**121**(12):2253-2263. DOI: 10.1182/blood-2012-06-435842

[29] Papageorgiou SG, Diamantopoulos P, Levidou G, Angelopoulou MK, et al. Isolated central nervous system relapses in primary mediastinal large B-cell lymphoma after CHOP-like chemotherapy with or without rituximab. Hematological Oncology. 2013;**31**(1):10-17. DOI: 10.1002/hon.2012

[30] Vorobiev AI. Guidelines for Hematology. 3rd ed. Vol. 3. Moscow: Newdiamed; 2003. pp. 40-69

[31] Gavrilina OA, Parovichnikova EN, Zvonkov EE, Troitskaya VV, et al. Diffuse large B-cell lymphoma with monoclonal immunoglobulin secretion. Therapeutic Archives. 2016;**88**(7):56-61. DOI: 10.17116/terarkh201688756-61

[32] Dorokhina EI, Magomedova AU, Kulikov SM, Kremenetskaya AM, et al. Long-term results of high-dose chemotherapy in patients with diffuse large B-cell lymphoma according to the modified NHL-BFM-90 program. Hematology and Transfusiology. 2016;**61**(1):44

Chapter 8

Primary Intraocular Lymphoma: The Masquerade Syndrome

Alessandro Lupi, Barbara Iaccheri, Davide Tucci, Carlo Cagini and Tito Fiore

Abstract

This chapter aims to provide a complete knowledge over the primary intraocular lymphoma (PIOL) and a correct clinical approach towards this rare condition, to avoid delays in diagnosis, which is considered the most important prognostic factor. A PIOL arises with no specific symptoms and could mimic both inflammatory and non-inflammatory ocular conditions. Also known as reticulum cell sarcoma in the past, PIOL is an ocular malignant condition, with a strong bond with primary central system lymphoma (PCNSL). This linkage is underlined by the fact that approximately 30% of the patients with PIOL have also PCNSL at presentation, while 45–90% will develop PCSNL in the following months. A correct diagnosis is currently achieved by the means of many different techniques: cytology, flow cytometry, immunohistochemistry, molecular analysis, and cytokines assay. Treatment of this condition has been completely revolutionized with the introduction of monoclonal antibodies directed against specific proteins present on the surface of lymphomatous cells.

Keywords: primary intraocular lymphoma (PIOL), primary vitreoretinal lymphoma (PVRL), masquerade syndrome, monoclonal antibodies

1. Introduction

An intraocular lymphoma is a heterogeneous group of malignant lymphoid neoplasia, which are divided into two main categories: those arising from vitreoretinal tissue (PVRL) and those deriving from uveal tract [1]. Lymphomas of the retina and/or vitreous are considered as a primary lesion, often with a concomitant central nervous system (CNS) involvement. Conversely, uveal lymphomas can be both primary diseases or metastasis of systemic non-Hodgkin lymphoma (NHL) [1, 2].

The most common form of PIOL is the vitreoretinal lymphoma, an extra nodal, non-Hodgkin, diffuse, large, B-cell lymphoma. Rare cases of primary T-cell vitreoretinal lymphoma can occur, but they are usually secondary to human T-cell lymphotropic virus type 1 infection or metastatic T-cell lymphoma [3–5]. Among immunocompetent individuals, the average incidence of vitreoretinal lymphoma is between 50 and 60 years, while in immunocompromised populations this condition develops earlier [6–8].

The most frequent pattern of presentation of PVRL is the infiltration of the sub-retinal pigment epithelium (RPE) in the form of lymphomatous aggregates and the presence of single neoplastic cells in the vitreous cavity [9, 10]. Although

 IntechOpen

less frequently than posterior segment involvement, some important findings in the anterior segment are: keratic precipitates, aqueous cells, flare, and iris nodules; however, these important elements are not specific for a correct diagnosis of intraocular lymphoma [8, 11].

Regarding the involvement of the central nervous system (CNS), the periventricular site is the most common way of presentation and would explain the tendency to spread to cerebrospinal fluid and leptomeninges.

The linkage between PVRL and PCNSL is variable, indeed CNS disease could occur before, following, or simultaneously with the ocular presentation; several previous studies show that 25% of patients with PCNSL will have the concomitant ocular disease at the time of diagnosis [12]. On the other hand 56–85% of individuals with PVRL will develop CNS involvement subsequently [13–16].

Therefore, PVRL is usually fatal. Despite its rare occurrence, PVRL remains a diagnostic and therapeutic challenge and the lack of effective therapeutic tools and delay in diagnosis may lead to a poor prognosis [17].

Previously misnamed as "reactive lymphoid hyperplasia" or "uveal pseudotumor", primary uveal lymphoma is a less common entity involving any region of the uveal tract, with a less-aggressive clinical course [18, 19]. Cockerham and associates re-evaluated pathological specimens of benign choroidal reactive lymphoid hyperplasia archived at the Armed Forces Institute of Pathology, and found out that 80% of these are low-grade, B-cell lymphomas [20] and that their subtype is of an extra-nodal, marginal zone or mucosa-associated, lymphoid tissue lymphoma [18]. Primary uveal lymphomas are typically quiescent, paucisymptomatic but with a marked propensity towards extraocular extension [18, 21].

Rarely they tend to turn into more malignant and aggressive tumors and, when treatment is necessary, they are very radiosensitive and carry a good prognosis [19, 20].

Despite the importance of the uveal form as well, we will exhaustively focus on the type of large B-cell intraocular lymphoma [1].

2. Epidemiology

Vitreoretinal lymphomas are rare tumors, with an annual incidence of 0.46 per 100,000 people, representing 4–6% of primary brain tumors and 1–2% of extra nodal lymphomas [12, 16, 22].

In the last 15 years, the incidence of this condition has tripled both in the US and in Europe. At the beginning, this increase in incidence was associated with the arise of immunocompromised persons due to AIDS condition, but since the introduction of highly active antiretroviral therapy, the development of intraocular lymphoma does not follow the decrease of patients with the acquired immune deficiency syndrome (AIDS) [23–26]. Iatrogenic immunosuppression may also lead to PIOL [27]. The cause for the increased incidence in immunocompetent patients is unknown [24].

3. Aetiology

The aetiology of PIOL/PCNSL is not very clear. Two theories have been implicated in PVRL development: infectious origin and hematological spread.

3.1 Infectious origin

According to the infectious theory, neoplastic transformation occurs into two steps: in the first one, viruses such as HIV or EBV, especially in immunocompromised people, attack the lymphoid cells while, in the second one, it happens neoplastic transformation, that occurs in the CNS and/or in the eye.

This theory is supported by the frequent isolation of the EBV virus in AIDS patients with intraocular lymphoma, which also shows more aggressive characteristics [28]. In rare cases the parasite *Toxoplasma gondii* has also been isolated in patients with B-cell lymphoma, although the connection is much less strong than that with EBV and HIV [29].

3.2 Haematological spread

In hematological spread, neoplastic cells from nodal and extra-nodal sites spread to ocular and CNS structures [30]. According to this theory, B-cell chemokines may selectively attract lymphoma cells from the choroidal circulation to the retinal pigment epithelium (RPE) and/or retina. This theory is supported by the fact that B-cell chemokine receptors CXCR4 and CXCR5 were detected in the lymphoma cells, whereas the ligands BLC and SDF-1 were detected only in the RPE [31]. On this basis, it has been suggested that inhibition of B-cell chemo-attractants could be a future strategy for the treatment of PIOL [31].

4. Clinical presentation

4.1 Ocular features

Because its presentation can mimic a wide variety of ocular diseases, PVRL has often been addressed as a masquerade syndrome. Signs vary significantly between patients and are usually bilateral (64–83%) but often asymmetrical at presentation [1, 2]. Symptoms of hazy vision and/or floaters are the most commonly reported by patients.

4.1.1 Anterior segment

Anterior segment findings are usually uncommon and specific, including few anterior chamber cells, keratic precipitates [32, 33], presence of pseudo-hypopyon [34, 35], and iris and trabecular meshwork [27, 36], which could cause, respectively, heterochromia and secondary angle closure.

4.1.2 Posterior segment

Posterior segment examination reveals vitritis, ranging from mild to severe.

Lymphomatous cells present in the vitreous cavity are homogeneous and tend to be larger than the reactive cells of the immune system and they rarely aggregate each other in clusters. Ophthalmoscopically it's possible to observe clumps, strands, sheets and membranes that cause mild-to-severe vitreous haze; these rows of cells along vitreous fibrils give it a similar appearance to the "aurora borealis". Involvement of the retinal layer and/or RPE is manifested by creamy lesions with a characteristic yellowish appearance on examination of the fundus of the eye [14]. This can result in a characteristic "leopard skin" pigmentation overlying the mass [10]. Other retinal findings include: isolated subretinal lesions [37], exudative retinal detachment [37], RPE atrophy with subretinal fibrosis, and disciform scarring at the macula. Optic nerve infiltration may also occur [38]. Cystoid macular oedema is usually absent.

4.2 Central nervous system features

At presentation, 16–34% of PVRL cases have neurological involvement and it has been estimated that between 42% and 92% of patients can develop intracranial lymphoma within a mean interval of 30 months [14].

Neurological symptoms may occur at any time during the disease course and can be focal and/or diffuse. Most common symptoms include behavioral changes, alteration in cognitive function, focal neurological deficits (like hemiparesis or ataxia) and new-onset seizures (which is a strong indicator of neurological involvement).

Infiltration of the meninges by malignant lymphoma cells without intracerebral involvement can also be noted [12].

5. Diagnosis

5.1 Diagnostic approach

When a PIOL is suspected, it's necessary to exclude other types of uveitis. Therefore, the patient's examination should include chest radiography, complete blood cell count, erythrocyte sedimentation rate, routine blood chemistries, and other laboratory studies.

The definitive diagnosis of PIOL is based on the identification of atypical lymphoid cells in the eye, usually sampling the vitreous. However, it's possible to reach a diagnosis by demonstrating the presence of lymphomatous cells in the cerebrospinal fluid (CSF), avoiding the vitreous biopsy, because PIOL is a subtype of PCNSL.

Furthermore, because PIOL is closely related to PCNSL, neuroimaging of the brain and orbits and a lumbar puncture are required, to exclude a neurological involvement [39–41].

5.2 Ocular examination

5.2.1 Optical coherence tomography (OCT)

OCT facilitates the detection of many retinal abnormalities whose presence is related to PVRL [42].

The most common alteration on OCT is the evidence of hyperreflective signals (nodules, bands, and nods) at the level of RPE, corresponding to homogenous semi-opaque greyish spots in fundus photography. Those findings are instrumental proof of invasion and proliferation of the lymphomatous cells inside the retinal tissue. Anyway, it's important to differentiate these hyper-reflective spots from those which can be detected in other clinical entities (e.g., diabetic retinopathy, age-related macular degeneration, etc.) [43–45].

Apart from this, a wide range of other OCT findings associated with PVRL has been reported, including hyper-reflective subretinal infiltration, hyper-reflective infiltrates in inner retinal layers, RPE undulation, clumps of vitreous cells, and sub-RPE deposits [46]. Conversely, cystoid macular oedema is a rare finding [47].

5.2.2 Fundus fluorescein angiography (FFA) and indocyanine green angiography (ICGA)

The positive and negative predictive value of the combined use of FFA and ICGA is 89% and 85%, respectively [48].

The most common alteration on FFA is the presence of hypo-fluorescent spots, presenting with the so-called "leopard-spot" appearance [49].

Apart from this, a wide range of other FFA findings associated with PVRL has been reported, including punctate hyper-fluorescent window defects (55%), round hypo-fluorescent lesions (34%), and vasculitis (14%) were reported. Cystoid macular oedema did not exceed 2%. In addition, fluorescein leakage along retinal vessels and peri-arteriolar staining may also be seen in eyes with PVRL [43].

The most common alteration on ICGA is the presence of small hypo-fluorescent lesions in the early stages of PVRL, that become less obvious in later stages of the disease [49].

5.2.3 Fundus autofluorescence (FAF)

FAF may facilitate the detection of the active status of PVRL.

The most common alteration on FAF is the presence of a granular pattern of hyper-auto-fluorescent spots encircled by a hypo-auto-fluorescent ring [46]. Granular patterns were detected in several retinal areas, but this finding was not restricted to visible tumor location. Usually, these hyper-auto-fluorescents spots on FAF corresponds to the hypo-fluorescence spots on FFA (36%) and the hyperreflective spots on OCT (43%) [43].

It is noteworthy, that, after intravitreal administration of methotrexate, these hyper-auto-fluorescents spots become hypo-auto-fluorescent [42, 43].

5.2.4 B-scan ultrasound

There are no specific features for PVRL in ultrasound B-scan. However, B-scan can be very useful when visualization of the posterior segment is difficult.

Findings include elevated chorioretinal lesions, retinal detachment, vitreous debris, and enlargement of the optic nerve shadow [49].

5.3 Neurological examination

5.3.1 Imaging

Intraocular lymphoma with CNS involvement is evidenced by computed tomography (CT) and magnetic resonance (MR).

On CT it appears as an isodense or hyperdense lesion while on MR it provides a hypodense signal in both TI and T2 sequences [50]. If the diagnosis is swift, it is probable to find a single lesion up to 70% of cases; with the delay of diagnosis grows the possibility of finding multiple lesions. The most affected regions are: basal ganglia, corpus callosum, or periventricular subependymal regions [51].

5.3.2 Invasive procedure

A lumbar puncture should be performed to obtain cerebrospinal fluid (CSF), and this should be sent for routine cytologic, chemical, and cytokine analysis. Lymphomatous cells can be identified in the CSF of up to 25% of patients with known lesions on MR [50].

If lymphoma cells are found in the CSF, then a diagnosis of PCNSL can be made and no further diagnostic procedures are necessary.

In the cases with suspected CNS lesions on neuroradiological images and with negative CSF cytology, patients should undergo a stereotaxic biopsy of the brain lesion to reach a certain diagnosis [52].

In cases of both negative neuroradiological images and CSF cytology, it is necessary to acquire histological material through diagnostic vitrectomy of the eye most affected by the neoplastic process or in the one with the least visual acuity [33].

5.4 Ophthalmic biopsy

5.4.1 Bioptic material sampling

5.4.1.1 Vitreous biopsy

Vitreous represent the preferred tissue to sample in case of chronic uveitis of unknown cause or when an intraocular malignancy/infection is suspected. Furthermore, vitrectomy can also be performed in case of suspected PCNSL, when lumbar puncture and cytologic analysis of CSF fail to reveal neoplastic cells [53]. A final diagnosis of PIOL allows clinicians to start the appropriate treatment [54, 55].

Cytologic examination of vitreous biopsy has been employed to make a diagnosis of PIOL since the mid-1970s. The technique for performing a complete pars plana vitrectomy in a suspected case of PIOL follows typical protocol:

- a standard three-port pars plana vitrectomy is performed
- a complete core vitrectomy is recommended because the cytological analysis is standard [56] and molecular analysis with polymerase chain reaction amplification (PCR) and cytokine-level analysis are commonly performed [41, 57]
- the first vitreous sample is used for cytological analysis
- the second vitreous sample is diluted to allow a subsequent analysis of cytokine levels
- the vitreous fluid is also studied for microbiological aspects
- aware of the easy tendency of tumor cells to deteriorate, the sample of vitreous fluid is mixed with Roswell Park Memorial Institute (RPMI) culture medium to allow better maintenance and a more complete analysis of cells.

These sample must be analyzed by expert pathologists in the shortest possible time to increase diagnostic possibilities because of the rapid deterioration of cancer cells [58]. It must be stressed out that timing is essential because lymphomatous cells rapidly begin to degenerate.

Vitreous samples may not always contain neoplastic cells and, thus, be negative for the diagnosis of PIOL. This might happen when there is minimal vitreal involvement or when cells have degenerated. In such events, it may be necessary to perform another vitrectomy and send it to a well-qualified cytological laboratory [15].

5.4.1.2 External chorioretinal biopsy

Failure to identify malignant cells in the vitreous can occur and may be due to degeneration of the cells in samples, paucity of cells into the vitreous cavity, or lack of vitreal involvement. Indeed, lymphomatous cells may be confined solely to the sub-RPE and, in this case, an external chorioretinal biopsy (pioneered by Peyman and colleagues) may lead to a definitive diagnosis of PIOL [59–62].

The technique for performing an external chorioretinal biopsy in a suspected case of PIOL follows typical protocol:

- first, if the fundus is visible, laser photocoagulation is applied 1–3 days before surgery in a zone of the area to be biopsied. When vitreous is too hazy, endo-laser is performed immediately after pars-plana-vitrectomy
- a three-port pars plana vitrectomy is performed (in addition to an endo-laser if it was not performed before the surgery)
- a nearly full-thickness scleral flap is made, leaving one side attached to act as a hinge; when the flap of the sclera is retracted, the surgeon can visualize the choroids
- penetrating diathermy is located across the chorioretinal layer along the inner choroidal side
- appropriate chorioretinal tissue is provided by two opening incisions parallel to the limbus
- then one blade of a 0.12 nipper is inserted for the entire chorioretinal thickness
- finally, to allow the correct removal of a block of chorioretinal tissue, two further incisions, perpendicular to the limbus, are made with Vannas scissors
- finally, the scleral flap is locked.

5.4.1.3 Internal chorioretinal biopsy

Internal chorioretinal (transvitreal retinochoroidal) biopsy is another approach by which chorioretinal tissue is acquired [63].

Biopsy should be carried out as follow:

- a standard three-port vitrectomy is performed (sending undiluted and diluted vitrectomy to the pathology laboratory for analysis)
- endo-diathermy is used to outline an area of the retina that is of interest
- the intraocular scissors are taken to the vitreous chamber where they dissect the marked area of the retina
- then the intraocular scissors carry retinal tissue out of the eye through the entry site.

5.4.2 Bioptic tissue examinations

5.4.2.1 Histochemical staining

The cytological study of lymphomatous cells represents a standardized technique that has greatly been improved by different types of histochemical staining, such as Giemsa, E-E (haematoxylin-eosin) or Diff-Quick [1].

The main cytological features are: big atypical lymphoid cells with considerable, irregular nuclei and one to several prominent nucleoli, basophilic cytoplasm, rare mitoses, and increased nuclear/cytoplasmic ratio [64]. The identification of lymphomatous cells is further complicated, in addition to their fragility, by the frequent reactive inflammatory infiltrate that accompanies the tumor response.

5.4.2.2 Immunophenotyping

Initial workup should always include immunophenotyping for B-cell markers (CD20, CD79a, PAX5) and T-cell markers (CD2, CD3), because atypical cells found in histochemical staining may also exist in certain reactive conditions, such as acute viral infection, leading to a misdiagnosis [65, 66].

Furthermore, immunophenotyping can detect the presence of monoclonality, which supports the diagnosis of lymphoma, because most PIOL are monoclonal B cell lymphomas that stain positively for B cell markers and show restricted expression of either kappa or lambda chain: indeed, a ratio of kappa/lambda light chains of >3 or <0.6 is considered as a reliable and useful marker for clonality expression [67].

Although most intraocular lymphomas arise from the B cell line, precursors from the T line can rarely be found.

This makes diagnosis much more difficult due to the lack of specific immunocytochemical markers.

Morphologically they can simulate a reactive inflammatory infiltrate but the immunohistochemistry for CD3 marker and the PCR for genetic rearrangements of TCR gene allow to discriminate these two different cell populations [68, 69].

In conclusion, cytology remains the diagnostic gold standard without forgetting, however, that flow cytometry guarantees important information for diagnostic purposes, indeed it can analyze several different markers simultaneously and has been used to confirm monoclonality in both B cell and T cell PIOL [1].

5.4.2.3 Cytokine's analysis

Although it's not diagnostic, analysis of the level of specific cytokines could give valuable information in the diagnosis of PIOL. Furthermore, it can be performed on the supernatant of the vitreous sample, sparing the main specimen for other exams.

The most useful cytokine is IL-10, which is an immune-suppressive cytokine, usually secreted by type-B lymphocytes, whose levels are elevated in both vitreous and aqueous humor (AH). Several studies have shown that interloquine 10 levels of at least 50 pg/mL in aqueous humor and 400 pg/mL in vitreous humor are strongly suspected for intraocular lymphoma.

Moreover, interloquine 10 levels into the vitreous became particularly valuable if compared to IL-6 levels (which is a pro-inflammatory cytokine commonly secreted by macrophages and T-cells): in fact, in other forms of uveitis (given the inflammatory nature of the process) IL-6 levels are lot higher than IL-10 ones, while in PIOL (due to the monoclonal proliferation of type-B lymphocytes) IL-10 levels became prominent. Therefore, also the relationship between the interloquine 10 and the interloquine 6 represents an effective method in placing the diagnostic suspicion of intraocular lymphoma; a ratio greater than 1 is very suggestive for tumor pathology.

On the other side, low interloquine 10 levels may be particularly helpful when a T-cell lymphoma is suspected [70].

5.4.2.4 PCR analysis

Molecular investigations of vitreous samples with PCR can be very useful in the research of lymphocytes' clonality, which is essential for the validation of PIOL diagnosis [70–76].

Detection of clonal immunoglobulin (IgH) and clonal T-cell receptor (TcR) genes rearrangements can contribute to the molecular diagnosis of B-cell and T-cell lymphoma, respectively [73–75].

However, obtain a significant result of genetic analysis, an adequate number of cells should be studied and this is not always possible due to the lack and fragility of lymphoma population [75, 77]. Moreover, with the aim of avoiding misinterpretation of minor clonal expansions as evidence of lymphoma, the results should be evaluated in the context of clinical and morphological features.

5.5 Differential diagnosis

PIOL is one of the most challenging masquerade syndromes. Due to its heterogeneous clinical features, diagnosis is often belated, inducing delayed therapeutic management with poor visual prognosis and life-threatening complications [14].

Differential diagnosis must consider the age of the patient and the clinical presentation. Further investigations will be mandatory to confirm the diagnosis, when possible.

5.5.1 Infectious entities

5.5.1.1 Viral retinitis

PIOL may masquerade as acute retinal necrosis (ARN), caused by a herpes virus infection, typically in immunocompetent patients. Necrosis usually starts at the peripheral retina, progresses rapidly towards the posterior pole, and is associated with vasculitis and dense vitritis. Retinal detachment may occur in 30–75% of cases during the disease.

PIOL may also masquerade as a CMV retinitis, that, conversely, typically occurs in immunocompromised patients.

In both cases, necrosis and hemorrhages can mimic a PIOL and differential diagnosis is confirmed only by AH or vitreous sampling and PCR analysis [78].

5.5.1.2 Severe ocular toxoplasmosis

The differential diagnosis with lesions caused by *Toxoplasma gondii* is very important; they are generally very characteristic already at the ophthalmoscopic examination in immunocompetent people but the greatest difficulties occur in immunocompromised patients because the involvement of anterior segment, vitreous cavity, and retinal scars can simulate the changes in RPE, typical of intraocular lymphoma.

It is therefore very important an appropriate analysis of the ocular fluid that allows isolating the parasite to differentiate the two conditions; nevertheless, in some cases of PIOL the parasite was isolated, suggesting a possible infectious origin of the lymphomatoid process [29].

5.5.1.3 Ocular lue

Syphilitic retinitis has very specific ophthalmoscopic and diagnostic characteristics that can allow to differentiate it from the forms of intraocular lymphoma.

It involves the peripheral retina and, more rarely, the posterior pole. It is associated with retinal vasculitis, moderate vitreous activity, and a modest spread to the anterior segment.

These lesions resolve without leaving any signs with appropriate antibiotic therapy and diagnosis is achieved thanks to serological examination.

5.5.1.4 *Whipple illness*

Whipple condition is a rare systemic disorder caused by *Tropheryma whipplei* which can present rare and late ocular manifestations such as uveitis and chorioretinitis with very disabling bleeding components [79]. Various neuro-ophthalmological manifestations have also been reported, such as ophthalmoplegia, supranuclear gaze palsy, nystagmus, myoclonus, ptosis, papilledema, or optic nerve atrophy.

Persistent vitritis along with retinitis may mimic PIOL. Specific antibiotics may cure the disease without corticosteroids.

5.5.2 *Non-infectious entities*

5.5.2.1 *Granulomatous processes*

The two conditions that mostly enter into differential diagnosis with intraocular lymphomas are sarcoidosis and TBC.

Both of these conditions affect older people and, specially, those with compromised immune defenses.

Although the presence of very specific elements such as posterior synechiae or cystoid macular edema enable an easy differential diagnosis with PIOL, in cases of the massive involvement of the posterior segment the clinical situation can be more difficult to define [80].

The further difficulty is given by the need to perform multiple tests to reach the correct diagnosis so that in some cases it is even necessary to analyze eye samples [81].

5.5.2.2 *Bechet's disease*

Bechet's disease occurs in young males more than females. Retinal necrosis is associated with dense vitritis, retinal vasculitis, and retinal vascular occlusion. Foci of retinitis may mimic areas of infiltration by PIOL and may resolve spontaneously.

Diagnosis is based on a set of criteria defined by the International Study Group for Bechet's disease.

5.5.2.3 *Atypical Fuchs iridocyclitis*

Fuchs iridocyclitis is typically unilateral disease that occurs in young adults and involves the anterior segment of the eye. Sometimes, it may also be associated with different types of intermediate uveitis as well as PIOL. Therefore, PIOL must be considered in atypical forms of FHC, especially when there is bilateral involvement.

5.5.2.4 *Cryptogenic inflammatory processes*

The presence of idiopathic inflammatory processes, especially in elderly and immunocompromised people, represents the most common and most difficult differential diagnosis.

These processes arise with completely nonspecific inflammatory affections, concerning the posterior segment.

In these cases, it's very important the diagnostic suspicion of lymphomatoid origin and clinicians should perform all the necessary analysis to discriminate this condition [82].

5.5.2.5 Miscellanea

Hodgkin's lymphomas can manifest themselves in the form of non-specific inflammatory processes of the posterior segment but, unlike PIOL, the vitreous involvement is much less evident [83].

Atypical uveo-meningitis that can mimic the clinical aspects of VKH syndrome and be resistant to common attack drugs should raise the suspicion of a lymphomatoid process [84].

Uveitis associated with the HTLV-1 virus provide ophthalmological characteristics very similar to PIOL; diagnostic investigations are therefore necessary for making a correct differential diagnosis [85].

6. Treatment

Optimal management for patients with PIOL requires a team of different specialists involving an ophthalmologist, The first line of treatment is high-dose systemic chemotherapy, associated with topical intravitreal chemotherapy and/or ocular radiotherapy, even in cases where no evidence of PCNSL is detected [2, 86].

6.1 Systemic chemotherapy

According to recent guidelines, systemic intravenous therapy with methotrexate represents the gold standard for the treatment of PIOL with a CNS and/or systemic involvement. Results show a very high remission rate, with an even better outcome when combined with other treatments [11, 87]. Several studies have also shown an increase in survival compared to treatments that did not include high doses of chemotherapy [88].

Among the many chemotherapic regimens including methotrexate, several studies reported that the MATRIX regimen (methotrexate, cytarabine, thiotepa, and rituximab) offers the best clinical outcome, with a higher success rate than methotrexate alone or any other form of a combination of drugs [89].

In cases with relapse or refractory response, treatment includes high dose chemotherapy with thiotepa, busulfan, and cyclophosphamide, followed by autologous peripheral blood stem cell transplantation [88].

6.2 Ocular chemotherapy

Ocular chemotherapy means the usage of specific chemotherapic agents administered intravitreally. Two local chemotherapic agents can be used in the treatment of PIOL: methotrexate and rituximab.

6.2.1 Intravitreal methotrexate

The use of intravitreal methotrexate, combined with systemic chemotherapy, has shown good results in the local control of PIOL. Currently, the dose is 400 μg in 0.1 mL and the plan assumes two injections per week during the first month, one injection per week in the next two months, and one injection per month during the following nine months, for a total of 1 year of therapy [90]. Same regimen is recommended in the treatment of relapsed PIOL [91–93], in the ocular relapse of PCNSL [94], and intrathecal chemotherapy [95].

Results show very high remission rates, while ocular complications are unlikely to happen and are essentially represented by transient changes in intraocular pressure and corneal epitheliopathy [96].

6.2.2 Intravitreal rituximab

The use of intravitreal Rituximab (an anti-CD20 monoclonal antibody) has recently been proposed for the treatment of CD20-positive PVRL [88]. The most studied treatment plan assumes one injection per week in four weeks.

Results show a high rate of the initial response to treatment, but there is still a high rate of tumor recurrence. In these cases, treatment can be with a new course of rituximab which has less toxicity than other chemotherapy drugs or by initiating therapy with methotrexate [97].

6.3 Radiation therapy

The use of radiation therapy for PIOL can vary according to various factors.

In forms of PIOL with exclusive ocular localization, local radiation exposure with external radiotherapy represents the current therapeutic standard, with an optimal dosage of 30–35 Gy administered in approximately 15 fractions [2, 98].

In cases, with concomitant involvement of both eyes and/or CNS and in cases in which systemic chemotherapy treatment has failed, panencephalic and ocular irradiation treatment can be added, but this could lead to complications both at the cerebral and ocular level, such as cognitive deterioration, ataxia, and, rarely, even death [98].

6.4 Rising treatments

In consideration of the continuous emerging of new resistance mechanisms put in place by cancerous cells against current therapies, there is a rising interest in developing new therapeutical approaches with engineered techniques.

One of the most studied strategies involves the use of FasL vesicles membranes, to stimulate the immune system to invade the eye (interrupting its situation as a privileged immune site) [99].

Another very promising strategy (tested only in animals) is the use of intraocular injection with recombinant immunotoxin HA22, which shows a very satisfactory response rate [100].

Other monoclonal antibodies (such as daclizumab, efalizumab, and alemtuzumab) have been tested and showed positive results in animal models [101].

Some authors described autologous stem cell transplantation as a possible therapeutic strategy in case of refractory and/or recurrent intraocular lymphomas, but, the lack of data does not allow to define of universal therapeutic standards as well as the correct chemotherapy regimen for transplant preparation [88, 102].

7. Prognosis

The diagnosis of PVRL is often delayed, due to late referral to an ophthalmologist: indeed, most patients present with unalarming symptoms, like persistent floaters but relatively preserved visual acuity.

The mortality rates between the various studies differ enormously.

This is partly due to the rarity of the disease which makes it impossible to identify a standardized and universally used therapeutic regimen, partly due to the clinical differences of the patients under examination.

Despite this, literature states that the rate fluctuates between 9 and 81%, guaranteeing an average survival of about 2 years from diagnosis [1, 98].

8. Conclusion

Management of PIOL is very challenging for the ophthalmologist because diagnosis is usually made difficult by the great capacity of this condition to masquerade other common ocular affections and treatment strategies that have poor clinical evidence (due to lack of cases). Anyway, in recent years the improvement of diagnostic techniques allowed a more rapid diagnosis and the development of new therapeutical strategies. The hope is that increasing in diagnostic efficiency and therapeutic perspectives could lead to the definition of univocal guidelines thanks to an increasing number of intraocular lymphomas to be subjected to various trials.

In conclusion, it's essential to create a multidisciplinary network of specialists involving an oncologist, onco-hematologist, and ophthalmologist to define the best diagnostic and therapeutic process.

Author details

Alessandro Lupi, Barbara Iaccheri*, Davide Tucci, Carlo Cagini and Tito Fiore
Department of Surgical and Biomedical Sciences, Section of Ophthalmology, University of Perugia, S. Maria della Misericordia Hospital, Perugia, Italy

*Address all correspondence to: barbaraiaccheri@gmail.com

References

[1] Coupland SE, Damato B. Understanding intraocular lymphomas. Clinical and Experimental Ophthalmology. 2008. DOI: 10.1111/j.1442-9071.2008.01843.x

[2] Chan C et al. Primary vitreoretinal lymphoma: A report from an international primary central nervous system lymphoma collaborative group symposium. The Oncologist. 2011. DOI: 10.1634/theoncologist.2011-0210

[3] Abrey LE et al. Primary central nervous system lymphoma: The memorial sloan-kettering cancer center prognostic model. Journal of Clinical Oncology. 2006. DOI: 10.1200/JCO.2006.08.2941

[4] Marshall AG et al. HTLV-I associated primary CNS T-cell lymphoma. Journal of the Neurological Sciences. 1998. DOI: 10.1016/S0022-510X(98)00111-7

[5] Coupland SE et al. T-cell and T/natural killer-cell lymphomas involving ocular and ocular adnexal tissues: A clinicopathologic, immunohistochemical, and molecular study of seven cases. Ophthalmology. 1999. DOI: 10.1016/S0161-6420(99)90492-X

[6] Babu K, Murthy KR, Krishnakumar S. Two successive ocular malignancies in the same eye of a HIV-positive patient: A case report. Ocular Immunology and Inflammation. 2010. DOI: 10.3109/09273940903374237

[7] Mathai A, Lall A, Jain R, Pathengay A. Systemic non-Hodgkin's lymphoma masquerading as Vogt-Koyanagi-Harada disease in an HIV-positive patient. Clinical & Experimental Ophthalmology. 2006. DOI: 10.1111/j.1442-9071.2006.01205.x

[8] Rajagopal R, Harbour JW. Diagnostic testing and treatment choices in primary vitreoretinal lymphoma. Retina. 2011. DOI: 10.1097/IAE.0b013e31820a6743

[9] Dean JM, Novak MA, Chan CC, Green WR. Tumor detachments of the retinal pigment epithelium in ocular/central nervous system lymphoma. Retina. 1996. DOI: 10.1097/00006982-199616010-00009

[10] Gass JDM et al. Multifocal pigment epithelial detachments by reticulum cell sarcoma: A characteristic funduscopic picture. Retina. 1984. DOI: 10.1097/00006982-198400430-00001

[11] Akpek EK et al. Intraocular-central nervous system lymphoma: Clinical features, diagnosis, and outcomes. Ophthalmology. 1999. DOI: 10.1016/S0161-6420(99)90341-X

[12] Hochberg FH, Miller DC. Primary central nervous system lymphoma. Journal of Neurosurgery. 1988. DOI: 10.3171/jns.1988.68.6.0835

[13] Peterson K, Gordon KB, Heinemann MH, De Angelis LM. The clinical spectrum of ocular lymphoma. Cancer. 1993. DOI: 10.1002/1097-0142(19930801)72:3<843::AID-CNCR2820720333>3.0.CO;2-#

[14] Cassoux N et al. Ocular end central nervous system lymphoma: Clinical features and diagnosis. Ocular Immunology and Inflammation. 2000. DOI: 10.1076/ocii.8.4.243.6463

[15] Char DH, Ljung BM, Miller T, Phillips T. Primary intraocular lymphoma (ocular reticulum cell sarcoma) diagnosis and management. Ophthalmology. 1988. DOI: 10.1016/S0161-6420(88)33145-3

[16] Freeman LN, Schachat AP, Knox DL, Michels RG, Green WR. Clinical features, laboratory investigations, and survival in ocular

reticulum cell sarcoma. Ophthalmology. 1987. DOI: 10.1016/S0161-6420(87)33256-7

[17] Fend F, Ferreri AJM, Coupland SE. How we diagnose and treat vitreoretinal lymphoma. British Journal of Haematology. 2016. DOI: 10.1111/bjh.14025

[18] Coupland SE et al. Extranodal marginal zone B cell lymphomas of the uvea: An analysis of 13 cases. The Journal of Pathology. 2002. DOI: 10.1002/path.1130

[19] Coupland SE, Joussen A, Anastassiou G, Stein H. Diagnosis of a primary uveal extranodal marginal zone B-cell lymphoma by chorioretinal biopsy: Case report. Graefe's Archive for Clinical and Experimental Ophthalmology. 2005. DOI: 10.1007/s00417-004-1050-4

[20] Cockerham GC, Hidayat AA, Bijwaard KE, Sheng ZM. Re-evaluation of 'reactive lymphoid hyperplasia of the uvea': An immunohistochemical and molecular analysis of 10 cases. Ophthalmology. 2000. DOI: 10.1016/S0161-6420(99)00025-1

[21] Neudorfer M, Kessler A, Anteby I, Goldenberg D, Barak A. Co-existence of intraocular and orbital lymphoma. Acta Ophthalmologica Scandinavica. 2004. DOI: 10.1111/j.1600-0420.2004.00354.x

[22] Aziz HA, Peereboom DM, Singh AD. Primary central nervous system lymphoma. International Ophthalmology Clinics. 2015. DOI: 10.1097/IIO.0000000000000055

[23] Goldberg DE, Smithen LM, Angelilli A, Freeman WR. HIV-associated retinopathy in the HAART era.Retina.2005.DOI:10.1097/00006982-200507000-00015

[24] Nasir S, DeAngelis LM. Update on the management of primary GNS lymphoma. Oncology. 2000

[25] Rivero ME et al. Acquired immunodeficiency syndrome-related intraocular B-cell lymphoma. Archives of Ophthalmology. 1999. DOI: 10.1001/archopht.117.5.616

[26] Sen HN et al. Intravitreal methotrexate resistance in a patient with primary intraocular lymphoma. Ocular Immunology and Inflammation. 2008. DOI: 10.1080/09273940801899764

[27] Chan SM, Hutnik CML, Heathcote JG, Orton RB, Banerjee D. Iris lymphoma in a pediatric cardiac transplant recipient: Clinicopathologic findings. Ophthalmology. 2000. DOI: 10.1016/S0161-6420(00)00172-X

[28] Margolis L, Fraser R, Lichter A, Char DH. The role of radiation therapy in the management of ocular reticulum cell sarcoma. Cancer. 1980. DOI: 10.1002/1097-0142(19800215)45:4<688::AID-CNCR2820450412>3.0.CO;2-F

[29] Shen DF et al. Detection of *Toxoplasma gondii* DNA in primary intraocular B-cell lymphoma. Modern Pathology. 2001. DOI: 10.1038/modpathol.3880424

[30] Buettner H, Bolling JP. Intravitreal Large-Cell Lymphoma. Mayo Clinic Proceedings. 1993. DOI: 10.1016/S0025-6196(12)62276-9

[31] Chan CC, Shen DF, Hackett JJ, Buggage RR, Tuaillon N. Expression of chemokine receptors, CXCR4 and CXCR5, and chemokines, BLC and SDF-1, in the eyes of patients with primary intraocular lymphoma. Ophthalmology. 2003. DOI: 10.1016/S0161-6420(02)01737-2

[32] Coupland SE, Heimann H, Bechrakis NE. Primary intraocular lymphoma: A review of the clinical, histopathological and molecular biological features. Graefe's Archive for Clinical and Experimental

Ophthalmology. 2004. DOI: 10.1007/s00417-004-0973-0

[33] Buggage RR, Chan CC, Nussenblatt RB. Ocular manifestations of central nervous system lymphoma. Current Opinion in Oncology. 2001. DOI: 10.1097/00001622-200105000-00001

[34] Corriveau C, Easterbrook M, Payne D. Lymphoma simulating uveitis (masquerade syndrome). Canadian Journal of Ophthalmology. 1986

[35] Lobo A, Larkin G, Clark BJ, Towler HMA, Lightman S. Pseudo-hypopyon as the presenting feature in B-cell and T-cell intraocular lymphoma. Clinical & Experimental Ophthalmology. 2003. DOI: 10.1046/j.1442-9071.2003.00624.x

[36] Velez G et al. Iris involvement in primary intraocular lymphoma: Report of two cases and review of the literature. Survey of Ophthalmology. 2000. DOI: 10.1016/S0039-6257(00)00118-1

[37] Levy-Clarke G, Byrnes GG, Buggage RR, Chan C-C. Primary intraocular lymphoma diagnosed by fine needle aspiration biopsy of a subretinal lesion. Retina. 2002. DOI: 10.1097/00006982-200208000-00026

[38] Hedayatfar A, Chee SP. Presumptive primary intraocular lymphoma presented as an intraocular mass involving the optic nerve head. Journal of Ophthalmic Inflammation and Infection. 2012. DOI: 10.1007/s12348-011-0045-7

[39] Hormigo A, DeAngelis LM. Primary ocular lymphoma: Clinical features, diagnosis, and treatment. Clinical Lymphoma. 2003. DOI: 10.3816/CLM.2003.n.010

[40] Bataille B et al. Primary intracerebral malignant lymphoma: Report of 248 cases. Journal of Neurosurgery. 2000. DOI: 10.3171/jns.2000.92.2.0261

[41] Tuaillon N, Chan C. Molecular analysis of primary central nervous system and primary intraocular lymphomas. Current Molecular Medicine. 2005. DOI: 10.2174/1566524013363915

[42] Egawa M, Mitamura Y, Hayashi Y, Naito T. Spectral-domain optical coherence tomographic and fundus autofluorescence findings in eyes with primary intraocular lymphoma. Clinical Ophthalmology. 2014. DOI: 10.2147/OPTH.S58114

[43] Folgar FA et al. Spatial correlation between hyperpigmentary changes on color fundus photography and hyperreflective foci on SDOCT in intermediate AMD. Investigative Ophthalmology and Visual Science. 2012. DOI: 10.1167/iovs.12-9813

[44] Ota M et al. Optical coherence tomographic evaluation of foveal hard exudates in patients with diabetic maculopathy accompanying macular detachment. Ophthalmology. 2010. DOI: 10.1016/j.ophtha.2010.06.019

[45] Barry RJ et al. Characteristic optical coherence tomography findings in patients with primary vitreoretinal lymphoma: A novel aid to early diagnosis. The British Journal of Ophthalmology. 2018. DOI: 10.1136/bjophthalmol-2017-311612

[46] Casady M et al. Fundus autofluorescence patterns in primary intraocular lymphoma. Retina. 2014. DOI: 10.1097/IAE.0b013e31829977fa

[47] Jiang T, Zhao Z, Chang Q. Evaluation of cytologic specimens obtained during experimental vitreous biopsy using B-cell lymphoma line. European Journal of Ophthalmology. 2014. DOI: 10.5301/ejo.5000488

[48] Fardeau C et al. Retinal fluorescein, indocyanine green angiography, and optic coherence tomography in non-hodgkin primary intraocular lymphoma. American Journal of Ophthalmology. 2009. DOI: 10.1016/j.ajo.2008.12.025

[49] Sagoo MS et al. Primary intraocular lymphoma. Survey of Ophthalmology. 2014. DOI: 10.1016/j.survophthal. 2013.12.001

[50] DeAngelis LM. Primary central nervous system lymphoma. Current Opinion in Neurology. 1999. DOI: 10.1097/00019052-199912000-00005

[51] Basso U, Brandes AA. Diagnostic advances and new trends for the treatment of primary central nervous system lymphoma. European Journal of Cancer. 2002. DOI: 10.1016/S0959-8049(02)00031-X

[52] Blumenkranz MS et al. Applications and limitations of vitreoretinal biopsy techniques in intraocular large cell lymphoma. Retina. 1992. DOI: 10.1097/00006982-199212031-00014

[53] Parver LM, Font RL. Malignant lymphoma of the retina and brain: Initial diagnosis by cytologic examination of vitreous aspirate. Archives of Ophthalmology. 1979. DOI: 10.1001/archopht.1979.01020020167016

[54] Klingele TG, Hogan MJ. Ocular reticulum cell sarcoma. American Journal of Ophthalmology. 1975. DOI: 10.1016/0002-9394(75)90453-5

[55] Michels RG, Knox DL, Erozan YS, Green WR. Intraocular reticulum cell sarcoma: Diagnosis by pars plana vitrectomy. Archives of Ophthalmology. 1975. DOI: 10.1001/archopht.1975. 01010020961005

[56] Whitcup SM et al. Intraocular lymphoma: Clinical and histopathologic diagnosis. Ophthalmology. 1993. DOI: 10.1016/S0161-6420(93)31469-7

[57] Wolf LA, Reed GF, Buggage RR, Nussenblatt RB, Chan CC. Vitreous cytokine levels. Ophthalmology. 2003. DOI: 10.1016/S0161-6420(03)00811-X

[58] Whitcup SM et al. Improving the diagnostic yield of vitrectomy for intraocular lymphoma. Archives of Ophthalmology. 2000

[59] Peyman GA, May DR, Ericson ES, Goldberg MF. Full-thickness eye wall resection: An experimental approach for treatment of choroidal melanoma. II. Homo- and heterograft. Investigative Ophthalmology. 1972

[60] Peyman GA, Meisels HI, Batko KA, Vlchek JK. Full thickness eye wall biopsy. I. An experimental approach to the tissue diagnosis and study of choroidal and retinal lesions. Investigative Ophthalmology. 1975

[61] Peyman GA, Homer P, Kasbeer R, Vlchek J. Full thickness eye wall biopsy. II. In primates. Investigative Ophthalmology. 1975

[62] Peyman GA, Juarez CP, Raichand M. Full-thickness eye-wall biopsy: Long-term results in 9 patients. The British Journal of Ophthalmology. 1981. DOI: 10.1136/bjo.65.10.723

[63] Nussenblatt RB, Davis JL, Palestine AG. Chorioretinal biopsy for diagnostic purposes in cases of intraocular inflammatory disease. Developments in Ophthalmology. 1992. DOI: 10.1159/000429641

[64] Araujo I, Coupland SE. Primary vitreoretinal lymphoma-A review. Asia-Pacific Journal of Ophthalmology. 2017. DOI: 10.22608/APO.2017150

[65] Coupland SE, Chan CC, Smith J. Pathophysiology of retinal lymphoma. Ocular Immunology and Inflammation. 2009. DOI: 10.1080/09273940903168696

[66] Kimura K et al. Clinical features and diagnostic significance of the

intraocular fluid of 217 patients with intraocular lymphoma. Japanese Journal of Ophthalmology. 2012. DOI: 10.1007/s10384-012-0150-7

[67] Davis JL, Ruiz P, Shah M, Mandelcorn ED. Evaluation of the reactive T-cell infiltrate in uveitis and intraocular lymphoma with flow cytometry of vitreous fluid (an American ophthalmological society thesis). Transactions of the American Ophthalmological Society. 2012

[68] White VA, Gascoyne RD, Paton KE. Use of the polymerase chain reaction to detect B- and T-cell gene rearrangements in vitreous specimens from patients with intraocular lymphoma. Archives of Ophthalmology. 1999. DOI: 10.1001/archopht.117.6.761

[69] Hoffman PM, McKelvie P, Hall AJ, Stawell RJ, Santamaria JD. Intraocular lymphoma: A series of 14 patients with clinicopathological features and treatment outcomes. Eye. 2003. DOI: 10.1038/sj.eye.6700378

[70] Merle-Béral H et al. Biological diagnosis of primary intraocular lymphoma. British Journal of Haematology. 2004. DOI: 10.1046/j.1365-2141.2003.04800.x

[71] Langerak AW et al. EuroClonality/BIOMED-2 guidelines for interpretation and reporting of Ig/TCR clonality testing in suspected lymphoproliferations. Leukemia. 2012. DOI: 10.1038/leu.2012.246

[72] Coupland SE, Hummel M, Müller HH, Stein H. Molecular analysis of immunoglobulin genes in primary intraocular lymphoma. Investigative Ophthalmology and Visual Science. 2005. DOI: 10.1167/iovs.05-0401

[73] Baehring JM et al. Analysis of clonal immunoglobulin heavy chain rearrangements in ocular lymphoma. Cancer. 2005. DOI: 10.1002/cncr.21191

[74] Wang Y, Shen D, Wang VM, Sen HN, Chan CC. Molecular biomarkers for the diagnosis of primary vitreoretinal lymphoma. International Journal of Molecular Sciences. 2011. DOI: 10.3390/ijms12095684

[75] Sugita S et al. Diagnosis of intraocular lymphoma by polymerase chain reaction analysis and cytokine profiling of the vitreous fluid. Japanese Journal of Ophthalmology. 2009. DOI: 10.1007/s10384-009-0662-y

[76] Coupland SE, Perez-Canto A, Hummel M, Stein H, Heimann H. Assessment of HOPE fixation in vitrectomy specimens in patients with chronic bilateral uveitis (masquerade syndrome). Graefe's Archive for Clinical and Experimental Ophthalmology. 2005. DOI: 10.1007/s00417-005-1166-1

[77] Montesinos-Rongen M et al. Interphase cytogenetic analysis of lymphoma-associated chromosomal breakpoints in primary diffuse large B-cell lymphomas of the central nervous system. Journal of Neuropathology and Experimental Neurology. 2002. DOI: 10.1093/jnen/61.10.926

[78] Balansard B et al. Necrotising retinopathies simulating acute retinal necrosis syndrome. The British Journal of Ophthalmology. 2005. DOI: 10.1136/bjo.2004.042226

[79] Drancourt M et al. Culture of tropheryma whippelii from the vitreous fluid of a patient presenting with unilateral uveitis. Annals of Internal Medicine. 2003. DOI: 10.7326/0003-4819-139-12-200312160-00025

[80] Evans M, Sharma O, LaBree L, Smith RE, Rao NA. Differences in clinical findings between caucasians and african americans with biopsy-proven sarcoidosis. Ophthalmology. 2007. DOI: 10.1016/j.ophtha.2006.05.074

[81] Lisa JF, Chan CC. Primary intraocular lymphoma. Archives of

Pathology and Laboratory Medicine. 2009. DOI: 10.5858/133.8.1228

[82] Gupta R, Murray PI. Chronic non-infectious uveitis in the elderly: Epidemiology, pathophysiology and management. Drugs and Aging. 2006. DOI: 10.2165/00002512-200623070-00001

[83] Towler H, De La Fuente M, Lightman S. Posterior uveitis in Hodgkin's disease. Australian and New Zealand Journal of Ophthalmology. 1999. DOI: 10.1046/j.1440-1606.1999.00224.x

[84] Pahk PJ et al. Intravascular lymphoma masquerading as Vogt-Koyanagi-Harada syndrome. Ocular Immunology and Inflammation. 2008. DOI: 10.1080/09273940802023810

[85] Buggage RR. Ocular manifestations of human T-cell lymphotropic virus type 1 infection. Current Opinion in Ophthalmology. 2003. DOI: 10.1097/00055735-200312000-00016

[86] Hoang-Xuan K et al. Diagnosis and treatment of primary CNS lymphoma in immunocompetent patients: Guidelines from the European Association for Neuro-Oncology. The Lancet Oncology. 2015. DOI: 10.1016/S1470-2045(15)00076-5

[87] Abdel-Reheim FA, Edwards E, Arber DA. Utility of a rapid polymerase chain reaction panel for the detection of molecular changes in B-cell lymphoma. Archives of Pathology & Laboratory Medicine. 1996

[88] Soussain C et al. Intensive chemotherapy with thiotepa, busulfan and cyclophosphamide and hematopoietic stem cell rescue in relapsed or refractory primary central nervous system lymphoma and intraocular lymphoma: A retrospective study of 79 cases. Haematologica. 2012. DOI: 10.3324/haematol.2011.060434

[89] Ferreri AJM et al. Chemoimmunotherapy with methotrexate, cytarabine, thiotepa, and rituximab (MATRix regimen) in patients with primary CNS lymphoma: Results of the first randomisation of the International Extranodal Lymphoma Study Group-32 (IELSG32) phase 2 trial. The Lancet Haematology. 2016. DOI: 10.1016/S2352-3026(16)00036-3

[90] Fishbume BC, Wilson DJ, Rosenbaum JT, Neuwdt EA. Intravitreal methotrexate as an adjunctive treatment of intraocular lymphoma. Archives of Ophthalmology. 1997. DOI: 10.1001/archopht.1997.01100160322009

[91] De Smet MD et al. Intraocular levels of methotrexate after intravenous administration. American Journal of Ophthalmology. 1996. DOI: 10.1016/S0002-9394(14)70444-1

[92] De Smet MD, Vancs VS, Kohler D, Solomon D, Chan CC. Intravitreal chemotherapy for the treatment of recurrent intraocular lymphoma. The British Journal of Ophthalmology. 1999. DOI: 10.1136/bjo.83.4.448

[93] Wang JK et al. An Asian patient with intraocular lymphoma treated by intravitreal methotrexate. Japanese Journal of Ophthalmology. 2006. DOI: 10.1007/s10384-005-0327-4

[94] Kim E, Kim C, Lee J, Cho Y. A case of primary intraocular lymphoma treated by intravitreal methotrexate. Korean Journal of Ophthalmology. 2009. DOI: 10.3341/kjo.2009.23.3.210

[95] Sou R, Ohguro N, Maeda T, Saishin Y, Tano Y. Treatment of primary intraocular lymphoma with intravitreal methotrexate. Japanese Journal of Ophthalmology. 2008. DOI: 10.1007/s10384-008-0519-9

[96] Chan CC, Sen HN. Current concepts in diagnosing and managing primary vitreoretinal (intraocular) lymphoma. Discovery Medicine. 2013

[97] Hashida N, Nakai K, Saitoh N, Nishida K. Association between ocular findings and preventive therapy with onset of central nervous system involvement in patients with primary vitreoretinal lymphoma. Graefe's Archive for Clinical and Experimental Ophthalmology. 2014. DOI: 10.1007/s00417-014-2584-8

[98] Berenbom A, Davila RM, Lin HS, Harbour JW. Treatment outcomes for primary intraocular lymphoma: Implications for external beam radiotherapy. Eye. 2007. DOI: 10.1038/sj.eye.6702437

[99] Gregory MS et al. A novel treatment for ocular tumors using membrane fasl vesicles to activate innate immunity and terminate immune privilege. Investigative Ophthalmology and Visual Science. 2005. DOI: 10.1167/iovs.05-0048

[100] Li Z et al. Eradication of tumor colonization and invasion by a B cell-specific immunotoxin in a murine model for human primary intraocular lymphoma. Cancer Research. 2006. DOI: 10.1158/0008-5472.CAN-06-1981

[101] Rodrigues EB et al. Therapeutic monoclonal antibodies in ophthalmology. Progress in Retinal and Eye Research. 2009. DOI: 10.1016/j.preteyeres.2008.11.005

[102] Soussain C et al. A single-center study of 11 patients with intraocular lymphoma treated with conventional chemotherapy followed by high-dose chemotherapy and autologous bone marrow transplantation in 5 cases. Leukemia & Lymphoma. 1996. DOI: 10.3109/10428199609054837

Section 2

Special Topics

Chapter 9

Primary Central Nervous System Lymphoma: Focus on Indian Perspective

Praful Pandey, Ahitagni Biswas, Saphalta Baghmar, Mukesh Patekar and Ranjit Kumar Sahoo

Abstract

Early suspicion, withholding steroids, stereotactic biopsy, and high-dose methotrexate (HD-MTX) are essential for the treatment of primary CNS lymphoma (PCNSL) making its management in lower-middle-income countries (LMIC) challenging. Novel radiological methods, clinician awareness about the disease, and utilization of drugs like thiotepa and ibrutinib which can be given on an outpatient basis may allow better management of these patients in resource-poor settings. Combined with a late presenting demographic, this results in poorer outcomes in the Indian subcontinent as compared to its western counterparts. In this review, we summarize the currently available data on PCNSL in the Indian subcontinent. We also review the current standard of care for PCNSL and present potential modifications or research areas that may potentially improve outcomes in LMIC.

Keywords: primary central nervous system lymphoma, PCNSL, lower middle income countries, LMIC, methotrexate, TEDDI, ibrutinib

1. Introduction

WHO 2016 classification for lymphomas [1] defines primary central nervous system lymphoma as a rare and aggressive form of extranodal diffuse large B-cell lymphoma (DLBCL) involving the brain, leptomeninges, or eyes without any systemic involvement. However, this entity responded poorly to conventional DLBCL regimens [2, 3] despite using radiotherapy or dexamethasone to enhance CNS efficacy. Further evidence supporting PCNSL as a distinct entity comes from studies showing unique GEP signatures [4] and transcriptomics (with heavy reliance on NF-KB) [5] compared to its nodal counterparts.

PCNSL is predominantly a disease of the elderly [6] and presents with focal deficits followed by features of raised intracranial pressure [7]. Initially suspected on MRI, it is typically diagnosed by a stereotactic biopsy or by cerebrospinal fluid evaluation in exceptional circumstances [8]. Modern management is based on HD-MTX based polychemotherapy followed by consolidative therapy in the form of WBRT, standard-dose chemotherapy or high-dose chemotherapy followed by stem cell transplantation. Rituximab addition may improve outcomes [9]. Novel ibrutinib-based combinations are used in relapsed settings and are being evaluated in the frontline settings as well [10].

In the LMIC, the lack of availability of HD-MTX and neurosurgical suites make management of PCNSL difficult. Novel MRI-based sequences, ibrutinib-based regimes, and utilization of consolidative WBRT may ease the burden. This review details the epidemiological, clinical, and radiological features of PCNSL with a focus on the Indian subcontinent. Furthermore, the current standard of therapy and potential modifications for easier delivery in the LMIC is also detailed.

2. Epidemiology

2.1 Incidence

Overall, the age-adjusted incidence rate (SEER database) of PCNSL is .47 cases per 10,000,000 people per year [11].

The incidence is increasing in elderly males for unclear reasons. Variations in CD4 subpopulations could be a likely cause [12].

From India, only two studies have reported temporal incidence trends. One study reported a 3.5× increase in the number of cases without any change in the proportion of all CNS neoplasms from 1980 to 2003 [13]. Another study done at a single center in northern India found no temporal variation in incidence [14].

2.2 Place in the lymphoma landscape

PCNSL accounts for 4% of all primary CNS tumors as per western data [15]. Two Indian studies, however, report a more conservative estimate of 0.92–0.95% [13] and 1.2% [14].

PCNSL is an uncommon NHL accounting for 4–6% of all extranodal lymphomas [11] and less than 1% of all NHLs as per western literature. A study from Southern India reports that PCNSL accounts for 9.6% of all primary extranodal lymphomas and roughly 3% of all NHLs [16].

2.3 Demographics

Table 1 contains the demographic details of PCNSL patients recruited in Indian studies.

In Western settings, non-HIV infected PCNSL is typically diagnosed at 45–65 years of age (median age of diagnosis in the fifth decade) with no gender predilection [6, 17–19]. However, the Indian demographic differs in having a younger affected population (median age at diagnosis ranging from 42 to 59 years) with slight male preponderance [13, 14, 20–31]. These changes are more likely from different population demographics rather than inherent disease biology, given that individuals aged more than 60 or 65 consistently amount to less than 9% and 7% of the total Indian population respectively [32].

HIV-infected individuals are also a younger cohort (Median age: 37 years) with a male preponderance [12].

Among transplant recipients: CNS involvement is present in 15% of all NHL cases [33] and is associated with a poorer prognosis [34]. However, amounting to only 0.9% of all PCNSL cases, this subset is not well studied [12].

2.4 Global vs. Indian burden of HIV in PCNSL

The prevalence of HIV in PCNSL patients is estimated to be 6.1% globally, with significant variation among nations [35]. Prevalence in India is significantly lesser

Study (n)	Demographics			Clinical presentation						Investigations			
	Median age (years)	Males (%)	HIV positive (%)	Median duration of symptoms (Months)	Most common presenting feature	Eye involvement (%)	Leptomeningeal involvement (%)	ECOG PS	Raised LDH (%)	Histopathology	Stereotactic biopsy (%)	Inadvertent resection (%)	Multiple lesions (%)
Patekar et al. (n = 99)	50	65.60	1.10	3.5	Neurological deficit	19.40	15.8	58.5% PS ≥ 3	19.40	DLBCL (97.7%)	49	40	81.80
Adhikari et al. (n = 22)	51.5	59	0	4	Neurological deficit	22.70	13.64	59.9% PS ≥ 3	45.45	DLBCL (100%)	50	50	75
Patel et al. (n = 73)	46	66	0	2.5	Raised ICP	—	—	—	—	DLBCL (95.9%)	54.80	45.20	64.40
Powari et al. (n = 40)	50	66	0	—	Raised ICP	—	—	—	—	DLBCL (100%)	—	100	87.50
Paul et al. (n = 56)	42	60	0.90	—	Raised ICP	—	—	—	—	DLBCL (93.2%)	—	—	21.40
Mahadevan et al. (n = 24)	53	58.33	0	—	Raised ICP	—	—	—	—	DLBCL (100%)	—	—	—
Dash et al. (n = 41)	52	53.40	0	—	Raised ICP	—	—	—	—	DLBCL (100%)	—	—	—
Sarkar et al. (n = 116)	44.4	69.30	0.80	—	—	—	—	—	—	DLBCL (100%)	—	—	—
Parischa et al. (n = 66)	46	50	0	—	Raised ICP	—	—	—	—	DLBCL (100%)	—	—	15
Sharma et al. (n = 65)	49	58.30	0	—	—	—	3	—	—	DLBCL (100%)	—	—	41.53

Study (n)	Demographics			Clinical presentation						Investigations			
	Median age (years)	Males (%)	HIV positive (%)	Median duration of symptoms (Months)	Most common presenting feature	Eye involvement (%)	Leptomeningeal involvement (%)	ECOG PS	Raised LDH (%)	Histopathology	Stereotactic biopsy (%)	Inadvertent resection (%)	Multiple lesions (%)
Yadav et al. (n = 32)	50	71	0	—	Raised ICP	0	0	—	—	DLBCL (100%)	—	—	68.80
Rudresha et al. (n = 26)	42.5	65.30		—	Raised ICP	0	4	—	30.70	DLBCL (96%)	46	54	38.50
Rudresha et al. (n = 53)	44	64	3.70	—	Raised ICP	0	6	—	32	DLBCL (100%)	49	51	30
Kumari et al. (n = 30)	47.8	60	0	—	Raised ICP	—	—	70% with PS ≥ 3	70	DLBCL (100%)	—	—	66
Puligundla et al. (n = 42)	46	68.70	4.70	—	Raised ICP	0	15.80	80.9% PS ≥ 2	—	DLBCL (97.6%)	42.80	57.10	23.80
Agarwal et al. (n = 26)	59	61.50	7.60	3	Neurological deficit	—	19.20	—	34.60	DLBCL (96.1%)	—	—	77

Table 1.
Demographic and clinical details of patients enrolled in Indian studies.

[35], with some studies not reporting even a single case [14, 25–27, 30]. Similarly, PCNSL accounts for 2.5% of all CNS lesions in HIV-positive patients compared to 10–17% in the western population [36]. Autopsy series show similar findings with the only published Indian series reporting no cases of PCNSL over 8 years [37] while western studies report the share to be between 1.4 and 3% [38, 39]. Shorter survival among AIDS patients in the Indian subcontinent could be the likely cause [40].

3. Clinical features and diagnosis

3.1 Presenting features

The most common presenting features reported are focal neurological deficits, neuropsychiatric symptoms, headache from raised intracranial pressure (ICP), seizures, and ocular symptoms [7]. Diagnosis may not be evident at presentation, with one study reporting a median time lag of 70 days from symptom onset to neuroimaging [41]. Personality changes and visual hallucinations are usually detected late, and a lower threshold to pursue neuroimaging is needed [41].

3.2 Clinical evaluation

Any suspected case of PCNSL should undergo neuroimaging in the form of a contrast-enhanced MRI of the brain and spine, CSF analysis unless contraindicated (ideally before stereotactic biopsy), slit-lamp examination, and testicular examination (in males) [42].

In some cases, pathological evaluation of ocular material or CSF may diagnose. In most cases, however, a stereotactic biopsy is needed [43]. The stark difference in the initial management of PCNSL, compared to high-grade gliomas, underlines the importance of early clinical suspicion and radiological expertise.

3.3 The Indian scenario

Table 1 contains the clinical features of patients enrolled in studies in Indian settings.

In the Indian subcontinent, delayed health-seeking behavior combined with high initial misdiagnosis rates leads to a high disease burden at presentation. Median time from symptom onset to diagnosis is reported around 3.5–5 months in Indian studies [20, 24, 29, 44], compared to 2.5–3 months in western studies [7, 41].

Delayed health-seeking behavior is evident if we compare clinicoradiological features at index presentation. While two studies report focal neurological deficits as the most common presenting feature [20, 29], most studies report headache from raised ICP as the index presentation [14, 21–23, 27, 28, 30, 31], which is typically a late feature in the western literature. Furthermore, while most western patients are ambulatory and capable of self-care at presentation [7], roughly 2/3rd of Indian patients are ECOG performance status (ECOG-PS) three or worse in retrospective [22, 25, 29] and prospective [44] studies. Similarly, multifocal lesions, reported in 25% of patients at presentation as per western literature [7], are seen in 30–82% of all patients presenting in the Indian settings [20, 22, 24–29, 31, 44]. However, some studies do give estimates nearing their western counterparts [14, 23, 30], perhaps highlighting differential health-seeking behavior.

Erroneous evaluation and emergent management are also common. Indian studies report misdiagnosis rates as high as 54% [20] to 100% [29], and inadvertent open surgical resection in 36-57% [20, 44] of PCNSL patients compared to 25% in western literature. In addition, inadvertent steroids are given before diagnosis in up to 2/3rd patients referred from primary care [20] although prospective studies document only 9% requiring corticosteroid therapy for life-threatening indications [44].

These delays and errors result in a patient population with advanced disease and a poorer prognosis. While the proportion of patients with LDH elevation (1/3rd) and CSF Protein elevation (2/3rd) are similar in Indian [22, 25, 28, 29, 31] and western studies [45], fewer patients are IESLG low risk in the Indian settings with concomitant better outcomes [22, 25, 29]. However, the MSKCC risk classification seems to underestimate the risk in the Indian population because of its weightage to older age [28, 31].

4. Treatment modalities and outcomes

Table 2 shows treatment details and outcomes of important studies from the Indian subcontinent.

4.1 Survival outcomes

4.1.1 Evolution of treatment modalities

Left untreated, PCNSL has a uniformly dismal prognosis (median OS = 2 months) [46]. Only marginally better are conventional DLBCL regimes with response rates ranging from 19 to 59% and less than half patients surviving at two years from diagnosis [2, 3]. A significant improvement in prognosis comes from modern multi-drug regimens incorporating high-dose methotrexate (HD-MTX) with appropriate consolidation (2 years OS of 80% and a five-year OS of 77%) [47]. More recent regimes utilizing autologous stem cell transplantation as consolidation report two-year OS as high as 81% [48].

4.1.2 Outcomes reported in India

Indian studies report modest outcomes. Up to 20% of PCNSL patients never receive therapy [20, 22, 29]. A single-institution reported a median EFS of 20.4 months and a median OS of 31.7 months at a median follow–up of 34 months with HD-MTX-based multiagent regimes and Rituximab and consolidative WBRT. [20] A prospective phase 2 trial evaluating response adapted radiotherapy showed a median OS of 19 months, underlining the necessity of consolidative WBRT to optimize outcomes [44]. A study evaluating the importance of HD-MTX therapy in the Indian setting [28] reported a median OS of 8 months, 13 months, and 23 months in WBRT, R-CHOP with WBRT, and HD-MTX with WBRT, respectively. Thus, there is a scope for improvement in the outcomes of PCNSL seen in the Indian sub-continent.

4.2 Long term toxicity

Studies using HD-MTX-based induction and WBRT consolidation report 15% long-term neurotoxicity rates [49]. However, no such delayed sequelae are documented in prospective studies using abbreviated WBRT [50, 51]. On the other hand, regimes using ASCT as consolidation report continuous cognitive improvement until 12–18 months after completion of therapy [48].

Study (n)	Pre-treatment details		Induction chemotherapy details				Post-induction chemotherapy	Long-term outcomes			
	IESLG low risk (%)	Treatment received (%)	Type of chemotherapy	Median induction cycles	Rituximab	Overall response rate, complete response rate (ORR/CR %)		Median follow-up duration (months)	Median event-free survival (months)	Median overall survival (months)	Severe late neurotoxicity (%)
Patekar et al. (n = 99)	7.10	77.70	MVP with Rituximab (94.8%) CHOP + HTMTX (2.6%) CHOP + IT MTX (1.3%) HD - MTX only (1.3%)	5	In affording patients	81.8% (46.8%)	WBRT in 54% (Ara - C in 86% of WBRT recipients) 11% HiDAC only	34	20.4	31.7	10
Adhikari et al. (n = 22)	—	100	MVP	5	In affording patients	93.7% (52.63%)	50% WBRT 50% reduced dose WBRT 68.18% post-WBRT HiDAC	11.25	Not reached	19	—
Parischa et al. (n = 66)	—	100	MPV followed by WBRT + HiDAC (DeAngelis protocol)	—	No	—	—	—	—	—	—
Yadav et al. (n = 32)	—	100	WBRT (36-50 Gy) followed by 6 cycles CHOP	6	No	87.5% (75%)	None	18	—	14 months	—
Rudresha et al. (n = 26)	—	100	DeAngelis protocol (92%), MTR followed by EA (8%)	5	No	ORR for DeAngelis: 92%, ORR for MTR regime: 100%	WBRT followed by HiDAC given in DeAngelis protocol, EA given to MTR recipients	—	—	20.5	—

Study (n)	Pre-treatment details		Induction chemotherapy details				Post-induction chemotherapy	Long-term outcomes			
	IESLG low risk (%)	Treatment received (%)	Type of chemotherapy	Median induction cycles	Rituximab	Overall response rate, complete response rate (ORR/ CR %)		Median follow-up duration (months)	Median event-free survival (months)	Median overall survival (months)	Severe late neurotoxicity (%)
Rudresha et al. (n = 53)	—	100	DeAngelis protocol (n = 31) CHOP + WBRT (n = 14) WBRT only (n – 6)	—	No	—	WBRT followed by HiDAC in DeAngelis protocol	—	—	23 months for DeAngelis protocol, 13 months for standard CHOP + WBRT treated, 6 months for WBRT only subset	26% in DeAngelis treated, 14% in CHOP + WBRT subset
Kumari et al. (n = 30)	10	100	40–52 Gy WBRT followed by 6 cycles of CHOP/PCV	—	No	—	—	—	—	—	—
Puligundla et al. (n = 42)	19	80.90	Modified DeAngelis (50%) Modified DeAngelis protocol + rituximab (29.4%) Steroids + radiotherapy (17.7%) BFM- NHL protocol (3%)	—	Given to 29.4% of patients	—	—	18	11	15.9	—
Agarwal et al. (n = 26)	36.3	84.60	MVP + Cytarabine	—	No	CR: 72.7%	WBRT in patients aged < 60 years (45%)	14.5	—	10	31.25%

Table 2.
Treatment administered and long term prognosis of PCNSL patients enrolled in Indian studies.

In the Indian setting, reliable estimates of long-term neurological toxicity are lacking given that most of the reported literature does not have adequate follow-up or assessment [22, 25–27, 30, 31]. However, limited studies report severe long-term neurotoxicity rates of 10–33%, with elderly patients and WBRT recipients at a higher risk [20, 28, 29].

5. How can we improve?

PCNSL requires multi-disciplinary care in resource-intense settings to optimize outcomes. However, in lower-middle-income countries (LMIC), the main barriers to applying modern evidence-based management of PCNSL are the lack of neurosurgical facilities and oncology units capable of handling HD-MTX.

5.1 Improving diagnosis

5.1.1 Better radiological support

Radiological differential diagnosis of PCNSL includes high-grade gliomas, tumefactive demyelinating lesions, metastasis, and granulomatous diseases/infections. Although, the radiological appearance of PCNSL is very distinctive with homogenous contrast enhancement, optic pathway, and cranial nerve infiltration, a predilection for deeper structures, lesser necrosis, and nearly no bleeding, many studies still report diagnostic difficulties while using conventional MRI only [52]. This differentiation is crucial because while PCNSL requires stereotactic biopsy followed by systemic chemotherapy, high-grade gliomas are usually treated with upfront gross total resection. With 40% of patients responding, prior steroid usage compounds this problem with high false-negative biopsy rates [53]. Thus, early radiological suspicion may allow many patients to undergo appropriate management in the form of no inadvertent steroid therapy, stereotactic biopsy, and early institution of HD-MTX-based therapy.

5.1.2 Conventional MRI sequences

Diffusion-weighted imaging is an essential diagnostic tool. PCNSL shows more restricted ADC than high-grade gliomas, given its higher cellular density and N: C ratio. However, solid portions of high-grade gliomas may mimic [52]. Therefore, a different measure," Relative minimum ADC," is often used given its reasonable diagnostic certainty [54]. Furthermore, dynamic contrast-enhanced MRI adds to ADC's diagnostic performance as well [55].

Another crucial diagnostic aid is the ^{1}H-magnetic resonance spectroscopy (^{1}H-MRS). Choline to creatine ratio, a marker of membrane turnover, is identical for PCNSL and high-grade gliomas. However, N-acetyl aspartate peaks (NAA), a marker of neuronal damage, may have variable results. The lipid peak arises from necrosis in GBM and release of fatty moieties via lymphocytes in PCNSL, making lipid resonance without necrosis the most specific finding [56].

^{1}H-MRS may allow assessment of other peaks as well. Conventional 1.5 T MRI cannot differentially assess glutamate (Glu) and glutamine (Gln) peaks, and there is no difference in Glutamate + Glutamine/ Creatinine peaks among PCNSL and high-grade gliomas. However, because of impaired Glutamate internalization in high-grade gliomas, glutamate to glutamine conversion is upscaled. Thus, 3 Tesla MRI machines which can differentially quantify glutamate and glutamine, allow assessment of Glu/Glu + Gln ratios which are reproducibly different in PCNSL and high-grade gliomas [57].

5.1.3 Newer MRI based modalities

Amide proton transfer weighted studies (based on 3 T MRI machines) also detect endogenous mobile proteins and peptides predominantly seen in the cytoplasm. PCNSL, with its high N:C ratio and thus, a low concentration of mobile proteins, shows much shows limited hyperintensities as compared to heterogenous hyperintensities much larger than the gadolinium-enhancing areas in high grade gliomas [55].

Dynamic susceptibility contrast-enhanced MRI can differentiate based on different tumor microenvironments. PCNSL lacks florid neovascularization compared to high-grade gliomas, as assessed by FVIII staining on resected specimens [58]. Contrast enhancement stems from breakage of the blood-brain barrier rather than increased vascularity resulting in a relatively lower rCBV than high-grade gliomas [59]. Neovascularization of surrounding infiltrated tissue can result in a specific shoulder-like pattern of signal intensity and enhance diagnostic performance [60]. Prospectively validated studies report an rCBV threshold of 2.56 having >90% sensitivity and specificity [54].

5.1.4 Machine learning: better analysis of conventional MRI meta-data

Fundamental differences of neovascularization and necrosis between PCNSL and high-grade gliomas may lead to subtle differences in imaging, which, although may not be evident to the human eye, are picked by metadata-based machine learning (ML) models. A recent meta-analysis assessing the utility of ML models for PCNSL diagnosis reports 0.878 as the lowest AUC across eight studies [61]. Another prospectively validated model reported an AUC of 0.978 using only T1 weighted images [62]. ML-based algorithms have advantages of being open access, easily accessible, and minimal reliance on novel machines or software. However, overfitting of models compromising external validity and prompting institute-specific algorithms is a challenge.

5.1.5 Metabolic imaging

Given its high cellular density, PCNSL shows intense homogenous FDG uptake (as opposed to heterogeneous uptake in high-grade gliomas) with SUVmax values around 12–14 (2.5 times of normal gray matter). However, surrounding physiological gray matter uptake hinders accurate assessment [63]. A study assessing the diagnostic utility of PET/CT for PCNSL reported an optimal SUVmax cut-off of 15 with only a single false positive [64]. Another study reported that a SUVmax cut-off of 12 had 86% accuracy as a standalone modality and 95% when combined with CE-MRI with DWI [65].

The tumor/normal (T/N) ratio overcomes the reliance of SUVmax on plasma glucose concentrations. A study reported good diagnostic performance with a cut-off 2.0. Prior Steroids may hinder both SUVmax, as well as T/N ratio [66]. PET/CT has additional utility in ruling out secondary CNS lymphoma and a 7% additional yield over CT and bone marrow examination [67].

5.2 Cerebrospinal fluid analysis

CSF analysis may allow diagnosis without neurosurgical procedures and its associated complications in up to 40% of patients. Therefore, patients without evidence of raised ICP should undergo CSF analysis with cytomorphology, flow-cytometry, and PCR for IGHV rearrangements either before or at least 1 week after the stereotactic biopsy [42].

A recent systematic review of 27 studies evaluating CSF cytomorphology and flow cytometry across different lymphoid neoplasms with meningeal involvement reported around 0.3-42.9% positive results with dual testing. Furthermore, 48% and 89% of studies reported samples positive on cytomorphology or flow cytometry alone, respectively, highlighting the importance of co-testing [68]. Another study assessing only PCNSL patients reported 13.3% and 23.3% positivity rates with CSF cytomorphology and flow cytometry, respectively [69].

CSF cell fragility impairs the diagnostic performance of cytomorphology and flow cytometry. However, PCR-based analysis of IGHV rearrangements to assess clonality does not require intact cells and may circumvent this problem. A study assessing IGHV rearrangement status in CSF among patients with PCNSL reported a sensitivity of 54% and specificity of 97% among the 84% patients having CSF with extractable DNA. The positive predictive value was 93%, with a further rise if only therapy naïve patients were considered [70]. However, a study prospectively evaluating CSF of 282 patients with PCNSL reported 10% samples with positive IGHV rearrangement PCR but negative cytomorphology and 12% samples with positive cytomorphology but negative IGHV rearrangement analysis [71]. Thus, IGHV rearrangement analysis may be better suited as an add-on than a replacement.

Novel approaches such as digital droplet PCR (ddPCR) analysis of MYD88 mutations [72], IL-10 levels [73], Osteopontin levels [74], neopterin levels [75], and miR-21 levels [76] may allow further diagnostic aid and potential negation of neurosurgical procedures in the future. Specifically, a meta-analysis reported that CSF IL-10 levels have a sensitivity of 81%, specificity of 97%, and an area under ROC of 0.95 at a cut-off of 6.88 pg/ml [77].

5.2.1 Slit lamp and intra-ocular biopsy

Like CSF analysis, Ocular involvement may also allow early diagnosis without reliance on neurosurgical procedures. Ocular involvement is seen in 15–25% of PCNSL patients, and slit-lamp examination is the diagnostic procedure of choice [78]. If involvement is suspected, a biopsy of vitreous fluid, choroid, or retina may allow histopathological diagnosis. Routine use of slit-lamp microscopy and a high index of suspicion is warranted given that more than 1/3rd of patients with ocular involvement are asymptomatic [79]. In cases with equivocal appearances, ocular ultrasound, fundus fluorescein angiography, and optical coherence tomography are adjunctive studies used for diagnosis [80].

Combined cytopathology, flow cytometry, and analysis of IGHV gene arrangement studies on multiple vitrectomy specimens have a combined sensitivity and specificity of 64% and 100%, respectively [81]. A chorioretinal biopsy is an option in suspicious cases with a normal vitreous biopsy [82].

Novel techniques may enhance diagnostic yields. For example, ARMS PCR-based MYD88 L265P mutation analysis is diagnostic in 86.7% FFPE samples of primary vitreoretinal lymphoma [83]. Techniques independent of DNA input such as ddPCR allow similar rates of MYD88 mutation detection from less invasive specimens like aqueous humor [72]. Lastly, elevated IL-10 levels or an IL-10/IL-6 ratio > 1 is suggestive but not diagnostic, and its utility as a standalone modality requires validation [78].

5.3 Improving therapy

5.3.1 Non-methotrexate containing induction regimes

High-dose methotrexate-based multiagent chemotherapy followed by consolidation with WBRT or autologous stem cell transplantation is the modern standard of care for PCNSL [42]. However, centers with facilities and experience for HD-MTX are lacking, necessitating the evaluation of alternative regime backbones.

Methotrexate doses of more than 3 g/m^2 are needed to cross the BBB and doses as high as 8 g/m^2 have been used without any guiding prospective randomized data. A recent observational study has reported higher CR rates and PFS with higher dose HD-MTX (8 g/m^2) [84]. An infusion time of 3 hours and 6 hours for doses of 3 g/m^2 and 8 g/m^2 respectively allows better CNS penetration per unit dose, allowing enhanced efficacy and an attenuated toxicity profile [85]. 5–7 cycles of HD-MTX-based polychemotherapy spaced at 2 weeks intervals rather than 3-week intervals are associated with optimal oncological outcomes [86]. Leucovorin rescue is typically started 24 h after infusion and at least 12 doses are given at 6-hour intervals [51]. The utility of therapeutic drug monitoring remains to be proven in these settings with a recommendation for assessment at 24 h, 48 h, and 72 h after initial infusion [87].

Thiotepa, a lipid-soluble organophosphorus-derived alkylator, is a potential answer. Evidence suggests that Methotrexate is optimally given in doses more than 3.5 g/m^2 over shorter infusion times (3 h) at a gap of 2–3 weeks for 5–8 cycles [42]. High dose cytarabine (Ara-C) addition to HD-MTX therapy led to more than doubling of responses, likely from prolonged exposure to S-phase cytostatics [88]. Subsequently, the IESLG32 study evaluated Rituximab addition and autologous SCT's utility in PCNSL and added Thiotepa to a third induction arm (MATRIx regime), which outperformed both combination chemotherapy and chemoimmunotherapy arms [9]. Thus, with a 100% plasma-to-cerebrospinal fluid ratio, 30-min infusion time, and synergy with anti-metabolites, Thiotepa might be a convenient alternative to HD-MTX, and the comparative efficacy of Thiotepa-high-dose Ara-C vs. HD-MTX is worth exploring. Notably, a study using high dose Ara-C with Thiotepa after initial HD-MTX showed an increase in responses [89].

Single-agent temozolomide [90], topotecan [91], and temsirolimus [92] have also shown modest activity in relapsed PCNSL settings, and different combinations may be worth evaluating.

Frequent mutations in the BCR subunit CD79B and Toll-like receptor adaptor protein MYD88 suggest addiction of PCNSL to BCR signaling [93], making Ibrutinib an attractive option. However, since Ibrutinib-driven responses in ABC DLBCL last for less than a year [94], cotherapy with blood-brain barrier crossing synergistic drugs is prudent. Recent studies have built on this, and Ibrutinib-based combination regimes are a promising HD-MTX-free approach. While Ibrutinib is antagonistic with most anti-folate drugs, it is synergistic with etoposide, doxorubicin, Ara-C, and mitomycin C [95]. Additionally, doxorubicin, a broad spectrum lymphocytic but BBB impermeable agent, may be given as a liposomal formulation that maintains CSF concentrations throughout therapy duration, likely from a reservoir-like effect [96]. On these lines, the dose-adjusted TEDDi-R regime given after a 14-day run-in of ibrutinib monotherapy showed 86% complete responses in a phase 1b study with 18 patients [97]. Notably, the activity of this regime did not become dependent on the presence of the specific MYD88 L265P mutation. However, severe adverse effects in the form of grade 4 neutropenia, grade 4 thrombocytopenia, and invasive fungal infections (most commonly aspergillosis) were noted in 53%, 30%, and 50%, respectively. These rates of invasive fungal infections are not found in other studies evaluating Ibrutinib (with or without steroids), and monocyte BTK inhibition may be causative [98]. Recognizing the need for prophylaxis, a recent phase 1b trial reported 75% CR rates and no invasive fungal infections with DA-TEDDi R with Isavuconazole prophylaxis [95]. In the Indian settings, concomitant dose reduction of both ibrutinib and liposomal doxorubicin [99] makes Voriconazole prophylaxis an attractive option offering maintained efficacy and reduced financial toxicity.

Lenalidomide may offer a potentially less intensive ibrutinib-based option. Given its capability to expand NK-cell pools, Lenalidomide is known to be synergistic with Rituximab (R^2-regimen) [100]. A proof-of-concept phase 2 study documented ORR and CR rates of 32% and 29%, respectively, in relapsed/refractory PCNSL with a tolerable safety profile [101]. Building on data from systemic DLBCL, ibrutinib and R^2 (IR^2) leads to complete responses in 1/3rd relapsed/ refractory PCNSL cases, and studies testing this regime in frontline settings are eagerly awaited [10].

Intrathecal delivery may enhance synergy between rituximab and lenalidomide. At conventional doses (375 mg/m^2), CSF compartment achieves only 0.1% of systemic rituximab concentrations [102]. Evidence suggesting that incorporation of systemic rituximab in lymphoma protocols does not impact the incidence of CNS relapse also points to potential inadequacy of intravenous rituximab in clearing the leptomeningeal compartment [103]. Given the acceptable safety profile of intrathecal rituximab in non-human primates [104], intrathecal rituximab-based combinations deserve consideration for further research. On these lines, a phase 1 study reported 25 mg as the optimal intraventricular dose (via ommaya reservoir) leading to an ORR of 60% and a CR rate of 40% with one parenchymal remission as well [105]. A subsequent study reported a CR rate of 43% in relapsed PCNSL when treated with a combination of intraventricular rituximab and methotrexate [106]. Thus, while intraventricular rituximab is an option with promising efficacy and cost benefits, larger studies are needed. Additionally, the utility of intrathecal rather than intraventricular therapy also requires consideration.

5.3.2 Optimizing consolidation therapy

More than 50% of PCNSL patients relapse within 5 years of therapy if treated with induction alone, necessitating some form of consolidation therapy [107]. The two largest comparative trials indicate comparable efficacy but lesser long-term neurotoxicity with HDT-ASCT than WBRT [108, 109]. While a longer follow-up may tell a different story [50], upfront HDT-ASCT for all PCNSL patients is not feasible for resource-limited settings.

In Indian settings, WBRT followed by HiDAC [107] remains the most common consolidation therapy. However, while western studies report comparable efficacy and lesser neurotoxicity by reduced dose WBRT [51, 110], studies in the Indian settings in our experience are less favourable [44].

Non-myeloablative chemotherapy may offer a balance of efficacy and cognition. For example, Etoposide-Cytarabine (EA regimen) showed efficacy comparable to historic WBRT treated cohorts in a single-arm phase 2 study. However, lack of randomized comparisons and high rates of grade ¾ hematological toxicity with the possible requirement of autologous stem-cell rescue are barriers to frequent utilization [111].

Maintenance with oral procarbazine, assessed in a phase 2 trial of elderly PCNSL patients, is a safe alternative, although randomized evidence is lacking [112]. Another study showed lesser relapse rates (non-randomized) with oral Temozolomide maintenance than WBRT, although atypical induction protocols used in this study negatively impact the external validity of findings [113]. Lenalidomide maintenance is also a safe option in elderly patients, although the efficacy in this setting is yet to be proven [114].

6. Conclusion

PCNSL, although morphologically like any other DLBCL, has distinct pathobiology and prognosis. The requirement of early radiological diagnosis and referral to a center equipped with neurosurgical facilities and safe administration of HD-MTX for every patient makes management of PCNSL challenging in resource-limited settings. Non-invasive methods of diagnosis and non-HD-MTX-based therapies need more research to allow PCNSL cases to be managed optimally in such settings.

Author details

Praful Pandey[1], Ahitagni Biswas[2], Saphalta Baghmar[3], Mukesh Patekar[4] and Ranjit Kumar Sahoo[1]*

1 Department of Medical Oncology, All India Institute of Medical Sciences, New Delhi, India

2 Department of Radiation Oncology, All India Institute of Medical Sciences, New Delhi, India

3 Department of Medical Oncology, Max Vaishali and Noida, India

4 Department of Medical Oncology, Fortis Memorial Research Institute, Haryana, India

*Address all correspondence to: drranjitmd@gmail.com

References

[1] Swerdlow SH, Campo E, Pileri SA, Harris NL, Stein H, Siebert R, et al. The 2016 revision of the World Health Organization classification of lymphoid neoplasms. Blood. 2016;**127**(20): 2375-2390

[2] Schultz C, Scott C, Sherman W, Donahue B, Fields J, Murray K, et al. Preirradiation chemotherapy with cyclophosphamide, doxorubicin, vincristine, and dexamethasone for primary CNS lymphomas: Initial report of radiation therapy oncology group protocol 88-06. Journal of Clinical Oncology: Official Journal of the American Society of Clinical Oncology. 1996;**14**(2):556-564

[3] O'Neill BP, O'Fallon JR, Earle JD, Colgan JP, Brown LD, Krigel RL. Primary central nervous system non-Hodgkin's lymphoma: Survival advantages with combined initial therapy? International Journal of Radiation Oncology, Biology, Physics. 1995;**33**(3):663-673

[4] Tun HW, Personett D, Baskerville KA, Menke DM, Jaeckle KA, Kreinest P, et al. Pathway analysis of primary central nervous system lymphoma. Blood. 2008;**111**(6): 3200-3210

[5] Courts C, Montesinos-Rongen M, Martin-Subero JI, Brunn A, Siemer D, Zühlke-Jenisch R, et al. Transcriptional profiling of the nuclear factor-κB pathway identifies a subgroup of primary lymphoma of the central nervous system with low BCL10 expression. Journal of Neuropathology and Experimental Neurology. 2007; **66**(3):230-237

[6] Miller DC, Hochberg FH, Harris NL, Gruber ML, Louis DN, Cohen H. Pathology with clinical correlations of primary central nervous system non-Hodgkin's lymphoma. The Massachusetts General Hospital experience 1958-1989. Cancer. 1994; **74**(4):1383-1397

[7] Bataille B, Delwail V, Menet E, Vandermarcq P, Ingrand P, Wager M, et al. Primary intracerebral malignant lymphoma: Report of 248 cases. Journal of Neurosurgery. 2000;**92**(2):261-266

[8] Green MR, Chowdhary S, Lombardi KM, Chalmers LM, Chamberlain M. Clinical utility and pharmacology of high-dose methotrexate in the treatment of primary CNS lymphoma. Expert Review of Neurotherapeutics. 2006;**6**(5):635-652

[9] Ferreri AJM, Cwynarski K, Pulczynski E, Ponzoni M, Deckert M, Politi LS, et al. Chemoimmunotherapy with methotrexate, cytarabine, thiotepa, and rituximab (MATRix regimen) in patients with primary CNS lymphoma: Results of the first randomisation of the International Extranodal Lymphoma Study Group-32 (IELSG32) phase 2 trial. Lancet Haematology. 2016;**3**(5):e217-e227

[10] Houillier C, Moluçon-Chabrot C, Moles M-P, Willems L, Ahle G, Waultier A, et al. Combination of Rituximab-Lenalidomide-Ibrutinib in relapsed/refractory primary Cns lymphoma: A Cohort study of the Loc network. Hematology & Oncology. 2021;**39**(S2):1. Available from: https://onlinelibrary.wiley.com/doi/abs/10.1002/hon.73_2880

[11] Villano JL, Koshy M, Shaikh H, Dolecek TA, McCarthy BJ. Age, gender, and racial differences in incidence and survival in primary CNS lymphoma. British Journal of Cancer. 2011;**105**(9): 1414-1418

[12] Shiels MS, Pfeiffer RM, Besson C, Clarke CA, Morton LM, Nogueira L, et al. Trends in primary central nervous system lymphoma incidence and

survival in the U.S. British Journal of Haematology. 2016;**174**(3):417-424

[13] Sarkar C, Sharma MC, Deb P, Singh R, Santosh V, Shankar SK. Primary central nervous system lymphoma—A hospital based study of incidence and clinicopathological features from India (1980-2003). Journal of Neuro-Oncology. 2005;**71**(2):199-204

[14] Powari M, Radotra B, Das A, Banerjee AK. A study of primary central nervous system lymphoma in northern India. Surgical Neurology. 2002;**57**(2): 113-116

[15] Hoffman S, Propp JM, McCarthy BJ. Temporal trends in incidence of primary brain tumors in the United States, 1985-1999. Neuro-Oncology. 2006;**8**(1): 27-37

[16] Arora N, Manipadam MT, Nair S. Frequency and distribution of lymphoma types in a tertiary care hospital in South India: Analysis of 5115 cases using the World Health Organization 2008 classification and comparison with world literature. Leukemia & Lymphoma. 2012:1008 (Table IV). Available from: https://www.meta.org/papers/frequency-and-distribution-of-lymphoma-types-in-a/22971239

[17] Braaten KM, Betensky RA, de Leval L, Okada Y, Hochberg FH, Louis DN, et al. BCL-6 expression predicts improved survival in patients with primary central nervous system lymphoma. Clinical Cancer Research: An Official Journal of the American Association for Cancer Research. 2003; **9**(3):1063-1069

[18] Herrlinger U, Schabet M, Clemens M, Kortmann RD, Petersen D, Will BE, et al. Clinical presentation and therapeutic outcome in 26 patients with primary CNS lymphoma. Acta Neurologica Scandinavica. 1998;**97**(4): 257-264

[19] Fine HA, Mayer RJ. Primary central nervous system lymphoma. Annals of Internal Medicine. 1993;**119**(11): 1093-1104

[20] Patekar M, Adhikari N, Biswas A, Raina V, Kumar L, Mohanti BK, et al. Primary CNS lymphoma in India: A 17-year experience from the all India institute of medical sciences. Journal of Global Oncology. 2019;**5**: JGO.18.00124

[21] Mahadevan A, Rao CR, Shanmugham M, Shankar SK. Primary central nervous system diffuse large B-cell lymphoma in the immunocompetent: Immunophenotypic subtypes and Epstein-Barr virus association. Journal of Neurosciences in Rural Practice. 2015;**6**(1):8-14

[22] Puligundla CK, Bala S, Karnam AK, Gundeti S, Paul TR, Uppin MS, et al. Clinicopathological features and outcomes in primary central nervous system lymphoma: A 10-year experience. Indian Journal of Medical and Paediatric Oncology: Official Journal of Indian Society of Medical & Paediatric Oncology. 2017;**38**(4):478-482

[23] Paul TR, Challa S, Tandon A, Panigrahi MK, Purohit AK. Primary central nervous system lymphomas: Indian experience, and review of literature. Indian Journal of Cancer. 2008;**45**(3):112

[24] Patel B, Chacko G, Nair S, Anandan J, Chacko AG, Rajshekhar V, et al. Clinicopathological correlates of primary central nervous system lymphoma: Experience from a tertiary care center in South India. Neurology India [Internet]. Available from: https://www.neurologyindia.com/article.asp?issn=0028-3886;year=2015;volume=63;issue=1;spage=77;epage=82;aulast=Patel

[25] Kumari N, Krishnani N, Rawat A, Agarwal V, Lal P. Primary central

nervous system lymphoma: Prognostication as per international extranodal lymphoma study group score and reactive CD3 collar. Journal of Postgraduate Medicine. 2009;**55**(4):247

[26] Sharma MC, Gupta RK, Kaushal S, Suri V, Sarkar C, Singh M, et al. A clinicopathological study of primary central nervous system lymphomas & their association with Epstein-Barr virus. The Indian Journal of Medical Research. 2016;**143**(5):605-615

[27] Yadav. Primary Central Nervous System Lymphoma: An Experience of a Regional Cancer Center from India [Internet]. Available from: https://www.journalrcr.org/article.asp?issn=2588-9273;year=2019;volume=10;issue=2;spage=104;epage=107;aulast=Yadav

[28] Rudresha. Evolution of the treatment of primary central nervous system lymphoma in a Regional Cancer Center of South India: Impact of high-dose methotrexate on treatment outcome [Internet]. Available from: https://www.cancerjournal.net/article.asp?issn=0973-1482;year=2020;volume=16;issue=1;spage=13;epage=17;aulast=Rudresha

[29] Agarwal PA, Menon S, Smruti BK, Singhal BS. Primary central nervous system lymphoma: A profile of 26 cases from western India. Neurology India. 2009;**57**(6):756

[30] Pasricha S, Gupta A, Gawande J, Trivedi P, Patel D. Primary central nervous system lymphoma: A study of clinicopathological features and trend in western India. Indian Journal of Cancer. 2011;**48**(2):199-203

[31] Rudresha AH, Chaudhuri T, Lakshmaiah KC, Babu G, Lokesh KN, Rajeev LK. Primary central nervous system lymphoma in immunocompetent patients: A regional cancer center experience. South Asian Journal of Cancer. 2017;**6**(4):165-168

[32] India—age distribution 2020 [Internet]. Statista. Available from: https://www.statista.com/statistics/271315/age-distribution-in-india/

[33] Buell JF, Gross TG, Hanaway MJ, Trofe J, Roy-Chaudhury P, First MR, et al. Posttransplant lymphoproliferative disorder: Significance of central nervous system involvement. Transplantation Proceedings. 2005;**37**(2):954-955

[34] Evens AM, Choquet S, Kroll-Desrosiers AR, Jagadeesh D, Smith SM, Morschhauser F, et al. Primary CNS posttransplant lymphoproliferative disease (PTLD): An international report of 84 cases in the modern era. American Journal of Transplantation: Official Journal of the American Society of Transplantation and the American Society of Transplant Surgeons. 2013;**13**(6):1512-1522

[35] Franca RA, Travaglino A, Varricchio S, Russo D, Picardi M, Pane F, et al. HIV prevalence in primary central nervous system lymphoma: A systematic review and meta-analysis. Pathology—Research and Practice. 2020;**216**(11):153192

[36] Sharma S, Dwivedi N, Kumar N, Bharti A, Meena L. Neurological manifestation of HIV infection in North-Eastern part of India. National Journal of Physiology Pharmacy and Pharmacology. 2014;**4**(1):4

[37] Lanjewar DN, Jain PP, Shetty CR. Profile of central nervous system pathology in patients with AIDS: An autopsy study from India. AIDS (London England). 1998;**12**(3):309-313

[38] Silva ACAL, Rodrigues BSC, Micheletti AMR, Tostes S, Meneses ACO, Silva-Vergara ML, et al. Neuropathology of AIDS: An autopsy review of 284 cases from Brazil comparing the findings pre- and

post-HAART (Highly Active Antiretroviral Therapy) and Pre- and Postmortem Correlation. AIDS Research and Treatment. 2012;**2012**: 186850

[39] Lang W, Miklossy J, Deruaz JP, Pizzolato GP, Probst A, Schaffner T, et al. Neuropathology of the acquired immune deficiency syndrome (AIDS): A report of 135 consecutive autopsy cases from Switzerland. Acta Neuropathologica. 1989;**77**(4):379-390

[40] Jha P, Kumar R, Khera A, Bhattacharya M, Arora P, Gajalakshmi V, et al. HIV mortality and infection in India: Estimates from nationally representative mortality survey of 1.1 million homes. BMJ. 2010; **340**:c621

[41] Haldorsen IS, Espeland A, Larsen JL, Mella O. Diagnostic delay in primary central nervous system lymphoma. Acta Oncologica. 2005; **44**(7):728-734

[42] Fox CP, Phillips EH, Smith J, Linton K, Gallop-Evans E, Hemmaway C, et al. Guidelines for the diagnosis and management of primary central nervous system diffuse large B-cell lymphoma. British Journal of Haematology. 2019;**184**(3):348-363

[43] Abrey LE, Batchelor TT, Ferreri AJM, Gospodarowicz M, Pulczynski EJ, Zucca E, et al. Report of an international workshop to standardize baseline evaluation and response criteria for primary CNS lymphoma. Journal of Clinical Oncology. 2005;**23**(22):5034-5043

[44] Adhikari N, Biswas A, Gogia A, Sahoo RK, Garg A, Nehra A, et al. A prospective phase II trial of response adapted whole brain radiotherapy after high dose methotrexate based chemotherapy in patients with newly diagnosed primary central nervous system lymphoma-analysis of acute toxicity profile and early clinical outcome. Journal of Neuro-Oncology. 2018;**139**(1):153-166

[45] Ferreri AJM, Blay J-Y, Reni M, Pasini F, Spina M, Ambrosetti A, et al. Prognostic scoring system for primary CNS lymphomas: The International Extranodal Lymphoma Study Group experience. Journal of Clinical Oncology: Official Journal of the American Society of Clinical Oncology. 2003;**21**(2):266-272

[46] Reni M, Ferreri AJ, Villa E. Second-line treatment for primary central nervous system lymphoma. British Journal of Cancer. 1999;**79**(3–4):530-534

[47] Yu J, Du H, Ye X, Zhang L, Xiao H. High-dose methotrexate-based regimens and post-remission consolidation for treatment of newly diagnosed primary CNS lymphoma: Meta-analysis of clinical trials. Scientific Reports. 2021;**11**(1):2125

[48] Omuro A, Correa DD, DeAngelis LM, Moskowitz CH, Matasar MJ, Kaley TJ, et al. R-MPV followed by high-dose chemotherapy with TBC and autologous stem-cell transplant for newly diagnosed primary CNS lymphoma. Blood. 2015;**125**(9): 1403-1410

[49] DeAngelis LM, Seiferheld W, Schold SC, Fisher B, Schultz CJ. Combination chemotherapy and radiotherapy for primary central nervous system lymphoma: Radiation therapy oncology group study 93-10. Journal of Clinical Oncology. 2002; **20**(24):4643-4648

[50] Correa DD, Rocco-Donovan M, DeAngelis LM, Dolgoff-Kaspar R, Iwamoto F, Yahalom J, et al. Prospective cognitive follow-up in primary CNS lymphoma patients treated with chemotherapy and reduced-dose radiotherapy. Journal of Neuro-Oncology. 2009;**91**(3):315-321

[51] Shah GD, Yahalom J, Correa DD, Lai RK, Raizer JJ, Schiff D, et al. Combined immunochemotherapy with reduced whole-brain radiotherapy for newly diagnosed primary CNS lymphoma. Journal of Clinical Oncology: Official Journal of the American Society of Clinical Oncology. 2007;**25**(30):4730-4735

[52] Malikova H, Koubska E, Weichet J, Klener J, Rulseh A, Liscak R, et al. Can morphological MRI differentiate between primary central nervous system lymphoma and glioblastoma? Cancer Imaging. 2016;**16**(1):40

[53] Paydas S. Primary central nervous system lymphoma: Essential points in diagnosis and management. Medical oncology (Northwood London England). 2017;**34**(4):61

[54] Wen J-B, Huang W-Y, Xu W-X-Z, Wu G, Geng D-Y, Yin B. Differentiating primary central nervous system lymphomas from glioblastomas and inflammatory demyelinating pseudotumor using relative minimum apparent diffusion coefficients. Journal of Computer Assisted Tomography. 2017;**41**(6):904-909

[55] Zhao J, Yang Z, Luo B, Yang J, Chu J. Quantitative evaluation of diffusion and dynamic contrast-enhanced MR in tumor parenchyma and peritumoral area for distinction of brain tumors. PLoS One. 2015;**10**(9):e0138573

[56] Harting I, Hartmann M, Jost G, Sommer C, Ahmadi R, Heiland S, et al. Differentiating primary central nervous system lymphoma from glioma in humans using localised proton magnetic resonance spectroscopy. Neuroscience Letters. 2003;**342**(3):163-166

[57] Aburano H, Ueda F, Yoshie Y, Matsui O, Nakada M, Hayashi Y, et al. Differences between glioblastomas and primary central nervous system lymphomas in 1H-magnetic resonance spectroscopy. Japanese Journal of Radiology. 2015;**33**(7):392-403

[58] Roser F, Saini M, Meliss R, Ostertag H, Samii M, Bellinzona M. Apoptosis, vascularity, and proliferation in primary central nervous system lymphomas (PCNSL): A histopathological study. Surgical Neurology. 2004;**62**(5):393-399; discussion 399

[59] Lee IH, Kim ST, Kim H-J, Kim KH, Jeon P, Byun HS. Analysis of perfusion weighted image of CNS lymphoma. European Journal of Radiology. 2010; **76**(1):48-51

[60] Blasel S, Jurcoane A, Bähr O, Weise L, Harter PN, Hattingen E. MR perfusion in and around the contrast-enhancement of primary CNS lymphomas. Journal of Neuro-Oncology. 2013;**114**(1):127-134

[61] Nguyen AV, Blears EE, Ross E, Lall RR, Ortega-Barnett J. Machine learning applications for the differentiation of primary central nervous system lymphoma from glioblastoma on imaging: A systematic review and meta-analysis. Neurosurgical Focus. 2018;**45**(5):E5

[62] Chen C, Zheng A, Ou X, Wang J, Ma X. Comparison of radiomics-based machine-learning classifiers in diagnosis of glioblastoma from primary central nervous system lymphoma. Frontiers in Oncology. 2020;**10**:1151

[63] Kawai N, Miyake K, Yamamoto Y, Nishiyama Y, Tamiya T. 18F-FDG PET in the diagnosis and treatment of primary central nervous system lymphoma. BioMed Research International. 2013;**2013**:247152

[64] Kosaka N, Tsuchida T, Uematsu H, Kimura H, Okazawa H, Itoh H. 18F-FDG PET of common enhancing malignant brain tumors. American Journal of Roentgenology. 2008;**190**(6): W365-W369

[65] Makino K, Hirai T, Nakamura H, Murakami R, Kitajima M, Shigematsu Y, et al. Does adding FDG-PET to MRI improve the differentiation between primary cerebral lymphoma and glioblastoma? Observer performance study. Annals of Nuclear Medicine. 2011;**25**(6):432-438

[66] Zhang Q, Gao X, Wei G, Qiu C, Qu H, Zhou X. Prognostic value of MTV, SUVmax and the T/N Ratio of PET/CT in patients with glioma: A systematic review and meta-analysis. Journal of Cancer. 2019;**10**(7):1707-1716

[67] Mohile NA, DeAngelis LM, Abrey LE. The utility of body FDG PET in staging primary central nervous system lymphoma. Neuro-Oncology. 2008;**10**(2):223-228

[68] Canovi S, Campioli D. Accuracy of flow cytometry and cytomorphology for the diagnosis of meningeal involvement in lymphoid neoplasms: A systematic review. Diagnostic Cytopathology. 2016;**44**(10):841-856

[69] Schroers R, Baraniskin A, Heute C, Vorgerd M, Brunn A, Kuhnhenn J, et al. Diagnosis of leptomeningeal disease in diffuse large B-cell lymphomas of the central nervous system by flow cytometry and cytopathology. European Journal of Haematology. 2010;**85**(6):520-528

[70] Ekstein D, Ben-Yehuda D, Slyusarevsky E, Lossos A, Linetsky E, Siegal T. CSF analysis of IgH gene rearrangement in CNS lymphoma: Relationship to the disease course. Journal of the Neurological Sciences. 2006;**247**(1):39-46

[71] Fischer L, Martus P, Weller M, Klasen HA, Rohden B, Röth A, et al. Meningeal dissemination in primary CNS lymphoma: Prospective evaluation of 282 patients. Neurology. 2008;**71**(14): 1102-1108

[72] Hiemcke-Jiwa LS, Leguit RJ, Snijders TJ, Jiwa NM, Kuiper JJW, de Weger RA, et al. Molecular analysis in liquid biopsies for diagnostics of primary central nervous system lymphoma: Review of literature and future opportunities. Critical Reviews in Oncology/Hematology. 2018;**127**:56-65

[73] Cerebrospinal Fluid IL-10 and IL-10/IL-6 as Accurate Diagnostic Biomarkers for Primary Central Nervous System Large B-cell Lymphoma | Scientific Reports [Internet]. 2021. Available from: https://www.nature.com/articles/srep38671

[74] Strehlow F, Bauer S, Martus P, Weller M, Roth P, Schlegel U, et al. Osteopontin in cerebrospinal fluid as diagnostic biomarker for central nervous system lymphoma. Journal of Neuro-Oncology. 2016;**129**(1):165-171

[75] Viaccoz A, Ducray F, Tholance Y, Barcelos GK, Thomas-Maisonneuve L, Ghesquières H, et al. CSF neopterin level as a diagnostic marker in primary central nervous system lymphoma. Neuro-Oncology. 2015;**17**(11):1497-1503

[76] Baraniskin A, Kuhnhenn J, Schlegel U, Chan A, Deckert M, Gold R, et al. Identification of microRNAs in the cerebrospinal fluid as marker for primary diffuse large B-cell lymphoma of the central nervous system. Blood. 2011;**117**(11):3140-3146

[77] Wang L, Luo L, Gao Z, Liu S-F, Liu C-J, Ma D-X, et al. The diagnostic and prognostic value of interleukin-10 in cerebrospinal fluid for central nervous system lymphoma: A meta-analysis. Leukemia & Lymphoma. 2017;**58**(10): 2452-2459

[78] Chan C-C, Wallace DJ. Intraocular lymphoma: Update on diagnosis and management. Cancer Control: Journal of the Moffitt Cancer Center. 2004;**11**(5): 285-295

[79] Grimm SA, McCannel CA, Omuro AMP, Ferreri AJM, Blay J-Y,

Neuwelt EA, et al. Primary CNS lymphoma with intraocular involvement. Neurology. 2008;**71**(17): 1355-1360

[80] Ursea R, Heinemann MH, Silverman RH, DeAngelis LM, Daly SW, Coleman DJ. Ophthalmic, ultrasonographic findings in primary central nervous system lymphoma with ocular involvement. Retina (Philadelphia PA). 1997;**17**(2):118-123

[81] Baehring JM, Androudi S, Longtine JJ, Betensky RA, Sklar J, Foster CS, et al. Analysis of clonal immunoglobulin heavy chain rearrangements in ocular lymphoma. Cancer. 2005;**104**(3):591-597

[82] Mastropasqua R, Thaung C, Pavesio C, Lightman S, Westcott M, Okhravi N, et al. The role of chorioretinal biopsy in the diagnosis of intraocular lymphoma. American Journal of Ophthalmology. 2015;**160**(6): 1127-1132.e1

[83] Raja H, Salomão DR, Viswanatha DS, Pulido JS. Prevalence of MYD88 L265P mutation in histologically proven, diffuse large B-cell vitreoretinal lymphoma. Retina (Philadelphia PA). 2016;**36**(3):624-628

[84] Li Q, Ma J, Ma Y, Lin Z, Kang H, Chen B. Improvement of outcomes of an escalated high-dose methotrexate-based regimen for patients with newly diagnosed primary central nervous system lymphoma: A real-world cohort study. Cancer Management and Research. 2021;**13**:6115-6122

[85] Hiraga S, Arita N, Ohnishi T, Kohmura E, Yamamoto K, Oku Y, et al. Rapid infusion of high-dose methotrexate resulting in enhanced penetration into cerebrospinal fluid and intensified tumor response in primary central nervous system lymphomas. Journal of Neurosurgery. 1999;**91**(2): 221-230

[86] Aoki H, Ogura R, Tsukamoto Y, Okada M, Natsumeda M, Isogawa M, et al. Advantages of dose-dense methotrexate protocol for primary central nervous system lymphoma: Comparison of two different protocols at a single institution. Neurologia Medico-Chirurgica (Tokyo). 2013; **53**(11):797-804

[87] Ramsey LB, Balis FM, O'Brien MM, Schmiegelow K, Pauley JL, Bleyer A, et al. Consensus guideline for use of glucarpidase in patients with high-dose methotrexate induced acute kidney injury and delayed methotrexate clearance. The Oncologist. 2018;**23**(1): 52-61

[88] Ferreri AJ, Reni M, Foppoli M, Martelli M, Pangalis GA, Frezzato M, et al. High-dose cytarabine plus high-dose methotrexate versus high-dose methotrexate alone in patients with primary CNS lymphoma: A randomised phase 2 trial. The Lancet. 2009; **374**(9700):1512-1520

[89] Illerhaus G, Marks R, Ihorst G, Guttenberger R, Ostertag C, Derigs G, et al. High-dose chemotherapy with autologous stem-cell transplantation and hyperfractionated radiotherapy as first-line treatment of primary CNS lymphoma. Journal of Clinical Oncology. 2006;**24**(24):3865-3870

[90] Reni M, Zaja F, Mason W, Perry J, Mazza E, Spina M, et al. Temozolomide as salvage treatment in primary brain lymphomas. British Journal of Cancer. 2007;**96**(6):864-867

[91] Fischer L, Thiel E, Klasen H-A, Birkmann J, Jahnke K, Martus P, et al. Prospective trial on topotecan salvage therapy in primary CNS lymphoma. Annals of Oncology. 2006;**17**(7): 1141-1145

[92] Korfel A, Schlegel U, Herrlinger U, Dreyling M, Schmidt C, von Baumgarten L, et al. Phase II trial of

temsirolimus for relapsed/refractory primary CNS lymphoma. Journal of Clinical Oncology. 2016;**34**(15): 1757-1763

[93] Davis RE, Ngo VN, Lenz G, Tolar P, Young RM, Romesser PB, et al. Chronic active B-cell-receptor signalling in diffuse large B-cell lymphoma. Nature. 2010;**463**(7277):88-92

[94] Wilson WH. Treatment strategies for aggressive lymphomas: What works? Hematology. 2013;**2013**(1):584-590

[95] Roschewski M, Lionakis MS, Melani C, Butman JA, Pittaluga S, Lucas AN, et al. Dose-adjusted Teddi-R induces durable complete remissions in relapsed and refractory primary CNS lymphoma. Blood. 2018;**132** (Supplement 1):4195-4195

[96] da Ros M, Iorio AL, Lucchesi M, Stival A, de Martino M, Sardi I. The use of anthracyclines for therapy of CNS tumors. Anti-Cancer Agents in Medicinal Chemistry. 2015;**15**(6): 721-727

[97] Lionakis MS, Dunleavy K, Roschewski M, Widemann BC, Butman JA, Schmitz R, et al. Inhibition of B cell receptor signaling by ibrutinib in primary CNS lymphoma. Cancer Cell. 2017;**31**(6):833-843.e5

[98] Grommes C, Younes A. Ibrutinib in PCNSL: The curious cases of clinical responses and aspergillosis. Cancer Cell. 2017;**31**(6):731-733

[99] de Jong J, Hellemans P, De Wilde S, Patricia D, Masterson T, Manikhas G, et al. A drug-drug interaction study of ibrutinib with moderate/strong CYP3A inhibitors in patients with B-cell malignancies. Leukemia & Lymphoma. 2018;**59**(12):2888-2895

[100] Hernandez-Ilizaliturri FJ, Reddy N, Holkova B, Ottman E, Czuczman MS. Immunomodulatory drug CC-5013 or CC-4047 and rituximab enhance antitumor activity in a severe combined immunodeficient mouse lymphoma model. Clinical Cancer Research: An Official Journal of the American Association for Cancer Research. 2005;**11**(16):5984-5992

[101] Ghesquieres H, Chevrier M, Laadhari M, Chinot O, Choquet S, Moluçon-Chabrot C, et al. Lenalidomide in combination with intravenous rituximab (REVRI) in relapsed/ refractory primary CNS lymphoma or primary intraocular lymphoma: A multicenter prospective 'proof of concept' phase II study of the French Oculo-Cerebral lymphoma (LOC) Network and the Lymphoma Study Association (LYSA)†. Annals of Oncology. 2019;**30**(4):621-628

[102] Petereit H, Rubbert-Roth A. Rituximab levels in cerebrospinal fluid of patients with neurological autoimmune disorders. Multiple Sclerosis Journal. 2009;**15**(2):189-192

[103] Feugier P, Virion JM, Tilly H, Haioun C, Marit G, Macro M, et al. Incidence and risk factors for central nervous system occurrencein elderly patients with diffuse large-B-cell lymphoma: Influence of rituximab. Annals of Oncology. 2004;**15**(1):129-133

[104] Rubenstein JL, Combs D, Rosenberg J, Levy A, McDermott M, Damon L, et al. Rituximab therapy for CNS lymphomas: Targeting the leptomeningeal compartment. Blood. 2003;**101**(2):466-468

[105] Rubenstein JL, Fridlyand J, Abrey L, Shen A, Karch J, Wang E, et al. Phase I study of intraventricular administration of rituximab in patients with recurrent CNS and intraocular lymphoma. Journal of Clinical Oncology. 2007;**25**(11):1350-1356

[106] Rubenstein JL, Li J, Chen L, Advani R, Drappatz J, Gerstner E, et al.

Multicenter phase 1 trial of intraventricular immunochemotherapy in recurrent CNS lymphoma. Blood. 2013;**121**(5):745-751

[107] DeAngelis LM, Hormigo A. Treatment of primary central nervous system lymphoma. Seminars in Oncology. 2004;**31**(5):684-692

[108] Ferreri AJM, Cwynarski K, Pulczynski E, Fox CP, Schorb E, La Rosée P, et al. Whole-brain radiotherapy or autologous stem-cell transplantation as consolidation strategies after high-dose methotrexate-based chemoimmunotherapy in patients with primary CNS lymphoma: Results of the second randomisation of the International Extranodal Lymphoma Study Group-32 phase 2 trial. Lancet Haematology. 2017;**4**(11):e510-e523

[109] Houillier C, Taillandier L, Dureau S, Lamy T, Laadhari M, Chinot O, et al. Radiotherapy or autologous stem-cell transplantation for primary CNS lymphoma in patients 60 years of age and younger: Results of the intergroup ANOCEF-GOELAMS randomized phase II PRECIS study. Journal of Clinical Oncology: Official Journal of the American Society of Clinical Oncology. 2019;**37**(10):823-833

[110] Morris PG, Correa DD, Yahalom J, Raizer JJ, Schiff D, Grant B, et al. Rituximab, methotrexate, procarbazine, and vincristine followed by consolidation reduced-dose whole-brain radiotherapy and cytarabine in newly diagnosed primary CNS lymphoma: Final results and long-term outcome. Journal of Clinical Oncology: Official Journal of the American Society of Clinical Oncology. 2013;**31**(31): 3971-3979

[111] Rubenstein JL, Hsi ED, Johnson JL, Jung S-H, Nakashima MO, Grant B, et al. Intensive chemotherapy and immunotherapy in patients with newly diagnosed primary CNS Lymphoma: CALGB 50202 (Alliance 50202). Journal of Clinical Oncology. 2013;**31**(25): 3061-3068

[112] Fritsch K, Kasenda B, Schorb E, Hau P, Bloehdorn J, Möhle R, et al. High-dose methotrexate-based immuno-chemotherapy for elderly primary CNS lymphoma patients (PRIMAIN study). Leukemia. 2017; **31**(4):846-852

[113] Pulczynski EJ, Kuittinen O, Erlanson M, Hagberg H, Fosså A, Eriksson M, et al. Successful change of treatment strategy in elderly patients with primary central nervous system lymphoma by de-escalating induction and introducing temozolomide maintenance: Results from a phase II study by The Nordic Lymphoma Group. Haematologica. 2015;**100**(4):534-540

[114] Rubenstein JL, Hwang J, Mannis G. Preliminary analysis of lenalidomide maintenance after methotrexate-temozolomide-rituximab induction in older patients with PCNSL. Hematological Oncology. 2017;**35**(S2): 343-344

Chapter 10

Breast Implant-Associated Anaplastic Large Cell Lymphoma (BIA-ALCL): Breast Imaging Perspective

Fernando Collado-Mesa

Abstract

Breast implant-associated anaplastic large cell lymphoma is a rare disease first described in 1997. Since then, its incidence has continued to increase. Current estimated lifetime risk in women with textured breast implants range from 1:1000 to 1:30,000. Most cases present with rapid and dramatic breast swelling resulting from peri-implant fluid collection. Palpable mass, pain, and skin lesions also occur. A high index of suspicion in patients who develop a seroma around the breast implant more than one year after implant placement is required. The combination of clinical history, physical exam findings, and appropriate imaging workup can lead to a timely and accurate diagnosis. The disease has excellent prognosis when it is diagnosed earlier, and complete surgery is performed. Radiologists, particularly those involved in breast imaging, can play an essential role in early diagnosis. This chapter presents an overview of the disease, including relevant imaging findings.

Keywords: breast implant-associated anaplastic large cell lymphoma, epidemiology, pathophysiology, diagnosis, treatment, prognosis, mammography, ultrasound, magnetic resonance imaging, fine needle aspiration, needle biopsy, positron emission tomography

1. Introduction

Breast implant-associated anaplastic large cell lymphoma (BIA-ALCL) is a rare disease first described in 1997 when Keech & Creech published the first case report of anaplastic T-cell lymphoma in proximity to a saline-filled breast implant [1]. Following the initial report, additional case reports and case series of this entity have been published [2–4].

A possible association between breast implants and anaplastic large cell lymphoma was announced by the Food and Drug Administration (FDA) in 2011 [5], and in 2016, the World Health Organization (WHO) added BIA-ALCL as a provisionally recognized lymphoma to the family of existing ALCL [6].

In 2019 the FDA issued a safety communication stating, "all individuals who are considering a breast implant of any type be informed of the risk of developing BIA-ALCL". At the time, most cases of BIA-ALCL were reported to have Allergan's Biocell textured breast implants, thus, following an FDA recommendation, Allergan initiated a worldwide voluntary recall of their breast implant products in July 2019 [7].

The incidence of the disease has continued to increase with current estimates of the absolute risk for development of BIA-ALCL ranging from 1 in 3,817 to 1 in 30,000 [8].

BIA-ALCL is characterized by the development of peri-implant fluid collection that occurs >1 year after breast implant placement, and/or by a solid mass arising within the implant's fibrous capsule [9]. Median time since implant placement at diagnosis is estimated at 8–10 years [9].

Overall, the disease has an excellent prognosis, particularly if diagnosed and fully treated at early stage [10]. It is therefore important to increase awareness about this disease amongst health care providers in general and amongst radiologists and provide them with the relevant information for early diagnosis, referral, and treatment.

2. Etiopathogenesis

Although the etiology of BIA-ALCL remains poorly understood, there is evidence demonstrating a preponderance of patients with BIA-ALCL to have been exposed to textured breast implants, developed in the 1980s to reduce implant contractures, which in turn provides clues as to the pathogenesis of this condition [11, 12].

Texturing of the implant shell may lead to a greater inflammatory response of the surrounding fibrous tissue capsule eliciting an increased chronic antigenic stimulation, which in turn could potentially be responsible for the development of ALCL [12]. Other potential causes of chronic inflammation which have been postulated include lipopolysaccharide endotoxin, trauma to the breast pocket, viral infection, and allergens [13].

Currently, there is not enough data to determine whether ALCL may be found more or less frequently in individuals with silicone-filled breast implants compared to individuals with saline-filled breast implants [14].

The presence of germline and somatic mutations, which can increase the susceptibility of the host to BIA-ALCL has been postulated as a contributing factor [12].

Recent molecular studies have identified novel, activating mutations in the Janus kinase (JAK), and signal transducer and activator of transcription factor (*STAT3*) pathway as a major risk factor for the development of BIA-ALCL (the presence of germline and somatic mutations, which can increase the susceptibility of the host to BIA-ALCL). Aberrant *STAT3* signaling has been established as a mechanistic link between chronic inflammation in non–BIA-ALCL cancers, including B- and T-cell lymphomas, and amongst the latter systemic anaplastic large cell lymphomas (the presence of germline and somatic mutations, which can increase the susceptibility of the host to BIA-ALCL) and persistent *STAT3* activation has been definitively linked to improved tumor survival and cell proliferation, increased angiogenesis, and tumor metastasis [13].

3. Epidemiology

Current estimates suggest that each year over 1.8 million people worldwide receive breast implants for cosmetic or reconstructive purposes [15]. In July of 2019 the number of BIA-ALCL reported cases worldwide reached 573, with 320 those cases reported in the US [16]. The estimated lifetime risk of BIA-ALCL in women with textured breast implants range from 1:1,000 to 1:30,000 [17]. A reported geographic variation of the risk is likely due to variable reporting and less likely to geographic or genetic predisposition [17].

4. Clinical features

Mean age at diagnosis is 53.2 ± 12.3 years [17]. Mean interval from implant placement to diagnosis is 10.7 ± 4.6 years [17]. However, this late-onset diagnoses may reflect delayed diagnosis or misdiagnosis.

Patients most commonly present with rapid onset of a spontaneous fluid collection (60–90%) or capsular mass (10–40%) [9]. Approximately 30% of patients report pain, and about 25% present with skin lesions, most commonly erythema, subcutaneous nodules, eruption, erosion, or ulcer [9].

Implant capsule contracture is present in approximately 30% of cases [9]. When this occurs, there is a preponderance of grade III and IV contracture, defined as clinically symptomatic and visible contracture of the implant capsule [18].

BIA-ALCL disseminates locally in a small proportion of cases [19]. When local dissemination takes place it most commonly involves the ipsilateral axillary lymph nodes [19]. The prevalence of lymphadenopathy at diagnosis ranges from 2–14% [19].

Distant disease is uncommon. There are case reports of and distant lymph nodes and bone marrow involvement [19]. Systemic symptoms, such as unexplained weight loss, fever, or night sweats, are also uncommon affecting approximately 8% of patients [19].

5. Radiologic features

5.1 Mammography

In general, mammography findings include nonspecific capsular thickening, and circumferential asymmetry around the implant (**Figures 1** and **2**) [19, 20].

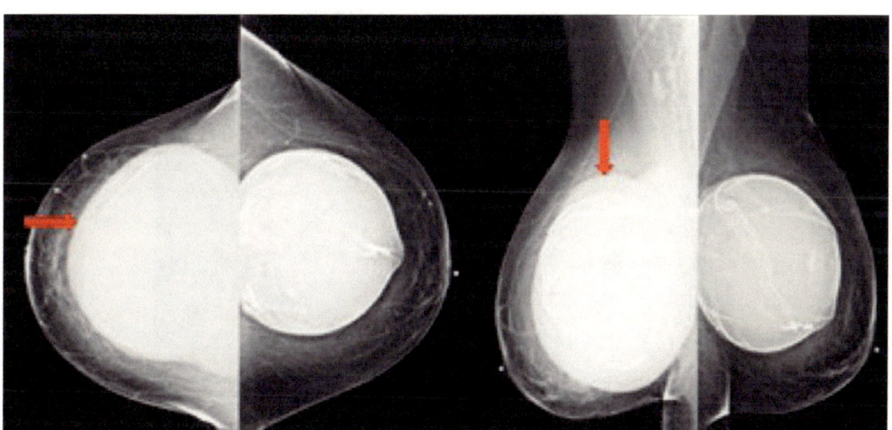

Figure 1.
63-year-old female with history of saline breast implants with textured surface placed 19 years ago presented with pain and swelling throughout the right breast and a palpable abnormality in the posterior third of the right breast at 7 o'clock for 1 month. Bilateral digital mammogram shows bilateral retro glandular saline breast implants. The right breast is larger than the left and shows a homogeneous and circumferential area of increased density (arrow) surrounding the implant, including the area of palpable abnormality noted by triangular marker in the posterior third of the right breast lower quadrants (source: Collado-Mesa et al. [20]).

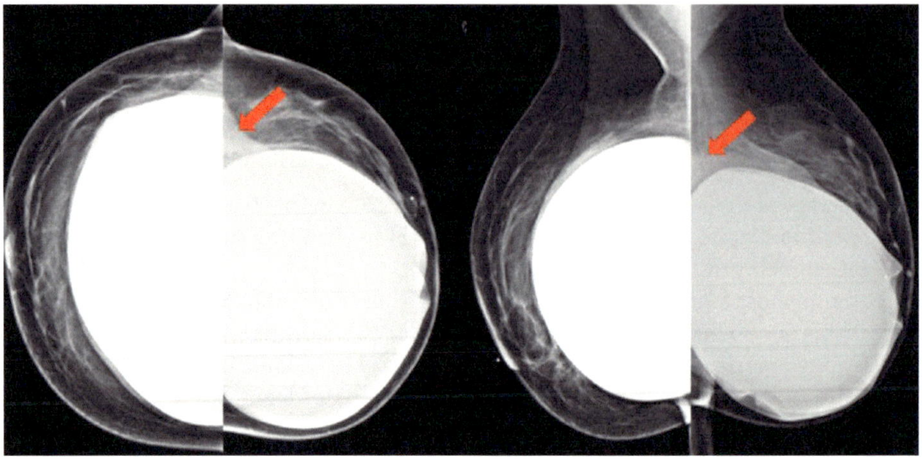

Figure 2.
54-year-old female status post left breast mastectomy for DCIS and right breast prophylactic mastectomy, followed by immediate bilateral breast silicone implant with textured surface reconstruction 11 years ago presented with sudden onset of right breast swelling and enlargement with associated discomfort. She denied fever or general symptoms. Bilateral mammogram shows irregular contours of the right breast silicone implant with associated focal-peri-implant increased density (arrows) (source: Collado-Mesa et al. [20]).

Unlike with primary breast cancer, mammography is not accurate for detection of either peri-implant effusion or mass-forming BIA-ALCL.

Overall, mammography has a lower sensitivity and specificity than both ultrasound and Magnetic Resonance Imaging (MRI) for any abnormality due to BIA-ALCL, at 73% and 50% respectively [21].

5.2 Ultrasound

Ultrasound (US) is the imaging exam of choice. Findings most commonly include a homogeneous peri implant effusion with inflammatory changes in the periprosthetic breast tissue (**Figures 3** and **4**).

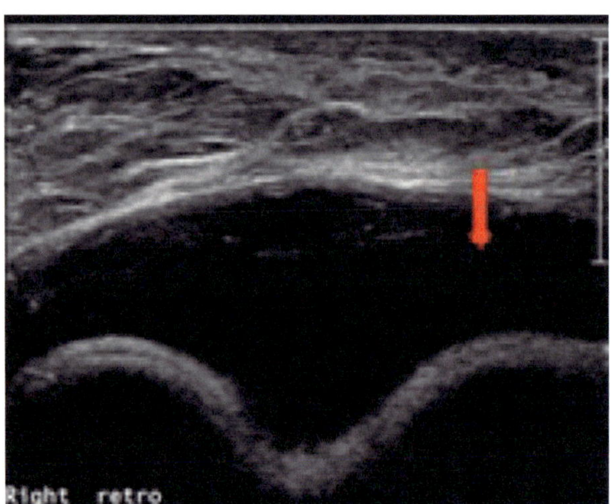

Figure 3.
63-year-old female with history of saline breast implants with textured surface placed 19 years ago presented with pain and swelling throughout the right breast and a palpable abnormality in the posterior third of the right breast at 7 o'clock for 1 month. Grey scale ultrasound shows right breast peri-implant fluid collection (arrow) (source: Collado-Mesa et al. [20]).

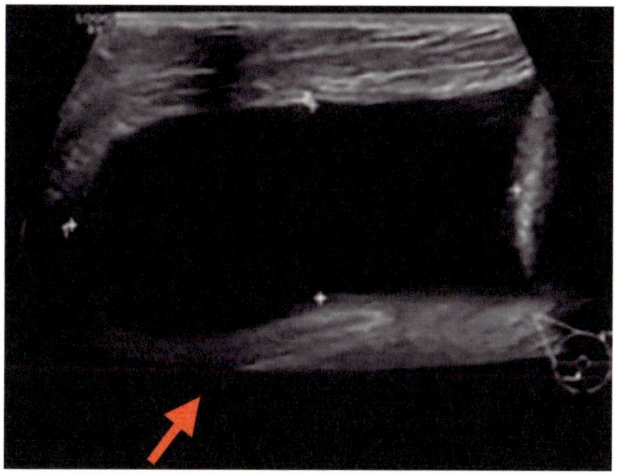

Figure 4.
Effusion-only BIA-ALCL in a 55-year-old woman after mastectomy for breast cancer. The initial breast implant was exchanged after 9 years; 7 years later, she experienced sudden new marked implant-associated swelling. Transverse US image shows a large seroma with septa surrounding the intact implant (arrow). US-guided fine-needle aspiration yielded cloudy yellow fluid, cytologic analysis of which demonstrated ALK-negative BIA-ALCL (source: Sharma B et al. [19]).

When a solid mass is present, it frequently appears as an oval, hypoechoic, circumscribed mass, without hypervascularity (**Figure 5**) [19, 20]. Less frequently, it appears as a complex cystic and solid mass [19, 20].

Some cases may present with abnormal ipsilateral axillary lymph nodes, including the presence of nodal cortical thickening or diffusely hypoechoic without evident fatty hilus.

Amongst the commonly used breast imaging modalities, the highest sensitivity for detection of peri-implant fluid collection is reported for ultrasound (84%) [21]. Ultrasound is also reported to have the highest specificity for detection of solid mass (100%) [21].

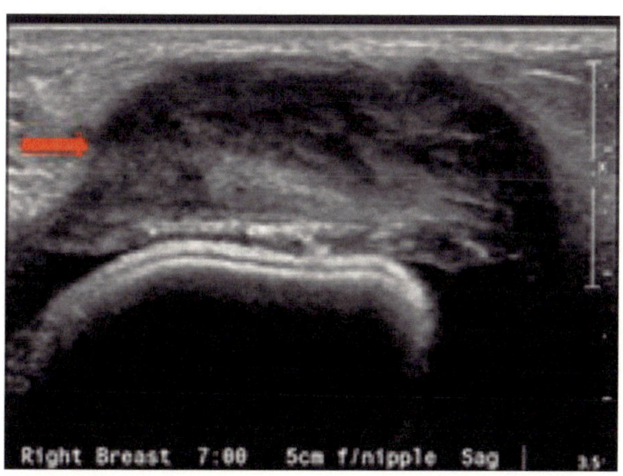

Figure 5.
63-year-old female with history of saline breast implants with textured surface placed 19 years ago presented with pain and swelling throughout the right breast and a palpable abnormality in the posterior third of the right breast at 7 o'clock for 1 month. Grey scale ultrasound shows a 4 × 1.4 × 2.4 cm mixed echogenicity, oval, partially, indistinct mass (arrow) abutting the fibrous capsule in the right breast at 7 o'clock, 5 cm from the nipple, corresponding to palpable abnormality (source: Collado-Mesa et al. [20]).

5.3 Magnetic resonance imaging

Breast Magnetic Resonance Imaging (MRI) is the imaging test of choice after US, and it particularly add value when US results are indeterminate.

MRI findings include peri-implant tissue edema and effusion, as well as peri-implant mass lesions, including small-volume mass components not detected with US. Enhancement with intravenous gadolinium contrast material may also help with characterization of some findings (**Figures 6–10**) [19, 20].

MRI also serves to evaluate for the presence of implant rupture when there is a silicone implant [19].

MRI is the imaging modality with the second highest sensitivity for peri-implant fluid collection at 82% and with the second highest specificity for mass at 93% [21].

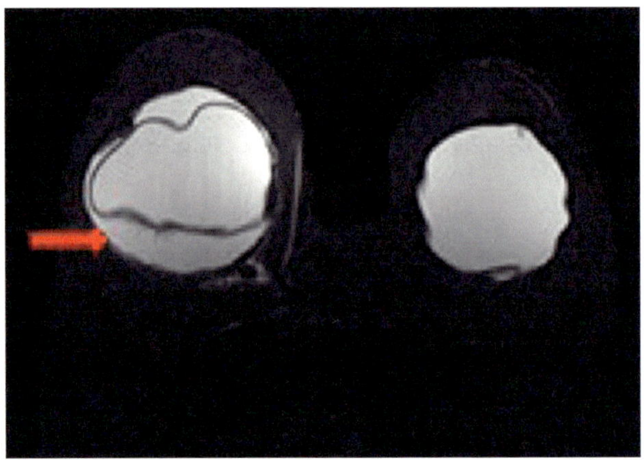

Figure 6.
63-year-old female with history of saline breast implants with textured surface placed 19 years ago presented with pain and swelling throughout the right breast and a palpable abnormality in the posterior third of the right breast at 7 o'clock for 1 month. Breast MRI axial T2-weighted fat-saturated sequence shows right breast peri-implant fluid collection (arrow) (source: Collado-Mesa et al. [20]).

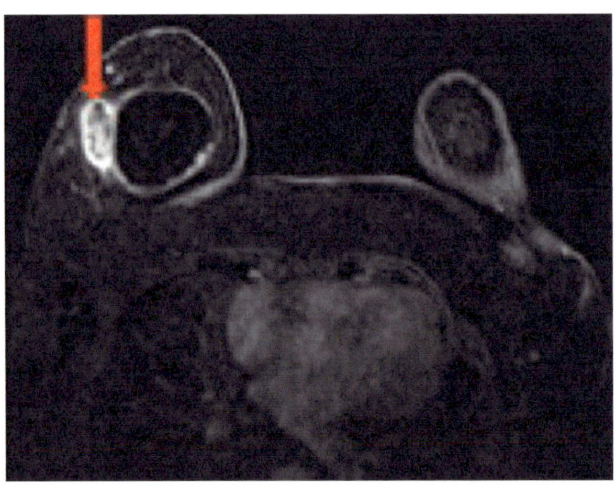

Figure 7.
63-year-old female with history of saline breast implants with textured surface placed 19 years ago presented with pain and swelling throughout the right breast and a palpable abnormality in the posterior third of the right breast at 7 o'clock for 1 month. Breast MRI axial T1-weighted fat saturated postcontrast subtraction shows a 4 × 1.7 × 2 cm oval heterogeneously enhancing mass (arrow) arising from the fibrous capsule in the right lower outer quadrant (source: Collado-Mesa et al. [20]).

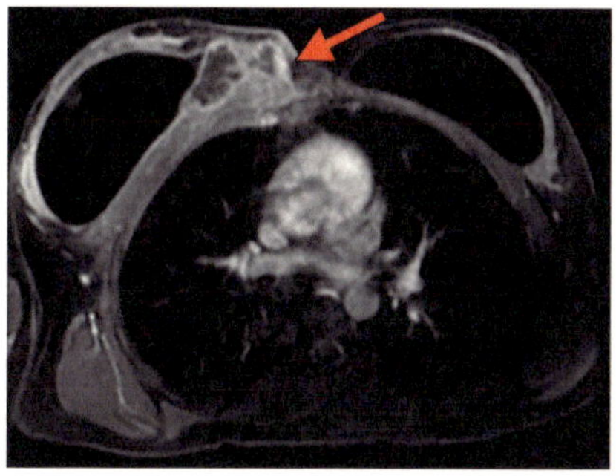

Figure 8.
Mass forming BIA-ALCL in a 29-year-old woman with a right upper inner breast mass 3 years after bilateral breast augmentation with TRF-520 implants (Allergan). Axial gadolinium enhanced fat-saturated breath-hold volume MR image shows a large implant-associated lobulated mass with a central necrotic area and intense rim enhancement (arrow) infiltrating the pectoralis major muscle and threatening the intercostal muscles. Biopsy demonstrated BIA-ALCL (source: Sharma B et al. [19]).

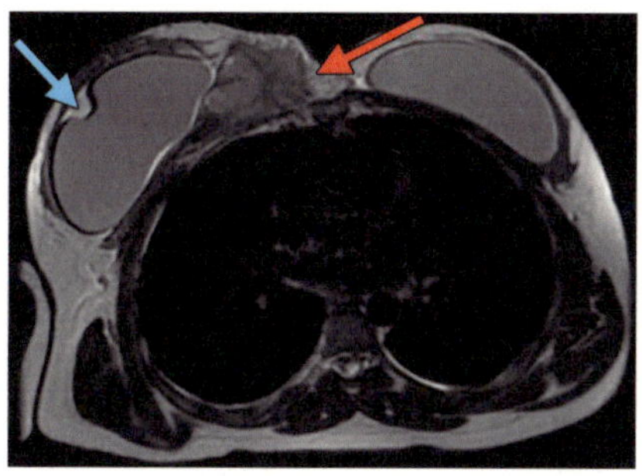

Figure 9.
BIA-ALCL with chest wall invasion in a 29-year-old woman who underwent bilateral breast augmentation with TRF-520 implants (Allergan) and developed a right upper inner breast lump 3 years after surgery. Axial fast spin-echo T2-weighted image with breath holding 4 months later shows irregular surface of the implant (blue arrow) and rapid enlargement (estimated at 7 cm axially) of the lobulated mass (red arrow), which is characterized by a central necrotic area. Biopsy demonstrated large atypical CD30-positive cells infiltrating the fibrous tissue. The final diagnosis was BIA-ALCL (source: Sharma B et al. [19]).

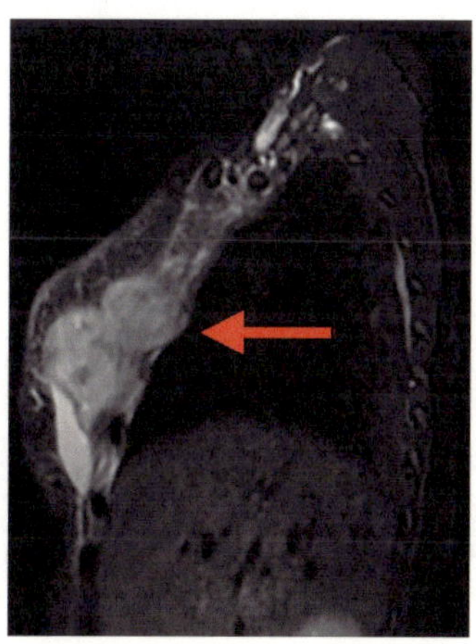

Figure 10.
BIA-ALCL with chest wall invasion in a 29-year-old woman who underwent bilateral breast augmentation with TRF-520 implants (Allergan) and developed a right upper inner breast lump 3 years after surgery. Sagittal short τ inversion-recovery (STIR) image obtained 4 months later shows the mass (arrow) infiltrating the pectoralis major muscle and threatening the intercostal muscles. Biopsy demonstrated large atypical CD30-positive cells infiltrating the fibrous tissue. The final diagnosis was BIA-ALCL (source: Sharma B et al. [19]).

6. Diagnosis and histologic features

A high index of suspicion of BIA-ALCL is required to allow a timely diagnosis.

Breast ultrasound should be obtained in patients with suspicious signs and symptoms such as breast swelling, palpable mass, pain, and skin lesions which have developed more than one year after implant placement (average 8–10 years).

If a peri-implant effusion is noted, then fine needle aspiration of at least 50 ml should be performed [22]. In cases where a peri-implant mass is present, either core needle biopsy or surgical excisional biopsy should be performed [22].

In cases with inconclusive findings on ultrasound, a breast MRI should be obtained [22].

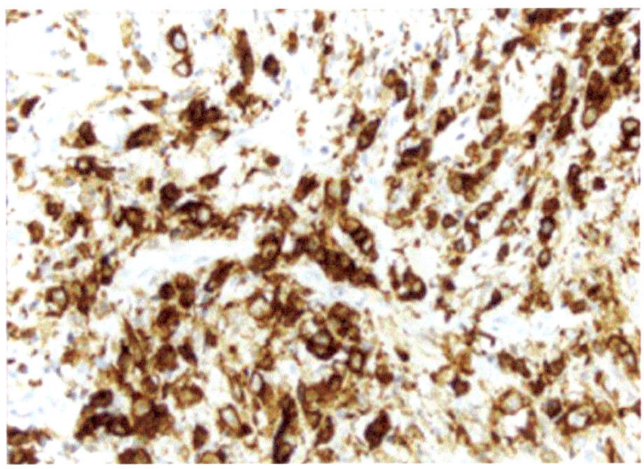

Figure 11.
Photomicrograph of ultrasound-guided core needle biopsy samples of solid mass showed in **Figure 5** *shows most of the cells to be strongly and uniformly positive for CD30 (CD30 immunohistochemistry, ×60) (Source: Collado-Mesa et al. [20]).*

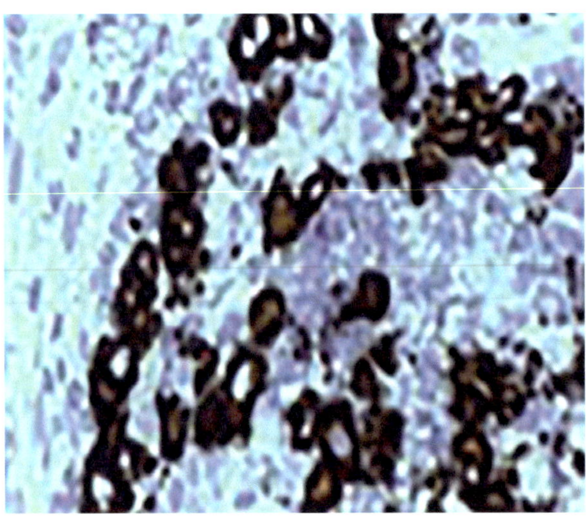

Figure 12.
Effusion-only BIA-ALCL in a 55-year-old woman after mastectomy, axillary node dissection, implant reconstruction, chemoradiotherapy, and immunotherapy. After 9 years, the implant was exchanged; 7 years later, sudden new marked swelling of the right breast developed. At US, a large seroma surrounded the intact right breast implant; diagnostic aspirate yielded cloudy yellow fluid, which was ALK-negative at cytologic analysis. Immunohistochemistry slides show that the infiltrate is positive for CD30 (source: Sharma B et al. [19]).

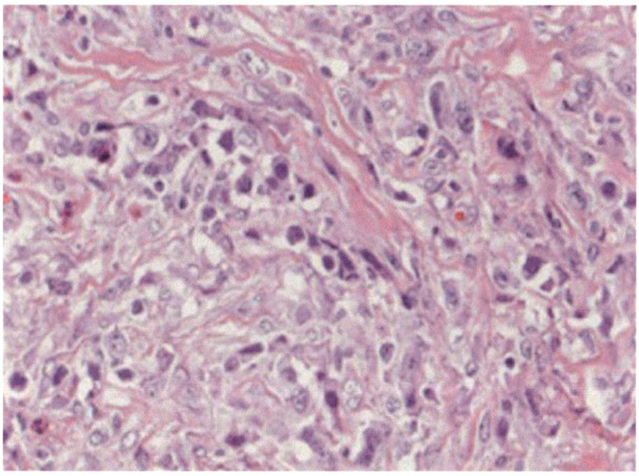

Figure 13.
Photomicrograph of ultrasound-guided core needle biopsy samples of solid mass showed in **Figure 5** *shows large and pleomorphic neoplastic cells with irregular nuclei, large prominent nucleoli, conspicuous mitotic activity, and moderate cytoplasm (hematoxylin and eosin [H&E], ×60) (source: Collado-Mesa et al. [20]).*

Samples should be sent for cytology, flow cytometry, immunohistochemistry for CD30 (**Figures 11** and **12**) and additional differentiation markers (CD2 – CD5, CD7, CD8, CD45, and ALK [19, 20, 22].

The presence of large neoplastic cells that have pleomorphic nuclei, abundant eosinophilic cytoplasm, and irregular cell membranes is required for diagnosis (**Figure 13**). Uniform CD30 expression, evidence of a single T-cell clone, and an absence of ALK expression are also observed [22]. Epithelial membrane antigen (EMA) is also often expressed by neoplastic cells [23]. "Hallmark cells" with eccentric kidney or horseshoe-shaped nuclei are not uncommonly seen [23].

If results are indeterminate, a referral to a cancer center is recommended. If results are negative, then it should be treated as a benign seroma. Patients with positive results require a disease workup [22].

7. Staging

The traditional staging for all lymphoma is the Ann Arbor classification. However, BIA-ALCL is not a classical non-Hodgkin lymphoma and it usually progress locally and/or regionally like a solid tumor; thus, it is better suited to the TNM system for staging solid tumors.

TNM	**Criteria**
T: Tumor extent	
T1	Confined to effusion or a layer on luminal side of capsule
T2	Early capsule infiltration
T3	Cell aggregates or sheets infiltrating the capsule
T4	Lymphoma infiltrates beyond the capsule
N: Lymph node	
N0	No lymph node involvement
N1	One regional lymph node involved
N2	Multiple regional lymph nodes involved

TNM	Criteria
M: Metastasis	
M0	No distant spread
M1	Spread to other organs/distant sites
Stage	TNM
IA	T1 N0 M0
IB	T2 N0 M0
IC	T3 N0 M0
IIA	T4 N0 M0
IIB	T1-3 N1 M0
III	T4 N1-2 M0
IV	T(any) N(any) M1

Modified from source: (Clemens et al. [22]).

Table 1.
TNM stage classification of BIA-ALCL.

The 2019 update of the National Comprehensive Cancer Network guidelines now include a TNM disease staging system based on clinical and pathological evaluation first proposed in 2016 by MD Anderson Cancer Center and which may be more applicable for predicting a prognosis and for evaluating treatment regimens in patients with BIA-ALCL [22].

In this TNM classification for BIA-ALCL the disease is considered extended (not localized) if there is tumor invasion beyond the fibrous capsule, spread to one or more regional lymph nodes, or spread to any organs/distant sites (**Table 1**).

8. Treatment

8.1 Surgical treatment

A surgical oncology consultation is not compulsory but may be beneficial for plastic surgeons unaccustomed to optimal surgical resection of a malignancy.

The goals of surgery are to remove the implant with the surrounding fibrous capsule and any associated capsule mass. Complete surgical excision prolongs both overall survival and event-free survival compared with all other therapeutic interventions [10].

All attempts should be made to gain complete surgical resection because retained or unresectable disease likely indicates the need for adjuvant treatments.

An estimated 2–4% of patients develop bilateral disease, and therefore surgeons may consider removal of the contralateral implant and capsule [10].

Currently, there is no clear role for radical mastectomy or sentinel lymph node biopsy. Full axillary dissection has been used rarely for gross involvement of multiple lymph nodes.

8.2 Adjuvant treatments

No data from prospective trials is available to guide management of patients with disseminated BIAS-ALCL. Current treatment is based on experiences from treating primary cutaneous and systemic ALCL.

Radiation therapy with 24–36 Gray (Gy) to the local or involved site is suggested for patients with local residual disease, positive margins, or unresectable disease with chest wall invasion [22].

Systemic therapy for patients with stage IIB-IV disease can be as combination anthracycline based chemotherapy or as a combination with brentuximab vedotin [22].

9. Surveillance and prognosis

In patients with complete response to treatment, surveillance should include history and physical exam and either a CT chest, abdomen, and pelvis with contrast or a whole-body PET-CT every 6 months for two years and then as clinically indicated (**Figures 14** and **15**) [22].

BIA-ALCL has shown to have an excellent prognosis when the disease is diagnosed earlier (localized disease), and when complete surgery, consisting of explantation, capsulectomy, and removal of any associated capsule mass, is performed [9, 10].

Compared to stage I disease, stage II and stage III disease have a rate of disease events and recurrence which are 2.6-fold higher and 2.7-fold higher respectively [10].

Patients with T1–T3 disease have 0% rate of disease events following complete surgical excision as compared to T4 disease have a 14.3% in patients with T4 disease [10]. Local recurrence is most common if incomplete resection or partial capsulectomy took place [10].

A study of causes of death in patients diagnosed with BIA-ALCL showed that all the patients who died had incomplete surgical excision or did not receive targeted therapy [24]. The study also reported delay in diagnosis or treatment for an average of 1–2 years [24]. Direct extension into the chest wall leading to respiratory failure was a common cause of death [24]. Other less commonly reported causes of death included stem cell transplant complication and development of a second unrelated lymphoma [24].

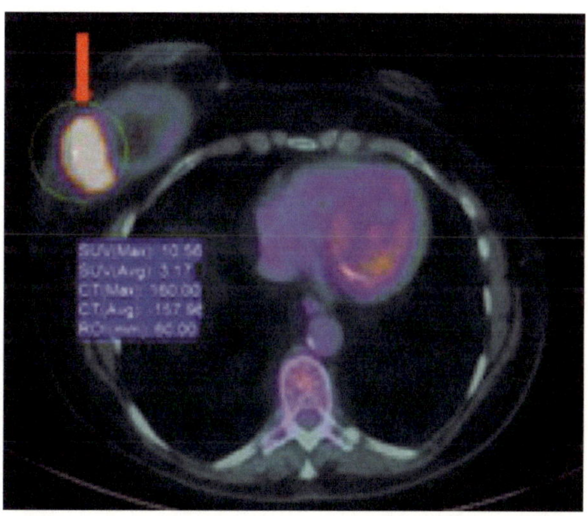

Figure 14.
63-year-old female with history of saline breast implants with textured surface placed 19 years ago presented with pain and swelling throughout the right breast and a palpable abnormality in the posterior third of the right breast at 7 o'clock for 1 month. Screen capture of a whole body 18F-FDG PET/CT shows FDG activity of SUV 10.56, corresponding to a soft tissue mass (arrow) in the lower outer quadrant of the right breast adjacent to the implant measuring 3.2 × 4.8 cm × 2.5 cm (source: Collado-Mesa et al. [20]).

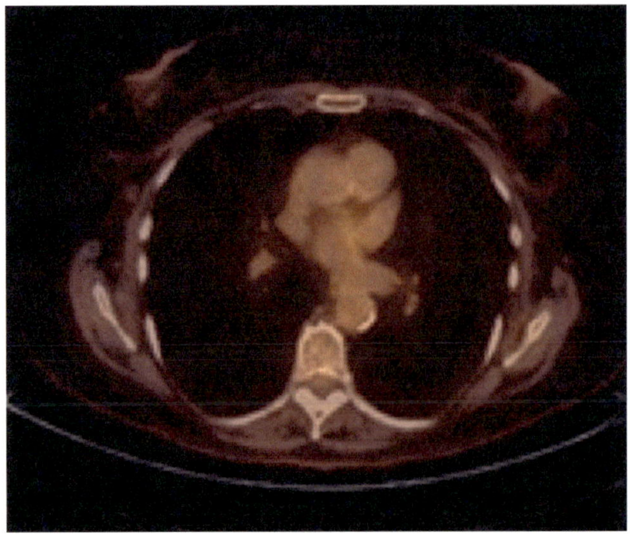

Figure 15.
63-year-old female with history of saline breast implants with textured surface placed 19 years ago presented with pain and swelling throughout the right breast and a palpable abnormality in the posterior third of the right breast at 7 o'clock for 1 month. Screen capture of a whole body 18F-FDG PET/CT obtained 6 months after bilateral breast explantation and total capsulectomy shows no abnormality (source: Collado-Mesa et al. [20]).

10. Conclusion

In the absence of infection or trauma, the development of a new peri-implant effusion more than one year after breast implant placement should prompt consideration for the diagnosis of BIA-ALCL As the clinical symptoms are often nonspecific, radiologists, particularly those involved in breast imaging, play an important role in its diagnosis,. While mammography may demonstrate subtle abnormalities, ultrasound and MRI have higher sensitivity and specificity. Diagnosis requires sampling of peri-implant fluid or mass and or lymph node. Suspicion of BIA-ALCL should be communicated to the pathologist, and immunohistochemistry for CD30 ordered. Once diagnosed, oncology referral and multi-specialty team care including plastic surgery and radiation therapy is recommended. Prompt diagnosis and complete treatment appear to lead to excellent prognosis.

Conflict of interest

The authors declare no conflict of interest.

Author details

Fernando Collado-Mesa
University of Miami Miller School of Medicine, Miami, Florida,
United States of America

*Address all correspondence to: fcollado@med.miami.edu

References

[1] Keech JA Jr, Creech BJ. Anaplastic T-cell lymphoma in proximity to a saline-filled breast implant. Plastic and Reconstructive Surgery. 1997;**100**:554-555

[2] Gaudet G, Friedberg JW, Weng A, Pinkus GS, Freedman AS. Breast lymphoma associated with breast implants: Two case reports and a review of the literature. Leukemia & Lymphoma. 2002;**43**(1):115-119

[3] Wong AK, Lopategui J, Clancy S, Kulber D, Bose S. Anaplastic large cell lymphoma associated with a breast implant capsule: A case report and review of the literature. The American Journal of Surgical Pathology. 2008; **32**(8):1265-1268

[4] Miranda RN, Lin L, Talwalkar SS, Manning JT, Medeiros LJ. Anaplastic large cell lymphoma involving the breast: A clinicopathologic study of 6 cases and review of the literature. Archives of Pathology & Laboratory Medicine. 2009;**133**(9):1383-1390

[5] Reports of Anaplastic Large Cell Lymphoma (ALCL) in Women with Breast Implants: FDA Safety Communication. 2011. Available from https://wayback.archive-it.org/7993/20170111070030/http://www.fda.gov/MedicalDevices/Safety/AlertsandNotices/ucm240000.htm [Accessed: 2021-08-02]

[6] Swerdlow SH, Campo E, Pileri SA, Harris NL, Stein H, Siebert R, et al. The 2016 revision of the World Health Organization classification of lymphoid neoplasms. Blood. 2016;**127**(20): 2375-2390

[7] US Food and Drug Administration. The FDA requests allergan voluntarily recall natrelle biocell textured breast implants and tissue expanders from the market to protect patients: FDA safety communication. Available from https://wayback.archive-it.org/7993/20191214045822/https://www.fda.gov/node/390731 [Accessed: 2021-08-02]

[8] US Food and Drug Administration. FDA In Brief: FDA updates public information about known risk of lymphoma from breast implants. Available from https://www.fda.gov/news-events/fda-brief/fda-brief-fda-updates-public-information-about-known-risk-lymphoma-breast-implants [Accessed: 2021-08-02]

[9] Clemens MW, Brody GS, Mahabir RC, Miranda RN. How to diagnose and treat breast implant-associated anaplastic large cell lymphoma. Plastic and Reconstructive Surgery. 2018;**141**(4):586e-599e

[10] Clemens MW, Medeiros LJ, Butler CE, et al. Complete surgical excision is essential for the management of patients with breast implant-associated anaplastic large cell lymphoma. Journal of Clinical Oncology. 2016;**34**(2):160-168

[11] Kadin ME, Deva A, Xu H, Morgan J, Khare P, MacLeod RA, et al. Biomarkers provide clues to early events in the pathogenesis of breast implant-associated anaplastic large cell lymphoma. Aesthetic Surgery Journal. 2016;**36**(7):773-781

[12] Rastogi P, Riordan E, Moon D, Deva AK. Theories of etiopathogenesis of breast implant-associated anaplastic large cell lymphoma. Plastic and Reconstructive Surgery. 2019;**143**(3S): 23S-29S

[13] DeCoster RC, Clemens MW, Di Napoli A, Lynch EB, Bonaroti AR, Rinker BD, et al. Cellular and molecular mechanisms of breast implant-associated anaplastic large cell lymphoma. Plastic and Reconstructive Surgery. 2021;**147**(1):30e-41e

[14] US Food and Drug Administration. Questions and answers about breast implant-associated anaplastic large cell lymphoma (BIA-ALCL). Available from https://www.fda.gov/medical-devices/breast-implants/questions-and-answers-about-breast-implant-associated-anaplastic-large-cell-lymphoma-bia-alcl [Accessed: 2021-08-02]

[15] International Society of Aesthetic and Plastic Surgery: International Survey on Aesthetic/Cosmetic Procedures performed in 2018. Available from https://www.isaps.org/wp-content/uploads/2019/12/ISAPS-Global-Survey-Results-2018-new.pdf [Accessed: 2021-08-02]

[16] US Food and Drug Administration. Medical device reports of breast implant-associated anaplastic large cell lymphoma. Available from https://www.fda.gov/medical-devices/breast-implants/medical-device-reports-breast-implant-associated-anaplasticlarge-cell-lymphoma [Accessed: 2020-02-18]

[17] Doren EL, Miranda RN, Selber JC, et al. U.S. epidemiology of breast implant-associated anaplastic large cell lymphoma. Plastic and Reconstructive Surgery. 2017;**139**(5):1042-1050

[18] Spear SL, Baker JL Jr. Classification of capsular contracture after prosthetic breast reconstruction. Plastic and Reconstructive Surgery. 1995;**96**(5): 1119-1123

[19] Sharma B, Jurgensen-Rauch A, Pace E, Attygalle AD, Sharma R, Bommier C, et al. Breast implant-associated anaplastic large cell lymphoma: Review and multiparametric imaging paradigms. Radiographics. 2020;**40**(3):609-628

[20] Collado-Mesa F, Yepes MM, Net JM, Jorda M. Breast implant-associated anaplastic large cell lymphoma: Brief overview of current data and imaging findings. Breast Disease. 2021;**40**(1): 17-23

[21] Adrada BE, Miranda RN, Rauch GM, Arribas E, Kanagal-Shamanna R, Clemens MW, et al. Breast implant-associated anaplastic large cell lymphoma: Sensitivity, specificity, and findings of imaging studies in 44 patients. Breast Cancer Research and Treatment. 2014;**147**(1):1-14

[22] Clemens MW, Jacobsen ED, Horwitz SM. NCCN consensus guidelines on the diagnosis and treatment of breast implant-associated anaplastic large cell lymphoma (BIA-ALCL). Aesthetic Surgery Journal. 2019, 2019;**39**(Suppl_1):S3-S13

[23] Pastorello RG, D'Almeida Costa F, Osório CABT, Makdissi FBA, Bezerra SM, de Brot M, et al. Breast implant-associated anaplastic large cell lymphoma in a Li-FRAUMENI patient: A case report. Diagnostic Pathology. 2018;**13**(1):10

[24] Abi-Rafeh J, Safran T, Al-Halabi B, Dionisopolous T. Death by implants: Critical analysis of the FDA-MAUDE database on breast implant-related mortality. Plastic and Reconstructive Surgery. Global Open. 2019;7(12):e2554

Chapter 11

Lymphoma and the Microenvironmental Cross-Talk between Sex Hormone Receptors and Epstein-Barr Virus in Predicting Lymphoma Clinical Status

Ahed J. Alkhatib

Abstract

Lymphoma is a significant clinical entity because of its high incidence and complicated etiology and pathology. In this chapter, we discussed lymphoma in general and made focus in our previous studies in which we found unique features linking the interaction of EBV with sex steroid hormones in lymphoma cells. Sex steroid hormones included estrogen receptor and progesterone receptors that were investigated for their expression in malignant lymphoid cells. The localization of EBV in malignant lymphoid cells was also investigated. The two main types of lymphoma, Hodgkin Lymphoma, and non-Hodgkin lymphoma, were investigated for the interaction of EBV with sex steroid hormones. Unique features were obtained in terms of a bridge-linking estrogen receptor with EBV in Hodgkin lymphoma and progesterone receptor with EBV in non-Hodgkin lymphoma. The interactions between EBV and lymphoma are classic, but the reasons beyond this are not well established. The results of our studies highlighted new features by the existence of expressed sex steroid receptors. We think that the dissociation of combination between sex steroid hormones and EBV bears the link to design new therapeutic strategies for lymphoma.

Keywords: lymphoma, Hodgkin lymphoma, non-Hodgkin lymphoma, EBV, estrogen receptor, progesterone receptor

1. Introduction

1.1 An overview of lymphoma

Lymphoma is a term used to describe a group of lymphoproliferative malignant disorders that arise from lymphatic T- and B-cells [1]. Lymphoma is a group of malignancies that affect the lymphatic system [2]. The organs, tissues, and veins of the lymphatic system are part of the immune system and are important for battling disease and infection throughout the body [3]. When lymphocytes (the lymphatic system's white blood cells) become malignant, they proliferate abnormally, forming tumors and squeezing out healthy cells [3].

1.2 Types of lymphoma

Lymphoma has traditionally been divided into the two types: Hodgkin lymphoma (HL) and non-Hodgkin lymphoma (NHL). However, it is now recognized that Hodgkin lymphoma is just one of many forms of lymphoma and that non-Hodgkin lymphoma is a largely meaningless phrase that encompasses all the disease's other subtypes [4]. Non-Hodgkin lymphoma is a diverse collection of over 40 lymphoproliferative tumors with varying patterns of behavior and treatment responses [5]. Non-Hodgkin lymphoma has a lower prognosis than Hodgkin lymphoma, and prognosis is determined by histologic type, stage, and treatment [6].

There are over 70 different forms of lymphoma. Some grow slowly (sometimes known as low-grade or indolent), while others grow quickly (referred to as high-grade or aggressive). Lymphoma has no known causes; however, several factors have been linked to an increased chance of having the disease. Hodgkin lymphoma and non-Hodgkin lymphoma are the two types of lymphomas. Hodgkin's lymphoma is a type of cancer that affects the lymphatic system [7, 8].

2. Hodgkin lymphoma

HL is a type of lymphoma that affects roughly 9000 adults and children in the United States each year. Hodgkin lymphoma can occur anywhere lymphocytes are detected in the body. However, lymph nodes in the chest, neck, and beneath the arms are where it usually starts. HL differs from all other kinds of lymphoma in several ways, the most notable of which is the existence of a cell known as the Reed-Sternberg cell. A Reed-Sternberg cell is a big, unusual cell that does not defend the body against infection. It is called for the two scientists who found it. When it multiplies improperly, it creates a tumor within a lymph node and attracts inflammatory cells. Chemotherapy and/or radiation therapy may be used to treat HL. A stem cell transplant may be considered in some circumstances, particularly if the disease does not respond to early treatment or returns after an initial response [9].

Hodgkin lymphoma is also known as Hodgkin's disease. It usually begins in a type of B cell that is found in the bone marrow. Hodgkin's disease is considered one of the most curable forms of cancer, especially if it is diagnosed and treated early. Several types of treatment can be used against Hodgkin lymphoma, including chemotherapy, immunotherapy, and stem cell transplantation [10]. Hodgkin lymphoma, often known as Hodgkin's disease, is a type of lymphoma. It usually starts in a specific type of B cell located in the bone marrow. Hodgkin's disease is one of the most treatable types of cancer, especially when detected and treated early [11]. Chemotherapy, immunotherapy, and stem cell transplantation are among the treatments available for Hodgkin lymphoma [12]. The presence of big aberrant tumor cells known as Hodgkin Reed-Sternberg cells distinguishes it. Hodgkin lymphoma can affect both children and adults; however, it is most diagnosed in young adults aged 20 to 34. Classic Hodgkin lymphoma and nodular lymphocyte-dominated Hodgkin lymphoma are the two primary subtypes of Hodgkin lymphoma. Classic Hodgkin lymphoma affects more than 90% of Hodgkin lymphoma cases [13].

Classical Hodgkin lymphoma is divided into five types as follows [14, 15]:

- Nodular sclerosis.
- Mixed cellularity.
- Hodgkin lymphoma.
- Hodgkin's disease.
- Hodgkin's disease with lymphocyte depletion.

3. Non-Hodgkin lymphoma (NHL)

Non-Hodgkin lymphomas (NHL) are a heterogeneous group of cancers, with B-cell origin in roughly 80% of cases (B-NHL). The presentation, clinical characteristics, prognosis, and therapeutic response of B-NHL are all different. Diffuse large B-cell lymphoma (DLBCL) is the most frequent histologic subtype, accounting for about a third of cases in the United States, followed by follicular lymphoma, which accounts for about a quarter of occurrences [16]. Other histologies are far less prevalent. Rituximab, cyclophosphamide, adriamycin, vincristine, and prednisone are used to treat about 60% of DLBCL patients (R-CHOP). Most patients who relapse after or are refractory to initial therapy, on the other hand, succumb to their condition. Over the last decade, new therapeutic research has concentrated on molecules that target the cell surface, internal pathways, and the microenvironment, rather than cytotoxic chemotherapy drugs. The chimeric anti-CD20 monoclonal rituximab changed B-NHL therapy, extending survival in the majority of subtypes. However, resistance builds with time, necessitating the use of additional techniques aimed at other targets [17].

3.1 Primary central nervous system lymphoma (PCNSL)

PCNSL (primary central nervous system lymphoma) is an uncommon extranodal non-Hodgkin lymphoma that is distinct from systemic diffuse large B-cell lymphomas. PCNSL is diagnosed at a median age of 65 years, and its prevalence is quickly increasing among the elderly. A total of 20% of all PCNSL patients are above the age of 80. Age, in particular, has been recognized as a poor prognostic factor for PCNSL. Elderly patients have a worse prognosis than younger patients and are more susceptible to iatrogenic toxicity; as a result, they are a distinct and vulnerable therapeutic class. The goal of this study was to provide a better understanding of the epidemiology, clinical features, diagnosis, prognosis, and therapy of PCNSL in the aged population by summarizing the current research. Notably, PCNSL is becoming more common in immunocompetent elderly patients, particularly men. Imaging guided stereotactic biopsy is the gold standard for the diagnosis of CNSL. Certain biomarkers have been described that can aid establish a diagnosis when stereotactic biopsy is not possible or conclusive. Even though numerous prognostic grading systems exist, and several prognostic markers have been discovered in PCNSL patients, the elderly have a very dismal prognosis. Furthermore, treating older individuals remains difficult; while a novel agent is unlikely to be utilized as a curative monotherapy, a combination of novel medicines with polychemotherapy or with other innovative therapies may have therapeutic potential [18].

3.2 Cutaneous lymphoma

Primary cutaneous lymphomas are a diverse category of extranodal non-Hodgkin lymphomas that are restricted to the skin at the time of diagnosis [19]. In 2005 [20], the European Organization for Research and Treatment of Cancer (EORTC) and the World Health Organization (WHO) developed a cutaneous lymphoma consensus classification, which was recently updated [21]. Unlike nodal non-Hodgkin lymphoma, which is mostly B-cell originated, about 75% of primary cutaneous lymphomas are T-cell derived, with two-thirds of them being categorized as mycosis fungoides (MF) or Sézary syndrome (SS) [20, 22, 23]. According to the Surveillance, Epidemiology, and End Results (SEER) registry, the incidence of cutaneous T-cell lymphomas (CTCL) has been growing and is now 6.4 per million people, with the greatest incidence rates seen among men and African Americans [23]. When compared to non-Black individuals with MF, there are several major distinctions, including a female predominance, a younger age of onset, and probably worse results [24, 25]. While CTCL can arise in adolescents and young adults, it is a rare occurrence that is generally linked to histopathologic MF variations [26].

4. Lymphoma diagnosis

Lymphoma is diagnosed primarily through pathologic examination of an acceptable tissue specimen in the right clinical situation, which may include morphologic, immunophenotypic, and cytogenetic studies as needed. Individual lymphomas are treated differently, necessitating an accurate and specific diagnosis to provide appropriate patient care [27]. The choice of biopsy procedure and place is a common practical challenge in patients suspected of having lymphoma. For initial diagnosis, surgical biopsy is preferred because the bigger tissue sample collected enables for investigation of processes that may involve the lymph node or extranodal mass in a variety of ways, as well as immunophenotypic, cytogenetic, and molecular analysis [28]. Fine needle aspiration may not allow for the study of histologic architecture, and it may not yield enough tissue for a thorough analysis, including the determination of biologic subtype [29]. In some cases, fine needle aspiration can confirm relapsed illness, although even in these cases, a core needle or surgical biopsy is preferred [30]. Core needle biopsy may allow for nodal architecture study, but it collects less tissue than surgical biopsy, perhaps missing a heterogeneous process and providing less material for thorough testing. Only in clinical scenarios where a surgical biopsy is not possible, a core needle biopsy is suggested for first diagnosis. Despite the WHO classification's established definitions, an experienced hematopathologist will modify about one-fifth of lymphoma diagnoses, with the rate varied among the different forms of lymphoma [31, 32]. Expert pathology review is recommended and should be regarded standard of care because proper therapy is fundamentally dependent on correct pathologic diagnosis. When the diagnosis of lymphoma is unclear, medical imaging can be helpful in staging, but a definitive diagnosis of lymphoma and determination of the histologic subtype require pathological examination [27]. Though not conclusive, [18F]-fluoro-2-deoxyglucose positron emission tomography (FDG-PET) imaging can identify aggressive from indolent lymphomas based on standard uptake value assessment and can help predict indolent lymphoma transformation (usually DLBCL). When transformation is suspected, PET can be used to choose an acceptable biopsy site where the standard uptake value is the highest and thus, transformation is most likely to be present; however, marked FDG avidity does not rule out transformation and does not eliminate the necessity for diagnostic biopsy [33].

5. Viruses and lymphoma

Hepatitis C virus (HCV) is well known for its role in the etiology of chronic non-A, non-B viral hepatitis, liver cirrhosis, and hepatocellular cancer; it has also been linked to a number of extra-hepatic "autoimmune" disease presentations. A causal link between HCV and non-Hodgkin lymphoma (NHL) was proposed just lately, and it has sparked a lot of research and debate. HCV appears to be implicated in the pathogenesis of at least a proportion of patients with NHL, based on epidemiological data, developing scientific investigations, and clinical observations. HCV-associated lymphomas are classified as marginal zone lymphoma (splenic, nodal, and extranodal), small lymphocytic lymphoma/chronic lymphocytic leukemia, lymphoplasmacytic lymphoma, lymphoplasmacytic lymphoma, and diffuse large B-cell lymphoma. Surprisingly, some HCV-associated NHLs appear to respond well to antiviral medication, giving clinical evidence for the link as well as the possibility of innovative therapeutic intervention [34].

Patients with HIV infection have a much higher rate of lymphoma than the normal population. Multiple factors appear to contribute to the increased risk of lymphoma, including the retrovirus's transforming properties, the disease's immunosuppression and cytokine dysregulation, and, most importantly, opportunistic infections with other lymphotrophic herpes viruses such as Epstein-Barr virus and human herpesvirus 8. Lymphomas are classified histologically into three groups: (1) those that occur in immunocompetent people, (2) those that occur more specifically in HIV-positive patients, and (3) those that occur in patients with various types of immunosuppression. The great majority of instances are aggressive lymphomas. They usually present with advanced stage, bulky cancer with a large tumor load and extranodal involvement. Clinical outcomes appear to be worse than those seen in the general population with similar severe lymphomas. The risk of developing lymphoma in the context of HIV infection has decreased, and the clinical result has improved since the advent of highly active antiretroviral therapy [35].

Epstein-Barr virus (EBV) is a common virus that affects over 90% of the world's population [36]. It was discovered to be linked to the development of EBV-associated lymphoproliferative diseases, hemophagocytic lymphohistiocytosis (HLH), and solid tumors, among other things, after being identified as an oncogenic virus in a Burkitt's lymphoma cell line [37]. *In vitro* infection and transformation of quiescent B cells into lymphoblastoid cell lines (LCLs) have proven EBV's carcinogenic potential [36]. The ability of EBV to create a lifelong latent infection in B-lymphoma cells has been established as a key mechanism of EBV-induced lymphomagenesis. During EBV latency, the expression of highly immunogenic proteins is suppressed, while viral lytic proteins are increased, impairing antigen processing by infected cells, and destroying the cellular molecular signaling machinery and metabolism, allowing tumor cells to escape immune surveillance and grow and survive. The most frequent indolent and second most common non-Hodgkin lymphoma subtype is follicular lymphoma (FL) [38]. Follicular lymphoma with EBV is a poorly understood disease that is infrequently reported [39]. Even though Asians have a higher incidence of EBV-associated cancers than Westerners, EBV-positive FL has been observed in the Chinese community on a rare basis. EBV is also the most frequent virus linked to HLH, a rare condition characterized by severe, life-threatening hyperinflammation. The decreased function of cytotoxic T lymphocytes and natural killer (NK) cells is the fundamental pathophysiology of HLH, resulting in uncontrolled immunological activation, hypercytokinemia, and macrophage proliferation. With a fatality rate of up to 50%, EBV-associated HLH is thought to be particularly common in Asia [40]. This may occur prior to, concurrently with, or after EBV-positive lymphoproliferative diseases [40]. T-cell and

NK-cell lymphomas account for the bulk of HLH-related cancers. The majority of B-cell lymphoma associated HLH cases have been observed in Asians [37].

6. Microenvironmental interactions between lymphoma and EBV and sex hormones

The hypothesis of cross-talks between hormone receptors such as the estrogen receptor (ER) and the progesterone receptor (PR) in breast cancer has recently been revealed to have major effects on breast cancer. Many researches, including ours, have previously proven the associations of Epstein-Barr virus (EBV) with lymphoma. We wanted to see if "EBV cross-talk with sex hormones plays a role in dictating the kind of lymphoma, Hodgkin's Lymphoma (HL) or non-Lymphoma Hodgkin's (NHL)" in this work. In lymphoma patients representing HL and NHL, we looked at the expression of sex hormones, ER, and PR, as well as EBV. The expression of these biomarkers in lymphoma cases was assessed using immunoperoxidase staining. Our data revealed that EBV cross-talk with ER is strongly linked with HL ($p < 0.05$), but its cross-talk with PR is significantly associated with NHL ($p < 0.05$). The findings of this study suggest that EBV acts as the conductor of an orchestra, orchestrating the events of lymphoma through various interactions with sex hormones. This could pave the way for novel lymphoma treatment options [41].

Grywalska and Rolinski [42] highlighted in their review study that the Epstein-Barr virus (EBV) has been linked to cancer pathogenesis. EBV is a member of the Herpesviridae family, and through the expression of multiple genes, it has developed ways to maintain the integrity of the viral genome and to escape from the host's immune system during the latent stage of infection. This expression promotes the development of cancers. EBV can infect a wide range of cells, resulting in a variety of diseases, including B-cell lymphoma [43].

Several studies have reported the link between EBV infection and Hodgkin Lymphoma (HL) [42], and the presence of EBV in Hodgkin/Reed-Sternberg (HRS) was confirmed by researchers such as Weiss et al. [44] and Takeuchi et al. [45]. On the other hand, non-Hodgkin Lymphoma (NHL) includes a variety of lymphomas such as Burkitt lymphoma (BL) and diffuse large B-cell lymphoma (DLBCL) [46, 47].

Dolcetti [48] stated in his work that EBV has the power to alter the microenvironment to make it more conducive to cell transformation. EBV can boost the synthesis of a variety of substances that help lymphoid cells grow and/or survive while also allowing them to avoid immune system reactions. There is a complicated interplay between EBV-infected lymphoid cells and the tumor microenvironment that has the therapeutic potential against EBV-driven lymphoid malignancies.

There are few therapeutic alternatives in the treatment of lymphomas caused by EBV that can affect the virus within malignant cells. However, in most instances, no variations in therapy options have been found based on whether EBV is present. As prospective therapeutic methods, existing therapeutic techniques have focused on interfering with biological components of EBV to target lymphomas associated with EBV [49]. EBV-explicit methodologies include reinforcing the antiviral-/antitumor-resistant reaction with antibodies or EBV explicit cytotoxic T-lymphocytes, initiating lytic viral qualities to render tumor cells immune to antiviral treatments, and inhibiting downstream prosurvival or antiapoptotic pathways that may be triggered by dormant EBV proteins. EBV-explicit cytotoxic T-cell imbuements have shown to be effective in EBV-related post-transplantation lymphoproliferative disorder (EBVPTLD) and extending such assenting immunotherapies to additional EBV-related cancers is a hot topic of investigation [49]. Other EBV-related lymphomas, in contrast to EBV-PTLD, have progressively constrained, less immunogenic kinds of viral antigens to restoratively target with assenting immunotherapy. Furthermore, the threatening EBV-positive tumor cells of HL are dispersed during a thick layer of administrative T-cells, macrophages, and other cells, which may compromise supportive immunotherapy's antitumor efficacy [50]. Continuous preclinical and clinical assessments are areas of continuous methodology to overcome these impediments. Some emerging approaches to treating EBV-related lymphomas include combining specialists that trigger lytic viral replication with anti-herpes virus operators or using small particle inhibitors to block deterioration pathways that are constitutively triggered by EBV. EBV antibodies appear to be generally promising for the treatment or prevention of EBV-related cancers, as opposed to required EBV contamination avoidance [51]. Preliminary EBV vaccination trials in patients with residual or low-mass EBV-related malignancies, or for the counteractive effect of EBV-PTLD in EBV-seronegative patients awaiting strong organ transplantation, are moving forward [52]. In many cases, the treatment of EBV-positive lymphomas is identical to that of EBV-negative lymphomas with similar histologies [53]. Special cases include experimental conventions and situations where a responsive immunotherapy method is available [54, 55]. When EBV-positive lymphomas appear in the context of immunosuppression, boosting the invulnerable deformities can help with lymphoma treatment [56, 57]. Antiretroviral treatment is routinely used in HIV-related lymphomas, but potential pharmaceutical interactions and the effects of chemotherapy on the ability to maintain HAART treatment in terms of sickness, heaving, and mucositis must be considered when antiretroviral treatment is planned [58, 59]. In any case, antiretroviral therapy alone is insufficient for the treatment of EBV-related lymphomas in HIV patients. This contrasts with AIDS-related Kaposi sarcoma, where initiating antiretroviral medication in patients who are asymptomatic or insignificantly symptomatic and antiretrovirally innocent is frequently a regular practice [60, 61]. Select instances with EBV-PTLD may benefit from immunosuppressive reduction as a stand-alone treatment or as part of a therapeutic plan [62, 63]. The therapeutic choices for lymphomas associated with EBV are like those for lymphomas that are EBV-negative. Existing therapy methods, on the other hand, include addressing biological elements of EBV and may require further research to be firmly established.

7. Conclusions

This study showed that new therapeutic strategies are of great potential based on the interactions of EBV, lymphoid malignant cells, and sex steroid hormones, ER or PR. Our studies showed interesting features by identifying the impacts of interaction of progesterone receptors with EBV leading to the development of NHL, while the interaction of EBV with ER led to the development of HL. These features are unique and give the bases of designing new therapeutic lines that inhibit the binding of EBV with sex steroid hormones to participate in lowering the incidence of lymphoma.

Author details

Ahed J. Alkhatib[1,2]

1 Department of Legal Medicine, Toxicology and Forensic Medicine, Jordan University of Science and Technology, Jordan

2 International Mariinskaya Academy, Department of Medicine and Critical Care, Department of Philosophy, Academician Secretary of Department of Sociology, Jordan

*Address all correspondence to: ajalkhatib@just.edu.jo; drahedalkatib@yahoo.com; ahed.alkhatib64@yahoo.com

References

[1] Chen C, Gu YD, Geskin LJ. A review of primary cutaneous CD30+ lymphoproliferative disorders. Hematology/Oncology Clinics. 2019;**33**(1):121-134

[2] Justiz Vaillant AA, Stang CM. Lymphoproliferative Disorders. 2021. [Updated 2020 Dec 30]. In: StatPearls [Internet]. Treasure Island (FL): StatPearls Publishing; 2021 Jan. Available from: https://www.ncbi.nlm.nih.gov/books/NBK537162

[3] britannica.com. 2021. Available from: https://www.britannica.com/science/lymphoid-tissue [Retrieved: 9-11-2021]

[4] Momotow J, Borchmann S, Eichenauer DA, Engert A, Sasse S. Hodgkin lymphoma—Review on pathogenesis, diagnosis, current and future treatment approaches for adult patients. Journal of Clinical Medicine 2021;10:1125. https://doi.org/10.3390/jcm10051125

[5] Bezombes C, Pérez-Galán P. Immunotherapies in non-Hodgkin's lymphoma. Cancers. 2021;**13**:3625. https://doi.org/. DOI: 10.3390/cancers13143625

[6] Pratap S, Scordino TS. Molecular and cellular genetics of non-Hodgkin lymphoma: Diagnostic and prognostic implications. Experimental and Molecular Pathology 2019;**106**:44-51. [CrossRef]

[7] Cheson BD, Fisher RI, Barrington SF, Cavalli F, Schwartz LH, Zucca E, et al. Recommendations for initial evaluation, staging, and response assessment of Hodgkin and non-Hodgkin lymphoma: The Lugano classification. Journal of Clinical Oncology. 2014;**32**:3059e68

[8] Ninkovic S, Lambert J. Lymphoproliferative disorders. Medicine. 2018;**45**(5):297-304

[9] uchicagomedicine. 2021. Available from: https://www.uchicagomedicine.org/cancer/types-treatments/lymphoma/types-of-lymphoma [Retrieved: 13-9-2021]

[10] Montes-Moreno S, Odqvist L, Diaz-Perez JA, Lopez AB, de Villambrosia SG, Mazorra F, et al. EBV-positive diffuse large B-cell lymphoma of the elderly is an aggressive post-germinal center B-cell neoplasm characterized by prominent nuclear factor-kB activation. Modern Pathology. 2012;**25**(7):968-982

[11] Marcus R. Lymphoma: Pathology, Diagnosis, and Treatment. 14th ed. Cambridge University Press; 2007:1- 277

[12] Travis LB, Hill DA, Dores GM, Gospodarowicz M, van Leeuwen FE, Holowaty E, et al. Breast cancer following radiotherapy and chemotherapy among young women with Hodgkin disease. JAMA. 2003;**290**(4):465-475

[13] Canadian Cancer Society's Steering Committee. Canadian Cancer Statistics. 2009. In: Special Topic: Cancer in Adolescents and Young Adults. Available from: http://www.cancer.ca/Canadawide/About%20cancer/Cancer%20statistics/~/media/CCS/Canada%20wide/Files%20List/English%20files%20heading/pdf%20not%20in%20publications%20section/Stats%202009E%20Special%20Topics.ashx2009

[14] Armand P, Engert A, Younes A, Fanale M, Santoro A, Zinzani PL, et al. Nivolumab for relapsed/refractory classic Hodgkin lymphoma after failure of autologous hematopoietic cell transplantation: extended follow-up of the Multicohort Single-Arm Phase II CheckMate 205 Trial. Journal of Clinical Oncology. 2018;**36**(14):1428-1439

[15] McKay P, Fielding P, Gallop-Evans E, Hall GW, Lambert J, Leach M, et al.

Guidelines for the investigation and management of nodular lymphocyte predominant Hodgkin lymphoma. British Journal of Haematology. 2016;**172**(1):32-43

[16] Cheson BD, Nowakowski G, Salles G. Diffuse large B-cell lymphoma: New targets and novel therapies. Blood Cancer Journal 2021;11:68. https://doi.org/10.1038/s41408-021-00456-w

[17] Crump M, Neelapu SS, Farooq U, Den Neste EV, Kuruvilla J, Westin J, et al. Outcomes in refractory diffuse large B-cell lymphoma: Results from the international SCHOLAR-1 study. Blood. 2017;**130**:1800-1808

[18] Liu Y, Yao Q, Zhang F. Diagnosis, prognosis and treatment of primary central nervous system lymphoma in the elderly population (Review). International Journal of Oncology. 2021;**58**:371-387

[19] Hristov AC, Tejasv T, Wilcox RA. Cutaneous T-cell lymphomas: 2021 update on diagnosis,risk-stratification, and management. American Journal of Hematology. 2021;**96**:1313-1328

[20] Willemze R, Jaffe ES, Burg G, Cerroni L, Berti E, Swerdlow SH, et al. WHO-EORTC classification for cutaneous lymphomas. Blood. 2005;**105**:3768-3785

[21] Willemze R, Cerroni L, Kempf W, Berti E, Facchetti F, Swerdlow SH, et al. The 2018 update of theWHO-EORTC classification for primary cutaneous lymphomas. Blood. 2019;**133**:1703-1714

[22] Bradford PT, Devesa SS, Anderson WF, Toro JR. Cutaneous lymphoma incidence patterns in the United States: A population-based study of 3884 cases. Blood. 2009;**113**:5064-5073

[23] Criscione VD, Weinstock MA. Incidence of cutaneous T-cell lymphoma in the United States, 1973-20 02. Archives of Dermatology. 2007;**143**:854-859

[24] Geller S, Lebowitz E, Pulitzer MP, Horwitz SM, Moskowitz AJ, Dusza S, et al. Outcomes and prognostic factors in African American and black patients with mycosis fungoides/Sezary syndrome: Retrospective analysis of 157 patients from a referral cancer center. Journal of American Academy of Dermatology. 2020;**83**:430-439

[25] Johnson WT, Kartan S, Sokol K, Nikbakht N, Porcu P. Clinical characteristics and outcomes of black patients with mycosis fungoides and Sezary syndrome: A subgroup analysis of the phase III MAVORICtrial. Leukemia & Lymphoma 2021;**62**(8):1877-1883. https://doi.org/10.1080/10428194.2021.1888376.HRISTOV ET AL. 1321

[26] Jung JM, Lim DJ, Won CH, Chang SE, Lee MW, Lee WJ. Mycosis fungoides in children and adolescents: A systematic review. Journal of the American Academy of Dermatology. 2021;**157**:431-438

[27] Word, Matasar M. Advances in the diagnosis and management of lymphoma. Blood Lymphat Cancer. 2012;**2**:29-55. https://doi.org/10.2147/BLCTT.S15554

[28] Zelenetz AD, Hoppe RT. NCCN: Non-Hodgkin's lymphoma. Cancer Control. 2001;**8**(6 Suppl 2):102-113

[29] Mourad WA, Tulbah A, Shoukri M, Al Dayel F, Akhtar M, Ali MA, et al. Primary diagnosis and REAL/WHO classification of non-Hodgkin's lymphoma by fine-needle aspiration: Cytomorphologic and immunophenotypic approach. Diagnostic Cytopathology. 2003;**28**(4):191-195

[30] Young NA, Al-Saleem TI, Ehya H, Smith MR. Utilization of fineneedle aspiration cytology and flow cytometry

in the diagnosis and subclassification of primary and recurrent lymphoma. Cancer. 1998;**84**(4):252-261

[31] LaCasce AS, Kho ME, Friedberg JW, Niland JC, Abel GA, Rodriguez MA, et al. Comparison of referring and final pathology for patients with non-Hodgkin's lymphoma in the National Comprehensive Cancer Network. Journal of Clinical Oncology. 2008;**26**(31):5107-5112

[32] Matasar MJ, Shi W, Silberstien J, Lin O, Busam KJ, Teruya-Feldstein J, et al. Expert second-opinion pathology review of lymphoma in the era of the World Health Organization classification. Annals of Oncology 2012;**23**(1):159-166

[33] Noy A, Schoder H, Gonen M, Weissler M, Ertelt K, Cohler C, et al. The majority of transformed lymphomas have high standardized uptake values (SUVs) on positron emission tomography (PET) scanning similar to diffuse large B-cell lymphoma (DLBCL). Annals of Oncology. 2009;**20**(3):508-512

[34] Viswanatha DS, Dogan A. Hepatitis C virus and lymphoma. Journal of Clinical Pathology. 2007;**60**:1378-1383

[35] Grogg KL, Miller RF, Dogan A. HIV infection and lymphoma. Journal of Clinical Pathology. 2007;**60**: 1365-1372

[36] Young LS. Epstein-Barr virus at 50-Future perspectives. Chinese Journal of Cancer. 2014;**33**(11):527-528. DOI: 10.5732/cjc.014.10208

[37] Xu H, Xu X, Cui G, Fang J, Chen W, Xue M, et al. Secondary hemophagocytic lymphohistiocytosis with Epstein–Barr virus-associated transformed follicular lymphoma: A case report and literature review. Frontier in Oncology. 2021;**11**:681432. DOI: 10.3389/fonc.2021.681432

[38] Mackrides N, Campuzano-Zuluaga G, Maque-Acosta Y, Moul A, Hijazi N, Ikpatt FO, et al. Epstein-Barr virus-positive follicular lymphoma. Modern Pathology. 2017;**30**(4):519-529. DOI: 10.1038/modpathol.2016.214

[39] Cahir McFarland ED, Izumi KM, Mosialos G. Epstein-Barr virus transformation: Involvement of latent membrane protein 1-mediated activation of NF-Kappab. Oncogene. 1999;**18**(49):6959-6964. DOI: 10.1038/sj.onc.1203217

[40] Smith MC, Cohen DN, Greig B, Yenamandra A, Vnencak-Jones C, Thompson MA, et al. The ambiguous boundary between EBV-related hemophagocytic lymphohistiocytosis and systemic EBV-driven T cell lymphoproliferative disorder. International Journal of Clinical and Experimental Pathology. 2014;**7**(9):5738-5749

[41] Alkhatib Ahed J. Does Epstein - Barr virus cross talks with sex hormone receptors on lymphoid cells differently to produce lymphoma? International Journal of Pharmacy. 2018;**8**(1):56-57

[42] Grywalska E, Rolinski J. Epstein-Barr virus–associated lymphomas. Seminars in Oncology. 2015;**42**(2): 291-303

[43] Frappier L. Epstein-Barr virus: Current questions and challenges. Tumour Virus Research. 2021;**12**:200218

[44] Weiss LM, Strickler JG, Warnke RA, Purtilo DT, Sklar J. Epstein-Barr viral DNA in tissues of Hodgkin's disease. The American Journal of Pathology. 1987;**129**(1):86-91

[45] Takeuchi H, Kobayashi R, Hasegawa M, Hirai K. Detection of latent Epstein-Barr virus (EBV) DNA in paraffin sections of nasopharyngeal carcinomas expressing no EBV-encoded small RNAs using in situ PCR. Archives of Virology. 1997;**142**:1743-1756

[46] Chabay PA, Preciado MV. EBV primary infection in childhood and its relation to B-cell lymphoma development: A mini-review from a developing region. International Journal of Cancer. 2013;**133**(6):1286-1292

[47] Rosenwald A, Ott G. Burkitt lymphoma versus diffuse large B-cell lymphoma. Annals of Oncology. 2008;**19**:67-69. DOI: 10.1093/annonc/mdn201

[48] Dolcetti R. Cross-talk between Epstein-Barr virus and microenvironment in the pathogenesis of lymphomas. Seminars in Cancer Biology. 2015;**34**:58-69

[49] Alkhatib Ahed J. The impact of Epstein Barr-Virus on therapeutic options of lymphoma. American Journal of Biomedical Science & Research. 2020;**8**(1):59-61. AJBSR.MS.ID.001240. DOI: 10.34297/AJBSR.2020.08.001240

[50] Shannon-Lowe C, Rickinson A. The Global Landscape of EBV-Associated Tumors. Front. Oncol. 2019;**9**:713. DOI: 10.3389/fonc.2019.00713

[51] Rezk SA, Zhao XI, Weiss LM. Epstein-Barr virus (EBV)-associated lymphoid proliferations, a 2018 update. Human Pathology. 2018;**79**:18-41

[52] Kanakry JA, Ambinder RF. EBV-related lymphomas: New approaches to treatment. Current Treatment Options in Oncology. 2013;**14**(2):224-236

[53] Duran-Struuck R, Huang CA, Matar AJ. Cellular therapies for the treatment of hematological malignancies; swine are an ideal preclinical model. Frontiers in Oncology 2019;**21**(9):418

[54] He J, Tang XF, Chen QY, Mai HQ, Huang ZF, Li J, et al. Ex vivo expansion of tumor-infiltrating lymphocytes from nasopharyngeal carcinoma patients for adoptive immunotherapy. Chinese Journal of Cancer. 2012;**31**(6):287-294

[55] Louis CU, Straathof K, Bollard CM, Gerken C, Huls MH, Gresik MV, et al. Enhancing the *in vivo* expansion of adoptively transferred EBV-specific CTL with lymphodepleting CD45 monoclonal antibodies in NPC patients. Blood. 2009;**113**(11):2442-2450

[56] Dharnidharka VR, Webster AC, Martinez OM, Preiksaitis JK, Leblond V, Choquet S. Post-transplant lymphoproliferative disorders. Nature Reviews Disease Primers. 2016;**2**:15088

[57] Morscio J, Finalet Ferreiro J, Vander Borght S, Bittoun E, Gheysens O, et al. Identification of distinct subgroups of EBV-positive post-transplant diffuse large B-cell lymphoma. Modern Pathology. 2017;**30**(3):370-381

[58] Biggar RJ, Jaffe ES, Goedert JJ, Chaturvedi A, Pfeiffer R, et al. Hodgkin lymphoma and immunodeficiency in persons with HIV/AIDS. Blood. 2006;**108**(12):3786-3791

[59] Carbone A, Cesarman E, Spina M, Gloghini A, Schulz TF, et al. HIV-associated lymphomas and gamma-herpesviruses. Blood. 2009;**113**(6):1213-1224

[60] Bigi R, Landis JT, An H, Caro Vegas C, Raab Traub N, et al. Epstein-Barr virus enhances genome maintenance of Kaposi sarcoma-associated herpesvirus. Proceedings of the National Academy of Sciences of the United States of America. 2018;**115**(48):E11379-E11387

[61] Moore PS, Chang Y. Why do viruses cause cancer? Highlights of the first century of human tumour virology. Nature Reviews Cancer. 2010;**10**(12):878-889

[62] Burkitt D. A sarcoma involving the jaws in African children. British Journal of Surgery. 1958;**46**(197): 218-223

[63] Shannon Lowe C, Rickinson A. The global landscape of EBV-associated tumors. Frontiers in Oncology. 2019b;**9**:713